Counseling and Motivational Interviewing

in Speech-Language Pathology

Counseling and Motivational Interviewing

in Speech-Language Pathology

Editor

Jerry Hoepner, PhD, CCC-SLP, ASHA Fellow

Professor of Communication Sciences & Disorders

University of Wisconsin, Eau Claire

Eau Claire, Wisconsin

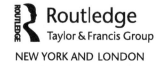
Routledge
Taylor & Francis Group

NEW YORK AND LONDON

First published in 2024 by SLACK Incorporated

Published 2024 by Routledge
605 Third Avenue, New York, NY 10017
4 Park Square, Milton Park, Abingdon, Oxon OX14 4RN

Routledge is an imprint of the Taylor & Francis Group, an informa business

© 2024 Taylor & Francis Group

Library of Congress Cataloging-in-Publication Data

Names: Hoepner, Jerry K., editor.
Title: Counseling and motivational interviewing in speech-language
  pathology / [edited by] Jerry Hoepner.
Description: Thorofare, NJ : SLACK Incorporated, [2023] | Includes
  bibliographical references and index.
Identifiers: LCCN 2023019626 (print) | ISBN 9781630917654 (paperback)
Subjects: MESH: Speech-Language Pathology--methods | Motivational
  Interviewing--methods | Counseling--methods | BISAC: MEDICAL / Audiology
  & Speech Pathology
Classification: LCC RC425 (print) | NLM WL 21 | DDC
  616.85/5--dc23/eng/20230614
LC record available at https://lccn.loc.gov/2023019626

ISBN: 9781630917654 (pbk)
ISBN: 9781003523345 (ebk)

DOI: 10.4324/9781003523345

Dedication

This textbook is dedicated to all of those individuals who taught me about the full spectrum of wellness and mental health. I have always been an optimist, who can see the backstory behind someone's behavior. If anything, I am prone to recognize challenging behaviors as a consequence of one's backstory. Not that I condone or excuse those behaviors, but I can understand why they occur. This enables me to be more empathetic and perhaps give them a mulligan from time to time. My weakness has been seeing the story behind eyes that appear to be just "fine" or even happy. I have learned through my personal and professional experiences that the quiet behaviors are just as important as the loud, in-your-face behaviors. Being sensitive and responsive to quiet behaviors can preempt both blow-ups and quiet withdrawals. This book is dedicated to the clients, colleagues, students, and family members who have taught me these important lessons. Thank you for your patience with me as I learn and continue to learn.

Contents

Extended Table of Contents

Acknowledgments

Special thanks to my youngest daughter, Madelyn Hoepner, for her photograph of Joshua Tree National Park which is featured on the textbook cover. Thanks as well to my oldest daughter, Mariah Hoepner, for numerous illustrations within the textbook. She is a medical illustrator whose illustrations have been featured in my neuroscience textbooks as well. I would like to acknowledge my friends and colleagues in the American Speech-Language-Hearing Association Special Interest Group 20: Counseling–Ying-Chiao Tsao, Anthony DiLollo, Christopher Constantino, Laura Plexico, and Rebecca Crowell. Thanks as well to my strengths-based counseling friends and colleagues, Laura Arrington, Jamie Azios, Michael Azios, Katelynn Carroll, Charlotte Clark, Audrey Holland, Jamie Maxwell, Ryan Nelson, and Jack Pickering.

About the Editor

Dr.Jerry Hoepner is a Professor at the University of Wisconsin - Eau Claire. He teaches courses in anatomy and physiology, neuroanatomy and neurophysiology, acquired cognitive disorders, dysphagia, and counseling. Jerry co-facilitates two community-based brain injury groups (Blugold Brain Injury Group and Mayo Brain Injury Group), a national poetry group for persons with brain injuries and aphasia (Thursday Night Poets), and the Chippewa Valley Aphasia Camp. His research addresses video self-modeling interventions for persons with acquired language or cognitive disorders and their everyday partners, aphasia camp outcomes for campers and students, motivational interviewing, counseling methods and training, undergraduate research outcomes, course-embedded clinical experiences, and instructional pedagogies. Dr. Hoepner is widely published in those clinical and academic research areas. He is a founding editor of Teaching and Learning in Communication Sciences and Disorders and editorial board member for Clinical Archives of Communication Disorders. In 2022, he co-founded the new ASHA SIG20 for counseling in Communication Sciences and Disorders. His poetry group the Thursday Night Poets published *I Don't Think I Did This Right*, a collection of poems by people with brain injuries and aphasia in 2021. Their second poetry book, *Poetry is Chocolate,* includes poems about their recoveries from brain injuries and aphasia is forthcoming in 2023. In 2018, he was awarded the University of Wisconsin – Eau Claire, Excellence in Mentoring in Research, Scholarship, and Creative activity. In 2020, he was awarded the University of Wisconsin Systems Regent's Teaching Excellence Award, the highest honor bestowed on University of Wisconsin faculty. In 2021, he was awarded Fellow of the American Speech-Language Hearing Association. In 2023, he was awarded the Council of Academic Programs in Communication Sciences and Disorders Distinguished Contribution Award for enriching education in CSD.

Contributing Authors

Rebecca H .Affoo, PhD, CCC-SLP, SLP-Reg, SLP(c) (Chapter 8c)
Assistant Professor
School of Communication Sciences and Disorders
Dalhousie University
Nova Scotia, Canada

Wendy and Nick Allen (Chapter 7)

Laura Arrington, PhD, CCC-SLP (Chapter 8a)
Assistant Professor
University of Louisiana at Lafayette
Lafayette, Louisiana

Miriam Carroll-Alfano, PhD, CCC-SLP (Chapter 8c)
Associate Professor
Midwestern University
Downers Grove, Illinois

Charlotte Clark, PhD, CCC-SLP (Chapter 8a)
Assistant Professor
University of Wisconsin, Eau Claire
Eau Claire, Wisconsin

Holly Damico, PhD, CCC-SLP (Chapter 8a)
Associate Professor
University of Louisiana at Lafayette
Lafayette, Louisiana

Jack Damico, PhD, CCC-SLP (Chapter 8a)
Professor
University of Colorado Boulder
Boulder, Colorado

Derek E .Daniels, PhD, CCC-SLP (Chapter 7)
Associate Professor
Department of Communication Sciences and Disorders
Wayne State University
Detroit, Michigan

Natalie Douglas, PhD, CCC-SLP (Chapter 8d)
Associate Professor
Department of Communication Sciences and Disorders
Central Michigan University
Mount Pleasant, Michigan

Julia M .Fischer, PhD , CCC-SLP (Chapter 8c)
Professor
Department of Communication Sciences and Disorders
University of Wisconsin Stevens Point
Stevens Point, Wisconsin

Deborah Hersh, PhD, FSPA (Chapter 8d)
Professor of Speech Pathology and Discipline Lead
Curtin School of Allied Health and enAble Institute
Chairperson
Australian Aphasia Association
Perth, Australia

Audrey Holland, PhD (Foreword)
Regents' Professor Emerita
University of Arizona

Dan Hudock, PhD, CCC-SLP (Chapter 8b)
Associate Professor
Idaho State University
Pocatello, Idaho

Rebecca L .Jarzynski, MS, CCC-SLP (Chapter 8a)
Clinical Instructor
University of Wisconsin-Eau Claire
Eau Claire, Wisconsin
PhD Student
Northern Illinois University
DeKalb, Illinois

Sandra Lever, MN, BHM, RN, CNC, NSLHD (Chapter 8e)
Clinical Lecturer
Susan Wakil School of Nursing and Midwifery
Faculty of Medicine and Health
University of Sydney
Sydney, Australia

Margaret McGrath, PhD, MSc, BSc (Chapter 8e)
Senior Lecturer
Sydney School of Health Sciences, Faculty of Medicine and Health
University of Sydney
Sydney, Australia

Ryan Nelson, PhD, CCC-SLP (Chapter 8a)
Associate Professor
University of Louisiana at Lafayette
Lafayette, Louisiana

Nancy Petersen, MSW (Chapter 8e)
Community Liaison and Medical Marketer
Ability KC
Kansas City, Missouri

Jack Pickering, PhD, CCC-SLP (Chapter 8b)
Professor
Communication Sciences and Disorders
College of Saint Rose
Albany, New York

Laura Plexico, PhD, CCC-SLP (Chapter 8a)
Professor and Department Chair
Department of Communication Sciences and Disorders
Auburn University
Auburn, Alabama

Robin Pollens, MS, CCC-SLP (Chapter 8e)
Adjunct Assistant Professor
Department of Speech, Language and Hearing Sciences
Western Michigan University
Kalamazoo, Michigan

Emma Power, PhD, BAppSc, CPSP MSPAA (Chapter 8e)
Associate Professor, Speech Pathology
Graduate School of Health, Faculty of Health
University of Technology Sydney
Sydney, Australia

Pamela Terrell, PhD, CCC-SLP (Chapter 8a)
Professor
University of Wisconsin—Stevens Point
Stevens Point, Wisconsin

Aspen Townsend, MS, CCC-SLP (Chapter 1)
Speech-Language Pathologist
Eau Claire Area School District
Eau Claire, Wisconsin

Eva van Leer, PhD, CCC-SLP (Chapter 8b)
Associate Professor
Dept. of Communication Sciences and Disorders
Director, Voice Research Lab
Georgia State University
Atlanta, Georgia

Christine Weill, PhD, CCC-SLP (Chapter 8a)
Clinic Director
University of Louisiana at Lafayette
Lafayette, Louisiana

CeCelia and Wayne Zorn (Chapter 7)

Preface

If I have seen further, it is by standing on the shoulders of giants . ~ Sir Isaac Newton

As I wrote this text and collaborated with brilliant colleagues, I was reminded of the expression "we stand on the shoulders of giants." This arose from Sir Isaac Newton's (1675) letter to fellow scientist Robert Hooke (yes, acoustics nerds, of Hooke's law fame): "If I have seen further, it is by standing on the shoulders of giants." This eloquent statement has deep meaning in the context of counseling in communication sciences and disorders. I believe we are on the cusp of a counseling revolution of sorts in our disciplines. There is rising interest and attention in counseling curriculum (Doud et al., 2020; McCarthy et al., 1986; Phillips & Mendell, 2008; Terrell & Osborne, 2020) thanks to growing acknowledgement of the centrality of counseling in our disciplines. Indeed, ASHA (2016) identifies counseling as one of the eight pillars of our profession, adding that wellness and collaboration (two key elements associated with counseling) make up nearly half of our service delivery domains. And yet, it is given little priority in curricular requirements and many students and practitioners feel ill equipped to deliver counseling in the moment. This should be shocking given the fact that most of those practitioners recognize the importance of counseling (Luterman, 2019). Giants, like David Luterman, a pioneer of counseling in audiology—and speech-language pathology for that matter—has addressed counseling methods and curricula for decades. Unfortunately, lack of required coursework and training has limited carryover of his brilliant foundational work. Likewise, Audrey Holland—even prior to publication of her widely used textbook on counseling, positive psychology, and wellness—has been a proponent of coaching and collaborative counseling in aphasia and more broadly in our profession for decades. Pioneers like Anthony DiLollo and Robert Neimeyer (inspired by the work of Julie Wolter) have moved our thinking about reconstructing personal narratives, in a manner so central to our discipline, across the lifespan. In recent years, I've had the privilege of collaborating (locking arms and shoulders, if you will) with Ying-Chiao Tsao, Anthony DiLollo, Christopher Constantino, and Laura Plexico in advocating for the addition of a 20th ASHA special interest group focused on counseling. This obvious, next step has the potential to promote counseling to its rightful place among the priorities in our profession. The renaissance has seen voices of clinician–researchers like Aspen Townsend (Doud), Deborah Hersh, Katarina Hilari, Sarah Northcott, Michael Biel, Jasvinder Sekhon, Brooke Ryan, Katarina Haley, Tyson Harmon, Scott Yaruss, Nina Simmons-Mackie, Jack Damico, Richard Adler, Jack Pickering, and many others expand our understanding of counseling approaches and applications. This is not to mention a burgeoning body of research about communication partner training across the lifespan, which is essentially a counseling intervention. Why is it important to highlight this history and these names? These people (and other newbees to come) make up a watchlist for counseling interventions and education. These are the folks you'll enter in your Google Scholar searches to stay up to date. These people are my heroes and I've been privileged to collaborate and learn from many of them. As for specifics, it will become clear that I have been strongly influenced by motivational interviewing. William Miller and Stephen Rollnick's seminal work in this area has become infused and inseparable from all of my speech-language pathology specific knowledge about assessment and intervention. Some years ago, in a pro sem during my doctoral training, fellow doctoral student and counseling innovator, Eva van Leer introduced me to motivational interviewing and the transtheoretical model of change. The seeds were planted, and it gelled so well with my thinking about cognitive rehabilitation (ala Mark Ylvisaker), that my paradigmatic counseling transformation was set into motion. Training sessions about motivational interviewing for healthcare professionals by Stephen Rollnick and a variety of motivational interviewing (MI) continuing education experiences and voracious consumption of MI articles strengthened this pathway. Strongly influenced by clinicians like Don MacLennan, Michael Biel, and Eva van Leer, I began to recognize the importance of training SLPs to feel comfortable in implementing and having explicit knowledge about counseling. Thank you to my counseling professor and mentor Linda Carpenter and to the many students, like Aspen Townsend (Doud), Erin Zigler, and countless others who have helped me to continue to learn alongside of them. Thank you to my clients and particularly my aphasia and brain injury group members who have taught me as much or more about counseling than any textbook or article I've read. I hope, in a small way, this textbook helps begin to amplify their voices and the lived experience (see Chapter 7). Thank you as well to all of the master-clinician contributors to Chapter 8, who bring a range of expertise that I cannot possibly replicate or possess. Special thanks go to Aspen Townsend, Deborah Hersh, and Katarina Haley for several formative conversations and feedback about this textbook. And so it is, we've arrived at this textbook, which I hope will serve as a compliment to the brilliant work of the giants who preceded and formed my thinking. With a little luck, I hope it moves the conversation about counseling even further.

With deep appreciation to these giants,

~ Jerry K .Hoepner, PhD, CCC-SLP

Foreword

As a field, we are becoming increasingly aware of the growing importance of counseling to the adequate delivery of services. Thus, I can only applaud this book. It provides a strong theoretical basis for the approach Dr. Hoepner takes to counseling. Dr. Hoepner is clearly committed to adequate training of both students and to clinicians currently at work in the field. In this sense it is a careful "how to" text, and will be a welcome addition to both readers and their instructors.

The second half of the book follows through as well. It is devoted to descriptions of how recognized, competent clinicians put their knowledge of counseling to work with real clients. It is strikingly important not only to teach "how to" but to take the next steps, demonstrating how that "how to" can be meaningfully applied in real clinical contexts. In his book, Dr. Hoepner as not only done each of these things well, but he has provided his readers with a well-rounded, holistic framework that underscores the importance of learning and applying principled counseling in the field of speech language.

~ *Audrey Holland, PhD*

How to Use This Textbook

Features

- Accessible, easy-to-read writing makes the topic approachable.
- BOXES include case examples, thinking exercises, podcasts, and potential assignments to aid readers' learning.
- Includes cases, examples, and content to address counseling across the lifespan, clinical settings, and disorders.
- Dialogue between the client/family and clinician are included in quotations. This is intended to demonstrate for readers some typical exchanges and model potential responses. While there is not *one* right way of saying things, readers get to see multiple models from multiple authors/master clinicians.
- Chapters 4 to 6 and some entries in Chapter 8 are focused on implementation of counseling techniques. This includes descriptions of how to implement specific techniques, case examples, dialogue examples to model potential wording, and specific modifications to make techniques accessible to individuals with communication or swallowing impairments.
- Chapters 1 to 6 and 8 make explicit connection to research evidence for counseling in speech-language pathology. Chapter 8 brings together content and clinical experts from 15 topic areas within speech-language pathology clinical practice who share clinical experiences and research evidence for specific disorders and special topics.

Chapter Features

- **Chapter 1** establishes scope of practice, referrals, and interprofessional collaborations, while dispelling common misconceptions of counseling in speech-language pathology. It includes a number of exercises designed to foster self-reflection, an important evidence-based tool for development of counseling skills. The "Notes for Supervisor" tool helps student clinicians to evaluate counseling skills and structure a conversation with their supervisor about current client caseloads. A podcast by Ian Kneebone about the Stepped Care Model is linked within the chapter.
- **Chapter 2** addresses approaches to learning counseling techniques. This includes specific approaches to learning and a framework for hands-on practice.
- **Chapter 3** addresses cultural humility and responsiveness, foundational counseling skills and principles, and educational counseling techniques. Stories are woven throughout that connect concepts to real individuals. Specific strategies and models for educational counseling are identified. Exercises include designing your own communicatively accessible written educational materials and drafting a discharge plan.
- **Chapter 4** includes structured interview approaches, collaborative goal setting, and screening of mental health. A number of specific structured interview tools for clients across the lifespan are reviewed, along with models for speech-language pathology wording and dialogue. Several approaches to facilitate collaborative goal setting and planning are addressed, allowing readers to align their approach with one that best suits their clientele. Communicatively accessible tools for screening mental health among adult and pediatric clients are addressed. A podcast about collaborative goal setting and the FOURC model with Katarina Haley is linked within the chapter.
- **Chapter 5** provides theoretical bases for motivational interviewing, along with detailed information about techniques and implementation, such as modifications for individuals with communication disorders. Specific examples and models of speech-language pathology wording and dialogue are included. Podcasts by Michael Biel (motivation) and Deborah Hersh (motivational interviewing and collaborative goal setting) are linked within the chapter. Case examples are used to model dialogue and implementation of motivational interviewing techniques.
- **Chapter 6** addresses other major counseling approaches in speech-language pathology, including cognitive behavioral therapy, positive psychology, acceptance and commitment therapy, solutions focused brief therapy, narrative approach, self-anchored rating scales, and group interventions. Each section includes detailed information about techniques and implementation, including modifications for individuals with communication disorders. A podcast on solutions focused brief therapy by Sarah Northcott and one on narrative approach by Katie Strong are linked in the chapter.
- **Chapter 7** addresses the lived experience from the perspectives of a partner (spouse), a parent, and an individual with a communication disorder. These provide unique insights into seeing clients and their families as the experts in living with a communication disorder and areas of deficit/needs for counseling. A podcast by Wayne and CeCelia Zorn on living with primary progressive aphasia is linked within the chapter.

- **Chapter 8** addresses specific disorders and topics. While it is not feasible to address each of the disorders or topics we encounter in speech-language pathology, this chapter attempts to address some key disorders and topics. Content and practical experts from the discipline and outside of the discipline (e.g., social work, nursing, occupational therapy) address topics across the lifespan. The chapter has five sub-chapters, including developmental, lifespan, acquired medical, acquired cognitive-communication, and important conversations. A podcast by Mary Kennedy on returning to college is linked within Chapter 8d.

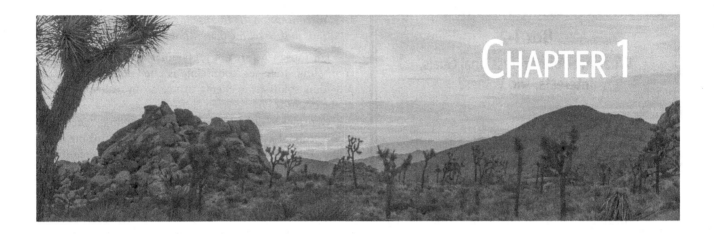

CHAPTER 1

What Is Counseling in Speech-Language Pathology?

Aspen Townsend, MS, CCC-SLP, and Jerry K. Hoepner, PhD, CCC-SLP

Anyone who willingly enters into the pain of a stranger is truly a remarkable person. ~ Henri Nouwen

Most of us have had some exposure to counseling or at least the idea of counseling—personally, through family, friends, television, or movies. As such, we may have a pretty good idea of what counseling is, or we may hold several misconceptions about it. Further, a variety of professionals deliver counseling, so our concept of counseling may be linked to a particular type of counseling. Before delving into counseling theories or approaches, let's begin by exploring your conceptualizations of counseling. Throughout this book, there are application boxes, which include exercises, cases, and other information. See Box 1-1 for the first of these applications.

Box 1-1

What Is Counseling?

Before starting, check in:

How would you define counseling? How and why do speech-language pathologists counsel in their practice?

Try to do this before reading the definitions. Begin with your intuitive definition.

Counseling Defined

Luterman (2019) defines counseling as "the components of the clinician-client relationship that promote self-enhancing behavior in the client through the judicious provision of information, while also allowing for the expression of painful feelings in an emotionally safe context" (p. 903).

DiLollo and Neimeyer (2022) define counseling as "those components of the clinician-client relationship that facilitate personal growth and empowerment for clients (and their families), with the goal of helping individuals and/or

Hoepner, J. K. (Ed.). *Counseling and Motivational Interviewing in Speech-Language Pathology* (pp. 1-14).

Box 1-2

What Are Your Professional Goals, Interests, and Values?

Check in:

Why do you want to become a speech-language pathologist?

families manage, adjust to, and cope with communication and swallowing disorders and the treatments for those disorders" (p. 5).

Holland and Nelson (2020) identify components of counseling in communication disorders as "trying to understand how the world looks to clients . . . encourage their expression . . . advising . . . and helping individuals to translate information into satisfying and successful actions" (pp. 12-13).

In the context of speech-language pathology, we define counseling as a collaborative relationship, whereby clinicians help to elicit client and/or family perspectives, feelings, goals, and solutions to challenges encountered within developmental and acquired communication and swallowing disorders and the treatment process. Clinicians are responsive to the client's ideas, culture, emotional status, readiness to learn, and focused on fostering meaningful participation within self-selected activity.

Addressing Misconceptions

We ask you to forget much of what you know or think you know about what counseling is. Many of the common perceptions of counseling are misconceptions or misinterpretations. Counseling, at its core, is about empowering, motivating, evoking, and uncovering a person's own solutions-values-beliefs, and suppressing our solutions-ideas-biases. It is about uncovering the backstory that explains the current behavior and inhibiting our human tendency to make judgments about the actions, beliefs, and thoughts of others. Consider your path to becoming a speech-language pathologist. How might that predispose you to having a fixer mentality? See Box 1-2 for a reflection exercise.

If your answer to the previous question is something along the lines of "I want to help other people be successful/communicate/have successful relationships/have a good quality of life," you're not alone. This is why many speech-language pathologists enter the field, but with it often comes a strong *fixer reflex*. Read on to learn why that fixer reflex might not be the best means toward your goal of helping others.

Misconception #1: Counseling is giving people solutions and/or telling them what they need to do.

For those who are not yet familiar with evidence-based counseling strategies, counseling is often conceptualized as providing solutions to clients' problems. In reality, it should be the opposite.

Consider a "direct" approach to counseling. Your client tells you about a problem they are facing. You think creatively and come up with a solution. You tell them the solution—easy fix! But they haven't followed your advice—it seems so easy; they can solve their problem if they just do this one thing. Why haven't they done it? Because it was your solution to the problem and not theirs. In many cases, advice elicits a pushback response. When we give advice, we make the arguments for change, which puts our clients in the position of arguing against change (Miller & Rollnick, 2013).

Or maybe they did follow your advice, and it worked. Great! You are the super speech-language pathologist and you swooped in, solved the problem, and made your client happy. Man, that feels good! But they eventually leave your caseload because we all know we can't work with our clients forever. Another problem comes up, except this time you're not around to give them the solution. Well, now what? Your client feels hopeless and doesn't know what to do. You gave them a one-time fix, but not the skills to fix future problems. You might not be around to see this part, but this doesn't feel so good. The super speech-language pathologist didn't help prepare the client to be independent after dismissal. Instead, you may have inadvertently created a false dependency.

This instinct to give our clients a solution to their problem is called the *fixer reflex*. As you continue to grow in your practice as a speech-language pathologist, you will have to learn how to actively inhibit your fixer reflex. The intentions of the fixer reflex are great, but the end result is not. It's also something that could get in the way of building a solid therapeutic alliance with your client (Hall et al., 2010; Lawton et al., 2016; Lieberman, 2018; Morrison & Smith, 2013; Pinto et al., 2012; Wolter et al., 2006). Imagine yourself as a *facilitator*, rather than a fixer. As a speech-language pathologist, you help facilitate clients' success toward their goals. You can evoke effective communication, reveal desires and motivation, and collaborate on a plan (Miller & Rollnick, 2013). In doing this, the client is solving their problem in a way that is manageable for them, while also developing the skills to continue to solve problems more and more independently.

It is important to be mindful and self-reflect to recognize when you are fixing rather than facilitating. If you can feel your fixer reflex trying to get through in a moment and aren't sure what to say in place of it, try just being silent. Leave room for your client to think, process, and say something first. Chapter 2 addresses some potential approaches to reflecting and learning from practice interactions.

Misconception #2: Counseling is more about talking than listening.

This misconception makes most speech-language pathologists uncomfortable because it can lead to silence and awkward pauses in conversations. We're speech-language pathologists because we generally like talking, right? The most valuable information a speech-language pathologist will get from a client often follows an awkward silence in the conversation. Especially if you take into consideration the fact that many of the clients we work with benefit from extended processing time.

Many of us have heard the term "active listening" but probably do not fully understand its meaning. Miller and Rollnick (2013) recoined this term as **reflective listening,** defined as "the skill of 'active' listening whereby the counselor seeks to understand the client's subjective experience, offering reflections as guesses about the person's meaning" (p. 412). The goal of reflective listening is to allow the client to reflect on their own experiences without interruption.

You'll learn more about specific listening and reflecting skills in the upcoming chapters. The important takeaway is that listening is likely more valuable than any advice you could ever give.

Give your client your undivided attention. Mirror their emotional expression. If a client shares something sad, you can have a sad expression on your face. This shows them that you are truly listening (Miller & Rollnick, 2013). If a pause occurs, sit in the silence with them and wait. That's where the magic happens.

Having considered this misconception (i.e., counseling is more about talking than listening), it is time to evaluate your current listening skills. See Box 1-3 for this exercise.

Misconception #3: Counseling is only needed for people with mental health diagnoses.

We utilize our communication skills to interact and connect with those around us. When communication is impacted in any way (articulation, language, cognition, voice, etc.), relationships are impacted.

Imagine this . . .

- You are no longer able to tell your partner that you love them.
- Speaking in public gives you incredible anxiety because you are worried what people will think if you stutter.
- You crave connection with people around you but don't understand neurotypical social norms essential to building relationships.
- You are just hearing for the first time that your child might not speak verbally.

These are situations that occur daily for many speech-language pathologists (Hoepner & Townsend, in press). These situations are all directly related to communication disorders. These situations can be incredibly intimidating if you don't have adequate counseling skills to address them. Speech-language pathologists recognize the need to proactively address mental health—one stated, "Go ahead

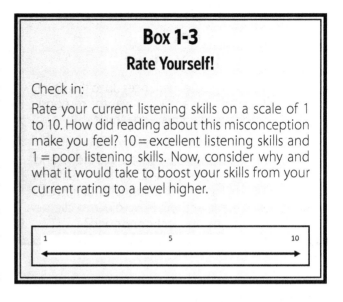

Box 1-3
Rate Yourself!

Check in:
Rate your current listening skills on a scale of 1 to 10. How did reading about this misconception make you feel? 10 = excellent listening skills and 1 = poor listening skills. Now, consider why and what it would take to boost your skills from your current rating to a level higher.

| 1 | 5 | 10 |

and [start] addressing their mental health right away, and the families' mental health right away because we know they're going to be struggling. We know they're going to be having hard times but yet we wait for them to reach out to us." Interviews of practicing speech-language pathologists revealed that they feel unprepared to handle many counseling moments, that they spent little time on counseling training in their graduate program, and they lack adequate skills to address grief and loss (Hoepner & Townsend, in press). Failure to address counseling moments occurs not only due to lack of comfort or preparation. One speech-language pathologist remarked, "Sometimes, I will literally just leave the room for 3 minutes because obviously we're timed in rehab with our, our care, so I will leave and then just come back in 3 minutes." Institutional factors, like productivity, can also impose a sense of constraint on time devoted to counseling. Others see counseling as a priority, "So, I think counseling is probably just as therapeutic as taking out your cognitive worksheets and doing some drill and practice exercises." Unfortunately, many speech-language pathologists do not employ specific, evidence-based counseling approaches, which has the potential to limit their intentionality and effectiveness. This is highlighted by this startling statement: "I feel pretty comfortable counseling them. I don't know if I am doing any structured counseling, and I don't know if I'm doing any evidence-based counseling." Our point is this: You will encounter counseling needs and thus you need specific training in counseling methods to respond to counseling moments.

Now that you have considered the misconception that counseling is only needed for those with mental health diagnoses, consider the types of counseling moments you have encountered with your clients and families (e.g., trouble communicating with loved ones, anxiety, trouble fitting in, loss and disruption to expectations). Complete the exercise in Box 1-4.

Box 1-4
Have You Ever?

Consider your clinical experiences up to this point. How did you interact and what was the response from your clients, partners, and families?

Check in:

Have you encountered clients, partners, and families who were experiencing the situations described previously? How did that situation go? What was your reaction? How did the clients, partners, and families react or respond?

Box 1-5
Reflections on Misconceptions

Check in:

What misconceptions did you hold prior to reading? How have your thoughts changed?

Self-reflection is a foundational step in building counseling skills. It's important to notice any biases you may hold, as they can easily come out during counseling moments. Recognizing these biases can help prevent them from arising while you are counseling clients. Reflection helps us to become more intentional about the way we counsel and the methods we use. It also helps us to develop our counseling voice, which we will discuss further in the upcoming chapters.

As a speech-language pathologist, when you have counseling skills you can rely on, these are the situations that make our job magical. Navigating and supporting clients and their families through these moments is where you will see real, tangible progress in daily communication (Hall et al., 2010; Lawton et al., 2016; Morrison & Smith, 2013; Pinto et al., 2012).

Communication does not happen out of context. We can't treat communication disorders without adequately recognizing the impact communication has on our daily lives. Speaking of which, let's talk about the "speech bubble."

Misconception #4: Counseling is not relevant to speech-language pathology.

It's not uncommon for speech-language pathologists to find comfort in their **speech bubble.** The speech bubble consists of targeting goals and monitoring progress all within your speech therapy room walls. The focus is on what the client is doing in an unnatural, decontextualized environment. When speech-language pathologists restrict their scope of practice strictly to therapy techniques addressing articulation, phonology, language, cognition, stuttering, voice, etc. in a controlled setting, it makes the job very easy. It can feel like everything is going well.

The trouble with this situation is that speech-language pathologists are looking at the communication disorder out of context. But in the real world, communication is all about context. How can we adequately treat a communication disorder without addressing the context for communication? How can we improve language skills in a client with aphasia without addressing how their reduced language ability has impacted their close relationships? How can we empower clients who stutter to speak confidently without addressing their experiences with bullying or anxiety related to speaking? How can we promote caregiver buy-in to helping a client use an AAC device without addressing how limited communication modes have impacted the family? We can't. Especially if our goals are measuring real life impact on communication skills, rather than arbitrary goals that keep us in our "speech bubble."

Now that you have read about several common misconceptions, identify which ones you held prior to this reading. Complete the exercise in Box 1-5 to identify your past misconceptions and any changes based upon this reading.

A New Beginning: A Baseline Assessment of Your Counseling Knowledge and Skills Status

Reflection is certainly a crucial part of developing as a clinician and counselor. We often use the mash-up term **preflection**, to think about expectations and questions heading into a new learning experience. The first **preflection** tool to consider is called the Notes to Supervisor assessment (Gottwald & Parris, 2006). See Box 1-6 for the Notes to Supervisor assignment. This is a great tool for beginning counselors, as they work with clients in parallel to their learning about counseling methods. Egan (2002) developed a checklist of **soft spots**, which identify an individual's tendencies in a counseling situation (Table 1-1). Being aware of your tendencies can help you be mindful of how to address them or preempt them in clinical contexts. For instance, I had a clinical supervisee who was very direct in her communication with me, other supervisors, and clinicians. Being clear in your communication is a tremendous asset, but it can sometimes be construed by others as abrasive or confrontational. After a difficult conversation, during which she of course shared that she had no idea she was coming across this way, we had a conversation about how she might deal with this "tendency." She identified that

Box 1-6

Notes to Supervisor: Exploration of Counseling Supervision Needs

For undergraduate or graduate students currently enrolled in a counseling course, concurrently with clinical experiences, we suggest completing this "assignment" and reviewing it with your clinical supervisor. If you are a practicing clinician, this reflection can help you frame learning goals and seek information or experiences to develop your counseling skills.

Supervisor: _____   Client type: _____

Providing supervisors with information about your background and experiences in the area of counseling will enable us to help you make the most of your clinical practicum and supervisory experiences. Please complete the following nine questions to guide us in facilitating your growth and development.

1. Describe any previous clinical experiences you have had where counseling was a component of the work with the client and/or their family.

2. Describe any coursework/training you have had that focused on or included information about counseling.

3. Write down three questions below that you have concerning the counseling components of your work with this client:

    a.

    b.

    c.

4. Using the rating scale below, rate your comfort level with each of the following activities:

    1. = Very Comfortable

    2. = Somewhat Comfortable

    3. = Neutral

    4. = Somewhat Uncomfortable

    5. = Very Uncomfortable

This set of questions and rating scale can be revisited periodically to reassess your level of comfort with your own counseling skills.

    How comfortable do you feel:

- Listening actively to your clients in an empathetic way?
- Providing your clients with reassurance and reinforcement?
- Restating what you hear your client saying?
- Reflecting feelings you hear your client expressing?
- Asking open-ended questions to encourage exploration?
- Sharing your own personal experiences with your client? Specifically, knowing when and when not to do so.
- Interpreting the underlying meaning of something your client says?
- Telling your client how you feel in the moment, such as annoyance at being interrupted or uncomfortable because of something they said?
- Challenging your client to identify their own discrepancies, contradictions, and/or irrational beliefs?

5. What do you think your greatest strengths and greatest needs are in becoming an effective speech-language pathologist in the area of counseling? See Egan's (2002) list of possible "soft spots" for ideas.

    a. Strengths:

    b. Soft spots:

(continued)

Box 1-6 (CONTINUED)
Notes to Supervisor: Exploration of Counseling Supervision Needs

6. What is your biggest concern about being in the role of counselor as a speech-language pathologist?

7. Put a hatch mark or X on the counseling continuum below, where you would place your current counseling skill level:

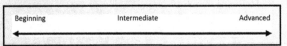

8. Questions to ask your supervisor:
   a. What potential counseling needs does this particular client(s) have?
   b. What is the supervisor's approach to counseling in general and specific to this client?

9. Any additional thoughts or comments?

You may wish to share this document with your supervisor or review it together.

---

she would try to be mindful of this tendency and soften her questions and statements to supervisors and peers. Further, we discussed the idea that she may want to disclose this about herself from the outset of a supervisory or collaborative relationship (e.g., "Sometimes when I'm unclear on something or need more information, I have a tendency to ask very direct questions or make statements that could be construed as questioning other's rationale or approach. I just want you to know that my intent is absolutely never to be disrespectful or put you on the defensive."). Simply disclosing this likely preempts any potential miscommunications, and her supervisors/peers will likely grow to appreciate her questions and statements of clarification. Likewise, recognizing and potentially disclosing or being mindful of our tendencies can be very important in our clinical relationships. These tendencies may affect not only how you say or do things, but how you react when others say or do things in their interactions with you (e.g., in this case, clients or their families or colleagues). As a "helper," you may not identify at all with some of these soft spots and may closely identify with others.

Distinguishing Professional Counseling (Psychotherapy) From Nonprofessional Counseling Practices

As we talk about counseling, it's important to recognize the difference between *professional counseling* practitioners (psychotherapists) and *nonprofessional counseling practices* (e.g., speech-language pathologists, nurses, occupational therapists, physical therapists). Licensed professional counselors (LPCs) and clinical social workers (CSWs) are two of the main professions that engage in professional counseling. According to the American Counseling Association (2011), "The practice of professional counseling includes, but is not limited to, the diagnosis and treatment of mental and emotional disorders, including addictive disorders; psychoeducational techniques aimed at the prevention of such disorders; consultation to individuals, couples, families, groups, and organizations; and research into more effective therapeutic treatment modalities."

These mental health professionals have the training and skills to assess and treat mental and emotional disorders. If you are working with a client who has or may have a mental health disorder, collaboration with an LPC or CSW is recommended. If your client is bringing forward social/emotional problems that are directly related to their communication disorder, or are a result of their communication disorder, then that counseling moment falls within your scope of practice.

TABLE 1-1	
Egan's Checklist of Soft Spots Summarized	
☑ **IF YOU DO THIS**	**SOFT SPOTS—YOUR TENDENCIES IN INTERPERSONAL INTERACTIONS**
	I'm shy and have trouble interacting with new people.
	I'm fairly compliant and sometimes let others push me around.
	I get angry pretty easily and sometimes let my anger show.
	I have trouble having enough energy to listen to others.
	I'm somewhat uncomfortable around/with people of a different gender.
	I can be somewhat insensitive or lack tact, although that is not my intent.
	I'm very covert with my emotions, not letting them show to others or even myself.
	I like to be in charge and exert control of situations.
	I have a strong need to be liked by others, so I'm careful not to disagree with or offend others.
	I have few positive feelings about myself and sometimes put myself down.
	I never stop to really examine my values and may flip flop on them.
	I feel deeply compelled to help others.
	I'm sensitive and easily hurt.
	My self-image is deeply rooted in what others think of me.
	Sometimes people see me as difficult, contradictory, and self-centered.
	I'm anxious a lot of the time.
	I'm a bit impulsive.
	I'm very stubborn and have fairly strong opinions.
	I'm not very reflective and don't really examine my own behaviors often.
	I'm pretty good at charming people to get them to do what I want.
	I don't often go out of my way to meet other people's needs.
	I'm somewhat lonely and question whether others like me.
	I'm awkward in social situations.
	I'm ditzy, sort of unaware, or naïve at times.
	I'm somewhat stingy or protective of my time.
	I have a tendency to defer to others or not stand up for what I think is right.
	I don't like (hate) conflict and tend to be a peace maker.
	I get defensive when others tell me what to do or question my approach.

Adapted from Egan, G. (2002). *Exercises in helping skills: A training manual to accompany the skilled helper* (7th ed.). Brooks/Cole Pub Co.

If you are ever uncomfortable or unsure whether a situation is in your scope or requires more support, it's always a good idea to reach out to a mental health professional. Many speech-language pathologists have found success in collaboration with these professionals (Attard et al., 2018; Boles & Lewis, 2000). When a situation moves out of your scope, counseling skills can benefit you in your response to the client and connecting them with more support.

Scope of Practice and Referrals

The American Speech-Language-Hearing Association (ASHA) outlines the scope of practice for speech-language pathology into eight main service delivery domains. One of these eight domains is counseling, and two of the other domains utilize counseling skills: collaboration and prevention and wellness (ASHA, 2016).

Therefore, counseling is a critical skill for speech-language pathologists. ASHA states, "The role of the SLP in the counseling process includes interactions related to emotional reactions, thoughts, feelings, and behaviors that result from living with the communication disorder, feeding and swallowing disorder, or related disorders" (p. 9). Speech-language pathologists directly address the impact the communication or swallowing disorder has on the individual through counseling.

Here are some specific ways speech-language pathologists can counsel, as outlined by ASHA (2016):

- Empower the individual and family to make informed decisions related to communication or feeding and swallowing issues.

- Educate the individual, family, and related community members about communication or feeding and swallowing disorders.

- Provide support and/or peer-to-peer groups for individuals with disorders and their families.

- Provide individuals and families with skills that enable them to become self-advocates.

- Discuss, evaluate, and address negative emotions and thoughts related to communication or feeding and swallowing disorders.

- Refer individuals with disorders to other professionals when counseling needs fall outside of those related to (a) communication and (b) feeding and swallowing.

Now that you have read ASHA's description of our scope of practice, consider your current understanding. Complete the exercise in Box 1-7.

Many speech-language pathologists do not feel prepared or competent in their counseling skills to regularly engage in counseling moments in practice (Pasupathy & Bogschutz, 2013; Phillips & Mendel, 2008). This is concerning, as ASHA regards counseling as a large part of speech-language pathology service delivery. Ineffective training in identifying and engaging in counseling moments could lead to speech-language pathologists implicitly avoiding sensitive topics their patients bring up (Simmons-Mackie & Damico, 2011). This is why Doud et al. (2020) argue for more consistent, effective counseling training across speech-language pathology graduate programs.

Because counseling in the scope of practice for speech-language pathologists is intentionally vague, many speech-language pathologists are uncertain as to when a situation falls within their scope or whether they should refer. Hoepner and Townsend (in press) interviewed speech-language pathologists across settings who worked with individuals with aphasia, and all of their participants commented on the ambiguity of the scope of practice in regard to counseling. One speech-language pathologist remarked that speech-language pathologists are often told, "'this is the psychologist's job,' but you're going to be in their shoes sometimes." Indeed, we do frequently find ourselves in this position, which is deeply related to our expertise in fostering communication and thus expression of emotions. Terrell and Osborne (2020) argue that our interventions themselves further prompt the need

Box 1-7
What Are the Bounds of Our Scope of Practice?

Check in:
Did you know counseling was included in the speech-language pathology scope of practice? How do you feel about the ways speech-language pathologists should counsel?

for counseling: "A patient's spontaneous expressions of emotion are often triggered by therapy itself, such as when the patient with word-finding difficulty is confronted, yet again, by the loss of facile speech and expresses deep concern about his ability to return to work. Similarly, a mother watching her young daughter unable to correctly answer questions on a language assessment may cry and worry aloud if her daughter will ever be able to graduate from high school. These are highly charged emotional scenarios that are completely within the scope of practice of speech-language pathologists" (p. 328). Speech-language pathologists need to have the skills to confidently address counseling moments when they arise (Simmons-Mackie & Damico, 2011). Having a strong relationship with the client helps the speech-language pathologist to be able to have these difficult conversations (Hall et al., 2010; Lawton et al., 2016; Morrison & Smith, 2013; Pinto et al., 2012; Worrall et al., 2011) and through these conversations, speech-language pathologists can determine whether the situations fit into their scope or if a referral is necessary. If it is beyond our scope, we need training in when and how to refer: "I think that there's probably some partnering that the SLP program needs to do with like psychology and counseling programs to better [improve] skills" (Townsend & Hoepner, 2021).

Knowing When and How to Refer to Mental Health Experts

Indications for referrals relate to our scope of practice, training and expertise, and the complexity of client needs. Here are some common reasons for making a referral to a mental health expert/counselor:

- The client presents with issues that are **not communication, cognition, or feeding and swallowing related.**

- The client presents with issues that go **beyond your expertise.**

- The client has issues that are communication, cognition, and swallowing related, but there are just **too many** to address while balancing with other treatment goals.

- You know that something is going on, and you're **not even sure** where to begin.

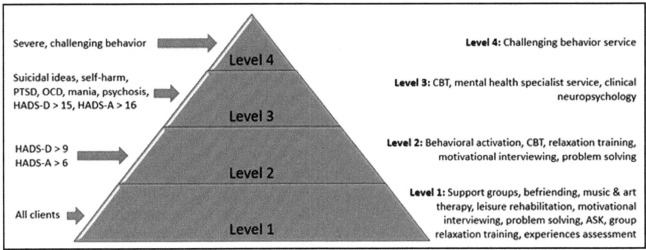

Figure 1-1. Stepped-Care Model of Collaborative Psychosocial Care (Reproduced with permission from Kneebone, I. I. (2016). Stepped psychological care after stroke. *Disability and Rehabilitation, 38*(18), 1836-1843. https://doi.org/10.3109/09638288.2015.1107764; Note: PTSD = posttraumatic stress disorder, OCD = obsessive compulsive disorder, HADS = Hospital Anxiety & Depression Scale, CBT = cognitive behavioral therapy, ASK = action success knowledge program.)

Box 1-8

The Stepped-Care Model

Check out this great podcast conversation on Aphasia Access Conversations, episode #34, with Dr. Ian Kneebone, as he discusses the Stepped-Care model and more.

https://aphasiaaccess.libsyn.com/34-in -conversation-with-ian-keebone

---

Your specific level of expertise relates to your individual training and competence in delivering counseling interventions. The Stepped-Care Model of Collaborative Psychosocial Care provides a guide for referrals and disciplinary expertise (Figure 1-1; Kneebone, 2016). For instance, most speech-language pathologists should have skills to carry out Level 1 interventions, including support groups, problem solving, and experiences assessment. Some speech-language pathologists, who have received training in techniques such as motivational interviewing or cognitive behavioral therapy, may have the competence and confidence to deliver Level 2 interventions. Behavioral activation techniques are similar to participation-based interventions, such as those delivered in the Life Participation Approach to Aphasia (Chapey et al., 2000). As a client's needs progress to Levels 3 and 4, referral is definitely warranted. Note that while the levels of intervention progress toward the need for specialized mental health professionals, this is not mutually exclusive from an integrated care model where mental health counselors collaborate across levels with speech-language pathologists. For more information about the Stepped-Care Model, see Box 1-8 for a link to a podcast on the topic with Ian Kneebone.

Once you determine that a referral is necessary, there are several considerations for that referral, including insurance options, network options, hometown options, and most important—client and family preferences. After you have helped clients and their families sort through those considerations, identify who is best prepared and positioned to help the types of clients on your caseload; which disciplines (in your facility, in your city/region) do the type of counseling you're looking for; and which providers are willing to learn communication techniques and to collaborate. Some individuals and their families prefer self-referral and others may already have a counselor, so be sure to explore these options as well.

As alluded to with regards to the collaborative, Stepped-Care Model, referral doesn't mean handoff. Our skill in supporting communication will continue to put our clients in a position to feel comfortable and capable of sharing with us. We may uncover things that others may not, even with a concerted training effort. Ongoing collaboration is key, so we can continue to address communication-related issues when they arise and communicate with professional counselors.

Forming and Maintaining Interdisciplinary Collaborations

A common challenge for initial referrals to professional mental health counselors is that they have limited training and skill in supporting communication for persons with developmental or acquired communication impairments. Consider a situation where you're working with an individual with a communication disorder, applying tools for supporting communication effectively, and they disclose a concern that warrants a referral to a professional counselor. One of the common challenges you may encounter, particularly following that counselor's first interactions with the client,

---

Box 1-9

Communication Partner Training Considerations for Mental Health Counselors

Skills to train:

- Broadly, multimodality communication techniques.
  - Supported conversation techniques (Kagan, 1998)
    - Written choice (Garrett & Beukelman, 1995)
    - Rating scales (Kagan, 1998)
    - Drawing (Lyon, 1995a, 1995b)
    - Keywords (Archer, 2016; Archer et al., 2019; Kagan, 1998)
    - Wait time
  - Self-generated photography as a means of expression. There is evidence from mental health nursing literature (Miller & Happell, 2006), as well as aphasia intervention literature (Baier et al., 2017; Brown et al., 2010; Germain, 2004; Hoepner et al., 2017) that self-generated photography can help individuals express complex ideas and feelings that are difficult to put into words.
  - Multimodal, visual sorts. Includes commercially available tools like Talking Mats (Bornman & Murphy, 2006), Activity Card Sort (Baum & Edwards, 2001, 2008), LIV Cards (Haley et al., 2010, 2013), and homegrown sorts.
  - Augmentative and alternative communication systems—no-tech, low-tech, and high-tech speech generative devices.

Training approach:

- Preferably hands-on, collaborative interactions with direct models and opportunities for practice.
- There are a number of communication partner training approaches to consider across the lifespan and disorders.

---

is that the counselor was unable to get anywhere with the client. Perhaps the client did not share any of their concerns with the counselor or the counselor simply lacked the communication skills necessary to have an effective counseling session. That may lead you to asking, "What does it take to nurture, support, strengthen, and maintain that collaboration?" Given the bounds of your counseling "jurisdiction," it may be useful to begin with a bit of grace. "You're the counseling expert. Here's where we overlap and where my expertise ends . . ." This type of a conversation may help to foster a sense of collaboration and avoid any territorialization. They are the mental health expert but you are the communication support expert. Our next role is to train them, following best practices for communication partner training, specifically those elements designed to train fellow professionals (see Box 1-9 for training content and methods).

Ideally, we should attempt to forge a collaboration, not a consultation. This can help to facilitate a two-way information exchange (as permitted, on a need-to-know basis, which likely varies with each client). They may share issues they're trying to work through and how we can help. Likewise, we share communication strategies and what you uncover given your skilled communication supports that they may or may not have uncovered.

Real-life issue: You will not only have to sort out how to maintain the synergistic collaborations . . .

- Some professional counselors can be territorial.
- Acknowledge your boundaries and scope.
- Emphasize your reliance on them for addressing deeper mental health concerns.

History and Direction— Why Speech-Language Pathologists?

Speech-language pathologists are experts in evoking a person's most effective modes of communication. Often times, speech therapy sessions are where clients are able to communicate to the best of their abilities. Therefore, it elicits the opportunity to communicate things that have been weighing heavy on their mind but are complicated to talk about. In this way, speech-language pathologists evoke feelings from clients naturally (Townsend & Hoepner, 2021). Consider your experiences addressing emotional adjustment

---

Box 1-10

Reflecting on Past Counseling Moments

Check in:

In your experiences to this point, have you had a situation where a client brought forward an emotional problem/situation? What did you do?

Box 1-11

Where Do You Stand?

Reflect on Chapter 1 as you begin to reshape your conceptions of counseling in speech-language pathology. This is a precursor to the Growth as a Counselor and "Self-Assessment of Counseling Skills" structured reflections that follow. You are encouraged to return to those structured reflections as you near the completion of your counseling course or your independent studies of this text. Reflect on your answers to these six questions.

1. How are you feeling right now? Label your emotions.
2. What stood out to you in this chapter?
3. What are your initial, honest reactions to the information in this chapter?
4. What do you want to get out of this text? Write at least two goals for yourself.
5. What are your goals as a speech-language pathologist? What do you value/want to pursue in your practice?
6. How do your past experiences, beliefs, values, culture, biases, knowledge, and skills influence the way you respond (internally or overtly) to your clients and their families?

---

moments with your clients. Complete the brief reflection in Box 1-10.

As a speech-language pathologist, you will encounter situations where clients share social emotional troubles with you on a regular basis. At the bare minimum, speech-language pathologists need the skills to navigate situations when these troubles arise. Ideally, speech-language pathologists possess counseling skills to adequately address how the communication disorder is impacting the client's life, and then use that conversation to transition to functional, client-centered therapy.

Through counseling skills, you can build a better therapeutic alliance with your client. This strong relationship and trust between speech-language pathologist and client has been proven to increase effectiveness of therapy (Attard et al., 2000; Lieberman, 2018; Wolter et al., 2006). Therefore, counseling is a critical skill needed to make effective growth in speech therapy.

Educational Versus Adjustment-Based Socioemotional Counseling

Speech-language pathologists require the skills to counsel in many different ways. It's important to make the distinction between educational counseling and socioemotional counseling. ASHA's practice portal makes the distinction between *informational counseling*, defined as "discussing with individuals and their families/caregivers the nature of a disorder or situation, intervention considerations and techniques, prognosis, and material and community resources," and *personal adjustment counseling*, defined as addressing "feelings emotions, thoughts and beliefs expressed by individuals and their families/caregivers (e.g., realization of the pervasive impact of a communication disorder on day-to-day life)" (ASHA, n.d.). Although many speech-language pathologists feel more comfortable with informational counseling (Townsend & Hoepner, 2021), both types of counseling are necessary for successful therapy.

You will learn more specific details on informational (educational) counseling and personal adjustment counseling later in this text. As a speech-language pathologist, you will have to determine what a client needs in the moment. Using counseling skills, you will be able to meet the client where they are. You can determine whether they are ready for extensive details of their communication disorder or if they can only handle the main points. You will need to determine if this is the time to give them information or if it should wait. Navigating these situations takes practice but will again lead to a better therapeutic alliance between you and your client, in turn increasing positive speech therapy outcomes (Hall et al., 2010; Lawton et al.; 2016, Morrison & Smith, 2013; Pinto et al., 2012).

Self-Reflection

Take a minute to process this information. Hopefully, you are beginning to understand how important counseling is to the field of speech-language pathology. Throughout this text you will gain specific, tangible knowledge to effectively incorporate counseling into speech therapy practice. These skills will change the way you approach your therapy as a speech-language pathologist. We want you to be ready to learn that information. In order to do that, check in with yourself now by completing the exercise in Box 1-11. Complete the following self-reflection:

Growth as a Counselor

The exercise in Box 1-12 landed here because it connects closely to concepts in this chapter; however, we would like you to revisit it at the end of your journey, so please bookmark this page and return to it at the end of your term (in the case of students) or when you finish reading this book.

Chapter Summary

Our conceptualization of "what counseling is" is likely to be based on our past experiences with counseling and exposure to counseling in popular media and our previous coursework. What counseling really is in the context of speech-language pathology may be something very different than what you had in mind. Reflecting upon and learning about yourself will strengthen your ability to deliver counseling effectively. We expect that your concept of "what counseling is" will evolve as you continue to read this text, engage in the exercises, and begin to incorporate counseling moments into your practice. You will develop a stronger understanding of the scope of practice for speech-language pathologists regarding counseling and how best to collaborate with and make referrals to other mental health professionals.

As speech-language pathologists, we are nonprofessional counselors. That doesn't mean we're not good at it; rather, it serves as a distinction between our scope of practice, where counseling is directly related to communication, cognition, or swallowing, vs. the roles of professional counselors. Part of feeling comfortable with our role in counseling as a speech-language pathologist is understanding when and how to make referrals along with how to collaborate with and train our professional counseling colleagues. The Stepped-Care Model is one tool to help frame our scope of practice and know when to refer.

Self-assessment and reflection are a crucial tool for developing clinical and counseling skills. A number of tools are available to help structure your reflections. We recommend that you reflect regularly and revisit structured self-assessment tools periodically.

Key Takeaways

- A speech-language pathologist's role in counseling may be different than your initial conceptualization of counseling.

- A speech-language pathologist's scope of practice for counseling includes informational and personal adjustment counseling delivered to individuals with communication disorders and their families/caregivers. Anything related to communication, cognition, and swallowing falls within our jurisdiction.
- The Stepped-Care Model helps define our counseling boundaries and when to refer to professional counselors.
- Regular reflection is important to development of clinical and counseling skills.
- Take some time to complete baseline and follow-up reflections as you continue to work through this text.

References

American Counseling Association. (2011). *Who are licensed professional counselors.* https://www.counseling.org/PublicPolicy/WhoAreLPCs.pdf

American Speech-Language-Hearing Association. (n.d.). *Counseling for Professional Service Delivery* (Practice Portal). https://www.asha.org/Practice-Portal/Professional-Issues/Counseling-For-Professional-Service-Delivery/

American Speech-Language-Hearing Association. (2016). *Scope of practice in speech-language pathology* (Scope of Practice). https://www.asha.org/policy/

Archer, B. (2016). Facilitated conversation groups for people with aphasia: A cognitive ethnographic study [Doctoral dissertation]. https://search.proquest.com/docview/1844992660

Archer, B., Azios, J. H., Tetnowski, J., Damico, J., Freer, J. C., Schmadeke, S., & Christou-Franklin, E. (2019). Key wording practices in three aphasia conversation groups: A preliminary study. *Aphasiology, 33*(10), 1248-1269. https://doi.org/10.1080/02687038.2019.1630596

Attard, M., Loupis, Y., Togher, L., & Rose, M. (2018). The efficacy of an inter-disciplinary community aphasia group for living well with aphasia. *Aphasiology, 32*(2), 105-138. https://doi.org/10.1080/02687038.2017.1381877

Baier, C. K., Hoepner, J. K., & Sather, T. W. (2017). Exploring snapchat as a dynamic capture tool for social exchange among individuals with aphasia. *Aphasiology, 32*(11), 1336-1359. https://doi.org/10.1080/02687038.2017.1409870

Barrett, S. E., Puryear, J. S., Westpheling, K., & Fund, C. (2008). *Health literacy practices in primary care settings: Examples from the field* (pp. 1-36). Commonwealth Fund.

Baum, C., & Edwards, D. (2001). *ACS: Activity Card Sort.* American Occupational Therapy Association, Incorporated (AOTA Press).

Baum, C., & Edwards, D. (2008). *ACS: Activity Card Sort.* American Occupational Therapy Association, Incorporated (AOTA Press).

Boles, L., & Lewis, M. (2000). Solution-focused co-therapy for a couple with aphasia. *Asia Pacific Journal of Speech, Language, and Hearing, 5*(2), 73-78. https://doi.org/10.1179/136132800805576988

Bornman, J., & Murphy, J. (2006). Using the ICF in goal setting: Clinical application using Talking Mats®. *Disability and Rehabilitation: Assistive Technology, 1*(3), 145-154. https://doi.org/10.1080/17483100612331392745

Brown, K., Worrall, L., Davidson, B., & Howe, T. (2010). Snapshots of success: An insider perspective on living successfully with aphasia. *Aphasiology, 24*(10), 1267-1295. https://doi.org/10.1080/02687031003755429

Chapey, R., Duchan, J. F., Elman, R. J., Garcia, L. J., Kagan, A., Lyon, J. G., & Simmons Mackie, N. (2000). Life participation approach to aphasia: A statement of values for the future. *The ASHA Leader, 5*(3), 4-6. https://doi.org/10.1044/leader.FTR.05032000.4

Box 1-12

Reflections on Your Growth as a Counselor

Whether you are reading this text as a part of your counseling class, as a resource about counseling methods you refer to in another course, or as a professional seeking to further develop your counseling skills, you are encouraged to revisit and reflect upon your counseling skills when you finish this text and/or at the end of your learning experience. To do so, we will draw upon a framework for **Reflecting on Growth as a Counselor** by Gottwald and Paris (2006; items 1 to 9) and modifications for addressing the motivational interviewing framework.

It may help to return to the **Self-Assessment of Counseling Skills** (Gottwald & Parris, 2006; items 1 to 9) and modifications for addressing the motivational interviewing framework (items 10 to 15), referred to earlier in this chapter in Box 1-6 but repeated and expanded here for easy access. In this case, we ask you to consider level of comfort and skill.

Key: 1 = novice, very uncomfortable; 2 = developing, somewhat uncomfortable, 3 = moderate, neutral; 4 = skilled, somewhat comfortable; 5 = very skilled, very comfortable

WHAT IS YOUR LEVEL OF COMFORT AND SKILL IN:	CIRCLE YOUR LEVEL				
1. Listening actively to your client in an empathetic way?	1	2	3	4	5
2. Providing your client with reassurance and reinforcement and/or affirming and validating your client?	1	2	3	4	5
3. Restating what you hear your client saying?	1	2	3	4	5
4. Reflecting feelings you hear your client expressing?	1	2	3	4	5
5. Asking open-ended questions to encourage exploration?	1	2	3	4	5
6. Sharing your own personal experiences with your client and knowing when to share/when not to share?	1	2	3	4	5
7. Interpreting the underlying (unspoken or covert) meaning from something your client says?	1	2	3	4	5
8. Telling your client how you feel in the moment, such as annoyance at being interrupted or uncomfortable because of something they said?	1	2	3	4	5
9. Challenging your client to identify their own discrepancies, contradictions, and/or irrational beliefs?	1	2	3	4	5
10. Eliciting information about your client's interests, values, and needs?	1	2	3	4	5
11. Collaboratively setting goals with your client?	1	2	3	4	5
12. Inhibiting your fixer reflex?	1	2	3	4	5
13. Inhibiting your righting reflex?	1	2	3	4	5
14. Evoking or eliciting your client's own solutions or reasons for change?	1	2	3	4	5
15. Helping your client to solidify their own concrete, actionable plan?	1	2	3	4	5

Note: For any items where your responses fall into the uncomfortable range, we encourage you to seek learning opportunities, mentorship and modeling, and continued reflection on your growth.

Reflecting on My Growth as a Counselor

1. What have I learned about helping people to change?

2. What have I learned about myself as a change agent/counselor?

3. What would I do differently with a given client, if I had to do it all over again? *[For students in a counseling class, you may wish to reflect on a specific client case from this semester. This could relate to a case summary assignment. For practicing professionals, you can reflect broadly on client successes and challenging clients or less than desirable outcomes.]*

4. The "nugget of gold" from this experience that I will remember.

DiLollo, A., & Neimeyer, R. A. (2022). *Counseling in speech-language pathology and audiology: Reconstructing personal narratives* (2nd ed.). Plural Publishing.

Doud, A., Hoepner, J. K., & Holland, A. (2019). A survey of counseling curricula among accredited CSD graduate student programs. *American Journal of Speech-Language Pathology, 29*(2), 789-803. https://doi.org/10.1044/2020_AJSLP-19-00042

Egan, G. (2002). *Exercises in helping skills: A training manual to accompany the skilled helper* (7th ed.). Brooks/Cole Pub Co.

Garrett, K. L., & Beukelman, D. R. (1995). Changes in the interaction patterns of an individual with severe aphasia given three types of partner support. *Clinical Aphasiology, 23*, 237-251.

Germain, R. (2004). An exploratory study using cameras and Talking Mats to access the views of young people with learning disabilities on their out-of-school activities. *British Journal of Learning Disabilities, 32*(4), 170-174. https://doi.org/10.1111/j.1468-3156.2004.00317.x

Gottwald, S. & Parris, D. (2006). *Helping people change: Teaching counseling skills in clinical practica.* American Speech-Language-Hearing Association Annual Convention.

Haley, K. L., Womack, J., Helm-Estabrooks, N., Caignon, D., & McCulloch, K. (2010). *Life interests and values cards.* University of North Carolina.

Haley, K. L., Womack, J., Helm-Estabrooks, N., Lovette, B., & Goff, R. (2013). Supporting autonomy for people with aphasia: Use of the Life Interests and Values (LIV) Cards. *Topics in Stroke Rehabilitation, 20*(1), 22-35. https://doi.org/10.1310/tsr2001-22

Hall, A. M., Ferreira, P. H., Maher, C. G., Latimer, J. & Ferreira, M. L. (2010). The influence of the therapist-patient relationship on treatment outcome in physical rehabilitation: A systematic review. *Physical Therapy, 90*(8), 1099-1110. https://doi.org/10.2522/ptj.20090245

Hoepner, J. K., Baier, C. K., Sather, T. W., & Clark, M. B. (2017). A pilot exploration of Snapchat as an aphasia-friendly social exchange technology at an aphasia camp. *Clinical Archives of Communication Disorders, 2*(1), 30-42. http://dx.doi.org/10.21849/cacd.2016.00087

Hoepner, J. K., & Townsend, A. K. (in press). Counseling practices of speech-language pathologists serving persons with aphasia: Examining training and preparedness within clinical practice. [Unpublished manuscript].

Holland, A. L., & Nelson, R. L. (2018). *Counseling in communication disorders: A wellness perspective.* Plural Publishing.

Kagan, A. (1998). Supported conversation for adults with aphasia: Methods and resources for training conversation partners. *Aphasiology, 12*(9), 816-830. https://doi.org/10.1080/02687039808249575

Kneebone, I. I. (2016). Stepped psychological care after stroke. *Disability and Rehabilitation, 38*(18), 1836-1843. https://doi.org/10.3109/09638288.2015.1107764

Lawton, H. M., Haddock, G., Conroy, P. & Sage, K. (2016). Therapeutic alliances in stroke rehabilitation: A metaethnography. *Archives of Physical Medicine and Rehabilitation, 97*(11), 1979-1993. https://doi.org/10.1016/j.apmr.2016.03.031

Lieberman, A. (2018). Counseling issues: Addressing behavioral and emotional considerations in the treatment of communication disorders. *American Journal of Speech-Language Pathology, 27*(1), 13-23. https://doi.org/10.1044/2017_AJSLP-16-0149

Luterman, D. (2020). On teaching counseling: Getting beyond informational counseling. *American Journal of Speech-Language Pathology, 29*(2), 903-908. https://doi.org/10.1044/2019_AJSLP-19-00013

Lyon, J. G. (1995a). Drawing: Its value as a communication aid for adults with aphasia. *Aphasiology, 9*(1), 33-50. https://doi.org/10.1080/02687039508248687

Lyon, J. G. (1995b). Communicative drawing: An augmentative mode of interaction. *Aphasiology, 9*(1), 84-94. https://doi.org/10.1080/02687039508248694

Miller, G., & Happell, B. (2006). Talking about hope: The use of participant photography. *Issues in Mental Health Nursing, 27*(10), 1051-1065. https://doi.org/10.1080/01612840600943697

Miller, W. R., & Rollnick, S. (2013). *Motivational interviewing: Helping people change.* Guilford Press.

Morrison, T. L., & Smith, J. D. (2013). Working alliance development in occupational therapy: A cross-case analysis. *Australian Occupational Therapy Journal, 60*(5), 326-333. https://doi.org/10.1111/1440-1630.12053

Pasupathy, R., & Bogschutz, R. J. (2013). An investigation of graduate Speech-Language Pathology students' SLP clinical self-efficacy. *Contemporary Issues in Communication Science & Disorders, 40*, 151-159. https://doi.org/10.1044/cicsd_40_F_151

Phillips, D., & Mendel, L. (2008). Counseling training in communication disorders: A survey of clinical fellows. *Contemporary Issues in Communication Science & Disorders, 35*, 44-53. https://doi.org/10.1044/cicsd_35_S_44

Pinto, R. Z., Ferreira, M. L., Oliveira, V. C., Franco, M. R., Adams, R., Maher, C. G., & Ferreira, P. H. (2012). Patient-centered communication is associated with positive therapeutic alliance: A systematic review. *Journal of Physiotherapy, 58*(2), 77-87. https://doi.org/10.1016/S1836-9553(12)70087-5

Simmons-Mackie, N., & Damico, J. S. (2011). Counseling and aphasia treatment: Missed opportunities. *Topics in Language Disorders, 31*(4), 336-351. https://doi.org/10.1097/tld.0b013e318234ea9f

Wolter, J. A., DiLollo, A., & Apel, K. (2006). A narrative therapy approach to counseling: A model for working with adolescents and adults with language-literacy deficits. *Language, Speech, & Hearing Services in Schools, 37*(3), 168-177. https://doi.org/10.1044/0161-1461(2006/019)

Worrall, L., Sherratt, S., Rogers, P., Howe, T., Hersh, D., Ferguson, A., & Davidson, B. (2011). What people with aphasia want: Their goals according to the ICF. *Aphasiology, 25*(3), 309-322. https://doi.org/10.1080/02687038.2010.508530

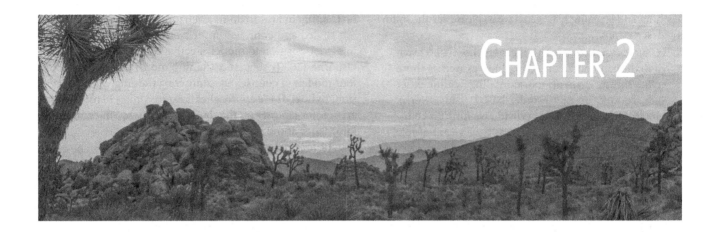

Learning to Counsel

Jerry K. Hoepner, PhD, CCC-SLP

A classroom should be a place where a mistake is not to be feared but viewed as a learning experience. ~ Proverb

As we learn, we teach. As we teach, we learn. ~ Latin Proverb

Our Charge

While the American Speech-Language-Hearing Association (ASHA; 2016) identifies *counseling* as one of the eight pillars of service delivery in speech-language pathology, there has been limited direction regarding how best to infuse counseling into curriculum and training programs. It is noteworthy that two of the remaining seven service delivery domains are *collaboration* and *prevention and wellness*, which are certainly complementary and interdependent skill sets to counseling. A clear understanding of our scope of practice and roles for counseling are essential to filling our place in educational (informational) and personal adjustment counseling, not to mention for making appropriate referrals. Unfortunately, there is a lack of uniformity and agreement across programs regarding how counseling is taught, what content and skills are included, and how counseling is implemented within the discipline. Luterman (2019) contends that

students and clinicians have insufficient training in personal adjustment counseling. Further, most students who do have access to counseling coursework primarily focus on informational/educational counseling (Luterman, 2019). Most practicing clinicians who received counseling training in their graduate program report little to no hands-on training about implementing counseling (Townsend & Hoepner, 2021). I would contend that hands-on practice is critical for learning counseling skills, regardless of your level of preparation or years in the profession. As we will discuss, empirical evidence of training approaches affirms that viewpoint.

This chapter will attempt to provide a clear discussion of evidence-based teaching and learning of counseling skills within speech-language pathology. Because the roles of course instructors, clinical supervisors, students, and practicing professionals intertwine, this content is pertinent to all readers. We are all placed in the role of teachers and learners when it comes to counseling. To gain a sense of the dif erent

Hoepner, J. K. (Ed.). *Counseling and Motivational Interviewing in Speech-Language Pathology* (pp. 15-25).

teaching and learning hats we all wear, please see the following descriptions.

Course instructors—This includes those who teach a dedicated course on counseling, as well as those who infuse elements of counseling within other coursework (e.g., disorder-based coursework). Instructors who directly provide training on counseling principles and techniques have a central role in teaching and learning. That being said, instructors of other courses in which discussions and training of counseling are embedded also have key roles in applying knowledge and skills to practice among the specific populations they address. As such, these other course instructors should have training in counseling.

Clinical supervisors—This includes those who supervise undergraduate or graduate student clinicians or practicing clinicians at a university setting or in the community, such as externship supervisors, clinical fellowship supervisors, and departmental supervisors. More loosely, it also includes peer mentors. Because supervisors provide instruction and feedback directly within context, they have the important role of transferring and applying counseling skill sets to those contexts.

Students—This includes students in the classroom and clinic contexts. While students are clearly a target audience of this text, lifelong learning and an understanding of one's approach to learning is crucial to ongoing development. Whether it be in a dedicated counseling course, addressing counseling in other coursework, or within clinical contexts, student learners need opportunities to implement counseling techniques with the guidance of more seasoned instructors, supervisors, and/or peers.

Practicing professionals—This includes speech-language pathologists in any clinical context (birth-to-3, schools, private practice, acute care hospitals, rehabilitation centers, long-term care, home care, etc.). This includes clinical fellows, who remain in a learning context with the support of their site supervisors. Note that some practicing professionals have had training in counseling within their graduate programs, some may have participated in continuing education, and others may have had little to no formal training.

Terrell and Osborne (2020) make a compelling case for counseling training to extend across academic and clinical experiences. This means, along with dedicated coursework to train counseling skills, clinical supervisors need to know what counseling knowledge their supervisees possess and have training in counseling themselves (Luterman, 2019; Terrell & Osborne, 2020). While clinical supervisors and community liaisons (practicing professionals) are expected to mentor students in counseling skills, most of them have

no training in how to do so. Even more important, if they are not skilled and confident in delivering counseling, they are in a poor position to model effective counseling. Terrell and Osborne (2020) suggest a training model that draws upon four models of counseling, counseling training, and supervision. In brief, these approaches create a comprehensive preparation for counseling that builds self-efficacy in counseling knowledge and skills.

Wellness/cognitive approach: This approach specifically addresses learning in the context of the potential impact of compassion fatigue and burnout (Williams, 2019). Perfectionism is common among speech-language pathology students and professionals. A cognitive approach helps to reframe cognitive distortions that hold us to a higher standard. Dismissing and reframing these irrational and unrealistic thoughts helps us reduce anxieties associated with counseling. Fitch and Marshall (2002) identified six common examples of anxious thinking among students, including concerns about how their current performance may affect their future career (unrealistic expectations of perfection while they're still learning), trying to live up to seasoned models from sessions viewed in class, concerns about the inadequacy of their counseling skills, stressors related to course and clinic demands, and other personal stressors. Refuting these self-defeating thoughts is an important part of becoming comfortable with implementing counseling in the moment. Breaking things down into small, achievable steps and accepting mistakes (particularly while learning counseling or any clinical skills) are the same tools they will use when counseling clients.

Reflective approach: This approach stems from the work of Geller and Foley (2009a, 2009b). It is a relationship-based, reflective model that focuses on uncovering, acknowledging, and considering how a client or family members' internal states influence therapeutic alliance and their readiness to change. Collaborating with clients and families, rather than doing therapy on them, empowers them as agents of change rather than passive recipients of therapy. Geller and Foley (2009a, 2009b) identify the following tenets of effective supervision and learning, (a) relationship-based learning (i.e., recognizing, appreciating, and developing an understanding of the relationship with the learner's intentions, emotions, comfort level) that creates a space for sharing and vulnerability, (b) forming a working alliance with the learner that reduces any power differential by demonstrating mutual respect and empathetically acknowledging their emotions, (c) fostering self-other awareness to shift the focus from learner to client, (d) transference-countertransference to emphasize how previous experience and history effects interactions (e.g., client-clinician and student-supervisor), (e) reflective practice to uncover assumptions, beliefs, biases, and motivation, and (f) use of self to construct knowledge about clinical experiences and reframe negative thoughts about self.

Triadic/peer approach: Hosting clinic supervision meetings with two or more student clinicians can strengthen student counseling skills. Because beginning counseling students are often self-focused, they miss opportunities (Borders et al., 2015). In this approach, early term feedback is one-to-one and peers are added at midterm, which decreases anxiety and develops readiness for peer feedback.

Explicit teaching approach: As the name implies, this approach uses explicit teaching of counseling skills. Kaderavek et al. (2004) used a three-session training sequence, including a lecture, followed by a three-person mock interview. This was coupled with reviewing video interactions and conducting and evaluating mock interviews. Throughout the process, students self-evaluate and debrief about their performance and associated feelings.

How We Learn to Counsel

Many of the skill sets we draw upon for counseling are nuanced and individualized. Beyond learning what counseling is, how it fits within our scope of practice, specific applications, and techniques, much of counseling is intangible. This includes establishing therapeutic alliance and professional relationships, finding our **counseling voice**, and situation-specific flexibility. We will expand upon each of these elements within the text but will focus here on the learning itself. Those intangible, nuanced skills are learned through doing (Holland & Nelson, 2020). Thus, teaching and learning in counseling must begin with doing.

Core elements of this learning through doing framework include:

- Self-assessment
- Practice and self-reflection
- Guided apprenticeship
- Peer discussions

Before we delve into how we learn, let's first examine what we believe. Before reading this text or taking a course in counseling, you might believe that counseling is about advice giving. That is a prominent world view of counseling but one that we will try to dispel in this text. Consider your existing definition of counseling; this is a great place to begin your self-assessment. Please complete the exercise in Box 2-1 regarding direct counseling vs. reflective listening.

Box 2-1
Direct Counseling Versus Reflective Listening

Learning experience #1: Have a simple conversation with a peer. In round #1, identify the peer's problem or question (e.g., "Since I started graduate school, I don't have time to work out as regularly as I did in undergrad"). Respond with an advice-giving, direct approach. After letting that play out for a few minutes, start over. This time, change your focus to active listening—drawing out their thoughts and ideas about the problem or question.

Self-Assessment

Examining one's beliefs, biases, knowledge, and skills is a crucial starting point for opening oneself to learning about counseling practices. Those who are unaware of or deny their beliefs and biases are prone to revealing those beliefs and biases to their clients. While disclosure of one's beliefs may hold some value, assuming the client or their family hold similar beliefs, those beliefs and biases can disenfranchise and break therapeutic alliance for those who implicitly or explicitly hold disparate values. As a simple demonstration, I often share a fairly benign illustration of this principle with my learners.

Several years back, when my youngest daughter was in middle school, I was giving my daughter and her friend (a nearby neighbor) a ride home from a school event. As we approached our neighborhood, I drove past a home that had a holiday lights scene projected on the side of their home. With the thought of breaking silence and making small talk, I nearly shared my bias, "Those lights are a bit gaudy and tacky." Something inside of me warned me not to put that out there, not knowing what my daughter's friend's opinion on such decorations was. A couple of blocks later, we turned the corner to her friend's home, revealing a similar projection of holiday lights on her home. Whew—I immediately felt a sense of relief that I had said nothing. That was followed by this comment from my daughter's friend, "Check out these new lights that my dad put up last night—lame." Now, you might think that statement—"lame"—is an invitation to respond with a "Yes, what a lame dad" sort of response but that is her statement to make not yours. Likely, if you make that statement, it will still evoke pushback.

While a fairly innocuous moment either way, this story illustrates the value of self-assessment while emphasizing the value of listening first. If you believe you hold the predominant opinions of those around you, not recognizing that others may have dif erent viewpoints, you place yourself at risk for disenfranchising those around you and showing your hand. In the context of this text, we will refer to those internal biases and opinions as "the righting reflex," referring to our very human tendency to want to respond with our own solutions, explanations, and ideas (Miller & Rollnick, 2013). There is much to be gained by recognizing your biases and beliefs, which allows you to inhibit that human nature that sometimes (perhaps often) compels us to share our views. There is a time and place for sharing our views, but counseling is rarely one of those moments.

Gottwald and Parris (2006) developed a number of tools designed to help learners develop counseling skills. The first of those tools is termed **Notes to Supervisor**, which was designed to help graduate students evaluate their current counseling-specific knowledge and skills and share them with their clinical supervisor (refer back to Box 1-6). The tool has potential implications for any clinician-supervisor context. This tool is accompanied by **Guiding Questions—Exploration-Insight-Action**, a framework to guide discussions between a supervisor and clinicians. It provides prompts for reflections on the interactions between clinician and client. Likewise, there is a more objective observational rating, **Self-Assessment of Counseling Skills** which can be completed by the clinician and a proxy (supervisor), refer back to Box 1-12. The final self-assessment tool is **Reflections on My Growth as a Counselor**, which prompts reflection on development of counseling skills (refer back to Box 1-12). While these tools are currently unpublished and have not been examined psychometrically, they can serve as a flexible framework for beginning self-assessment and communication with clinical supervisors. Please complete the exercise in Box 2-2, referring back to Box 1-12 for the **Self-Assessment of Counseling Skills** tool.

Regardless of what prompts or framework one follows, initial and ongoing self-assessment is a crucial skill set for developing and refining counseling skills. English et al. (1999), in one of the few published studies in communication sciences and disorders to directly examine instruction of counseling skills, identified self-assessment and reflection as crucial to the development of counseling skills.

Self-assessment is tied to self-efficacy and self-perceptions of comfort with one's **counseling voice**. Bandura (1991) defines self-efficacy as "people's beliefs about their capabilities to exercise control over their own level of functioning and other events in their lives" (p. 257). Self-efficacy is deemed to be a critical characteristic of an ef ective counselor, whether the counselor is seasoned or still in training (Beutler et al., 1994). Larson and Daniels (1998) found that counselors-in-training who had high self-efficacy regarding implementing counseling experienced more positive expectations and demonstrated less anxiety. This is important, as anxiety or discomfort can compromise one's ability to make clinical judgments and perform counseling techniques.

Box 2-2
Baseline Counseling Skills and Comfort Level

Learning experience #2: Complete the *Self-Assessment of Counseling Skills* document found at the end of Chapter 1 (Box 1-12). These will serve as your "baseline" comfort and skill levels for counseling skills.

Counselors-in-training who feel uncomfortable, stilted, or uncertain of their approach may struggle with finding a counseling voice that feels natural. As such, gains in development of counseling skills, coupled with modeling of techniques, and positive feedback are likely to strengthen self-efficacy (Larson & Daniels, 1998). Ultimately, a counselor's ability to identify their skills and have confidence in using them predicts the quality of counseling they provide (Bradley & Fiorini, 1999). Counseling training can have a positive influence on self-efficacy (Melchert et al., 1996).

While empirical evidence of counseling training approaches is scarce in our discipline, evidence is prominent in professional counseling training disciplines. Several studies have examined the Skilled Counselor Training Model (SCTM; Crews, 1999; Downing et al., 2001; Smaby et al., 1999; Urbani et al., 2002; Zimmick et al., 2000) for one-to-one training and the Skilled Group Counseling Training Model (SGCTM; Smaby et al., 1999). The SCTM and SGCTM approaches teach mastery of counseling skills, modeling, and persuasion; promote accurate self-appraisal; and foster counseling practice to learn and apply counseling techniques. The training framework follows a three-stage process (Hill & O'Brien, 1999). Training begins with learning and assessing basic attention and reflection skills, such as establishing appropriate eye contact, proximity, and reflecting/summarizing client statements. This can be accomplished initially through role plays and review of video models of those foundational skills. SCTM refers to this stage as **exploring**. Next, more intuitive and personalized counseling skills are practiced. This includes empathy, self-disclosure, and confrontation skills. In this **understanding** stage, learners are self-appraising, identifying areas for improvement but focusing heavily on their successes. Recognition of success promotes confidence. The final stage, **acting**, focuses on developing decision-making skills. Acting in-the-moment requires mastery and self-efficacy. Research shows that SCTM trained students acquired more skills than those trained solely by lections and role plays. Further, those students were able to transfer counseling skills to actual sessions with clients. Those with better self-monitoring skills were more likely to reach mastery. Thus, self-assessment, practice, and authentic contexts appear to be crucial for development and transfer of counseling skills.

To summarize, the three SCTM training steps include:

1. **Exploring**—training foundational skills such as appropriate eye contact, proximity, reflection, and summarization to mastery
2. **Understanding**—intuitive and personalized skills such as empathy, self-disclosure, and confrontation
3. **Acting**—developing skills to prompt decision making

Teachers and learners may wish to evaluate development of self-efficacy, as an indication of preparedness to deliver counseling skills in clinical contexts. The Counseling Self-Estimate Inventory is a self-report measure designed to address one's beliefs about one's own capacity to effectively counsel a client (Larson & Daniels, 1998). The 37-item self-assessment uses a six-point Likert scale to indicate degree of agreement or disagreement across statements (1 = strongly disagree to 6 = strongly agree). Victorino and Hinkle (2019) adapted the Counselor Activity Self-Efficacy Scale to assess self-efficacy of counseling skills among graduate students and early career speech-language pathologists. They emphasized that we need to learn how to address emotional support and insight skills within coursework and clinical supervision in order to increase confidence in delivering these skills. Improved self-efficacy for delivering counseling is correlated with increased comfort in counseling sessions, increased motivation to work with more challenging clients and families, improved emotional intelligence and empathy, problem solving, and in-the-moment decision making when counseling (Victorino & Hinkle, 2019).

If you are interested in learning more about self-efficacy, you are encouraged to review information in Box 2-3.

Practice and Self-Reflection

Beyond broad self-examination to consider beliefs and biases, self-reflection is best when connected to experiences. In the process of learning counseling skills, engaging in practice is crucial, whether it be in role plays, low-stakes practice, or collaborative-supported contexts with real clients. Because counseling can sometimes be a high-stakes skill set, early practice often takes the form of role plays and/or authentic but low-stakes interactions with peers. As with any flexible and individualized skill set, the closer the interaction comes to being authentic, the better. While there is no magic bullet for practice and reflection along this continuum, a gradual move from more contrived to more authentic is the general progression. In an effort to describe this incremental continuum clearly, potential implementation is listed in the following and depicted in Figure 2-1 (Hoepner & Zigler, 2021).

Hoepner and Zigler (2021) described an incremental process in four stages for developing counseling skills, drawn from literature reviewed previously in this chapter:

1. **Observation and discussion**—Learners engage in discussions and joint review of videos of counseling moments. This may include staged role plays, selected moments from recorded clinical sessions, or training videos where expert counselors model interactions in structured role-plays. These collaborative discussions may identify negative practices, such as consequences or behaviors during a direct, prescriptive counseling session or positive models during successful implementation of a constructive counseling session. Sometimes discussions compare and contrast approaches. The intent is to expose learners to models of counseling, demonstrate that even seasoned counselors make missteps, and to collaboratively identify specific counseling strategies in context. Freeze framing is used throughout joint video review, in order to pause and identify effective and ineffective strategies and interactions.

2. **Most contrived, structured role plays**—Learners engage in practice role plays of prescribed case scenarios with peers. Learners take on different roles, from client to family to clinicians. By taking on roles of the client or family, learners have the opportunity to take the perspective of those individuals, an important step in learning about counseling. In the role of clinician, learners respond in the moment to questions, frustrations, and even attacks by the client or family members. Because the scenarios are fully contrived (although often based on real clinic cases), this provides opportunities to freeze-frame moments for immediate discussion and to reflect on all aspects of the interaction. While it is tempting for the instructor to point out what went well and what could have gone better, the point is to create an opportunity for learners to self-evaluate. Like the process of counseling itself, it is sometimes necessary for the instructor to identify what went well and what could have gone better, as that knowledge is helpful when trying to cue learners to recognize those elements themselves.

3. **Contrived but infusing authentic moments, low-stakes counseling practice**—Learners engage in one-to-one interactions with peers, preferably based on low-stakes, real-life issues. Often those low-stakes issues are things like wanting to work out more consistently/regularly, wanting to eat a healthier diet, wanting to study more proactively, or the like. Such scenarios are a reasonable starting place for learners with limited counseling skill sets to try out techniques and hone their counseling voice. We will discuss the counseling voice more in future chapters, but it basically refers to a way of interacting with which the "counselor" feels comfortable and confident in delivering. While a given counselor may say something in a particular way and look/feel confident and competent doing so, others may feel stilted or uncomfortable using the same words or delivery. In low-stakes, authentic interactions, learners can set goals for what they hope to include or accomplish

Box 2-3
Foundations in Self-Efficacy

Self-efficacy has relevance to all of us as learners of counseling and to our clients.

Biel et al. (2018) summarized strategies to enhance self-efficacy around Bandura's (1997) four sources of self-efficacy (pp. 408-409). Small modifications are made here for broader application and to address this author's perspectives.

Mastery Experiences

- Provide early opportunities for success to build upon before addressing more challenging goals.
- Encourage clients to set achievable goals and task difficulty.
- Use a progression of highly achievable short-term goals to meet long-term goals.
- Break complex skills into smaller skills.
- Move toward practicing skills in progressively more challenging and representative contexts.
- Promote self-regulation to reduce barriers to success.
- Frame small successes as an expected indication of potential.
- Encourage attribution of success to client efforts and abilities, rather than clinician (or in the case of students/learners, rather than co-clinicians or supervisors).

Vicarious Experiences

- Capitalize on vicarious models of success, particularly early on or with new goals, to show that success is achievable.
- Vicarious models are best when they appear similar in type of injury, shared history of onset, age, etc. (or, in the case of students, students on their own level are better models than supervisor or instructor models). This relates to achievability of models—for instance, I don't get my cooking models from Martha Stewart.
- Use audio or video self-modeling to recognize and draw from their own successes (Haley et al., 2021; Hoepner & Olson, 2018; Hoepner et al., 2021).
- Provide exposure to achievable and positive recovery models, through group therapy and/or peer mentoring (Behn et al., 2018).
- Role play in groups to practice skills and strategies.

Verbal Persuasion

- Use verbal persuasion cautiously (sparingly) and only once strong rapport and trust have been established. Better yet, foster self-persuasion.
- Verbal persuasion and feedback should be genuine, specific-objective, and bring attention to success, avoiding vague knee-jerk praise (e.g., good job).
- Provide feedback about self-regulatory efforts (e.g., self-monitoring, patience, planning).
- Configure interactions so that feedback comes from other credible sources as well.

Physiological and Affective Experiences

- Guide clients away from misattributions of unsuccessful attempts to negative states like fatigue, stress, or anxiety. Instead foster accurate attribution to developing ability (e.g., "I need more practice").
- Encourage reflection on physiologic and affective states that affect their performance (e.g., "When I'm tired, I struggle more or it takes longer"). Note the subtle difference between blaming those factors for something that is actually a matter of ability or skill development.
- Identify physiological and affective barriers to success and develop strategies to manage them (e.g., using mindfulness and deep breathing to reduce anxiety prior to sessions).
- Consider using stress management techniques like progressive relaxation and mindfulness.
- Communicate with clients' or learners' physicians about potential physiological or affective issues that interfere with confidence (e.g., sleep disturbances, pain, mood disorders).

within the interaction. Often, we suggest that learners record those interactions for direct review after completion. Following the interaction and review of the video, learners are asked to reflect on what went well, what could be improved, and goals for their next low-stakes interaction. This provides a context for instructors to evaluate the learners use of counseling techniques, level of comfort and confidence with their counseling voice, and goals for future interactions. Instructors can use counseling frameworks to help provide further feedback to the learner about refining their approach. Like the counseling techniques we discuss in detail in this text, a fair amount of feedback prompts the learner to further reflect upon an approach. This indirect feedback is paired with more direct positive and constructive feedback.

4. **Collaborative, in-the-moment practice**—There is no substitute for the real thing. Regardless of how authentic planned practice interactions become, they do not compare to real-life moments. Unlike professional counselors, speech-language pathologists fill the role of nonprofessional counselors. As such, we do not typically begin a session intentionally with a counseling moment. Yes, sometimes counseling moments happen at the outset of sessions, even walking to an office but that is not typically part of the speech-language pathologists' initial game plan. But more often, counseling moments arise in the context of communication and/or swallowing therapy. As such, many counseling moments in our discipline are unpredictable and require an in-the-moment response. This may be why research has shown that some speech-language pathologists actively avoid responding to such counseling moments (Simmons-Mackie & Damico, 2011). Obviously, learning such a crucial skill on-the-spot poses some challenges and potential ethical concerns. As such, instructors and clinical supervisors should have a plan for how to support and scaffold learners to provide the support the client needs in the moment, while also providing opportunities for the learner to carry out as much of the support as they can. Following the framework of guided apprenticeship (Brown et al., 1989; Collins et al., 1989; Hautemo & Dalvit, 2016), instructors-supervisors-mentors collaboratively deliver in-the-moment counseling, ramping up support when the learner needs support to provide the necessary response and dialing down support when the learner has the skills to deliver that response independently. I strongly believe that learners will not reach a level of competence and confidence to deliver counseling in-the-moment without such guided opportunities to implement it in authentic contexts. While they may never feel fully confident to deliver counseling, as every counseling scenario is unique, they may reach a level of competence and confidence that allows them to address counseling moments, rather than avoid them.

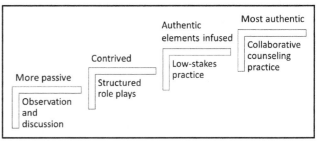

Figure 2-1. Stepwise continuum of counseling practice elements.

The collaborative counseling method has been examined in classroom settings, where graduate counseling students work together alongside the instructor to deliver counseling supports to persons with communication disorders (Hoepner, 2018; Hoepner & Zigler, 2021). In that approach, the students and instructor interview and interact with a client and/or partner who brings a goal or problem that they would like help addressing. Students are charged with finding out about the client, engaging with them to build rapport, focusing the conversation on the reason the client is present, evoking the client's potential solutions to the problem or to move toward meeting the particular goal, and collaboratively building a plan for the client to carry out. As long as the students are effectively implementing the counseling techniques practiced previously in role plays and low-stakes-authentic contexts, the instructor does not intervene. Rather, the instructor documents and outlines what the client has shared and the next steps in the process (e.g., moving from engaging to focusing, focusing to evoking, or evoking to planning; using open-ended questions, affirmations, reflections, or summary). Figure 2-2 depicts room set-up, including position of students, client, and instructor. Note the instructor's position at the white board, where they can document and outline important information and/or scaffold next steps. A shared Google document is used to provide this type of scaffolding in the online, video conferencing context. Figure 2-3 provides actual images of collaborative counseling sessions. Figure 2-4 provides an example of white board notes. When students reach a stuck point and/or show signs that they are uncertain about next steps, the instructor steps in to model an appropriate next step. Assuming that support moves the interaction forward, students are encouraged to retake the reigns. Hoepner and Zigler (2021) used five to six collaborative counseling sessions across the last half of the semester. Generally, more support was provided from the instructor in early collaborative counseling sessions and less in later sessions. Students became more independent and competent from initial to final sessions.

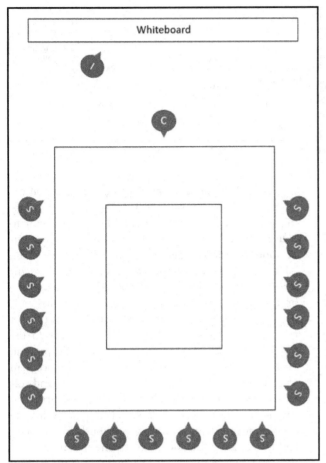

Figure 2-2. Classroom layout for collaborative counseling. (Used with permission from Hoepner (2018). Key: I = Instructor, S = Students, C = Client).

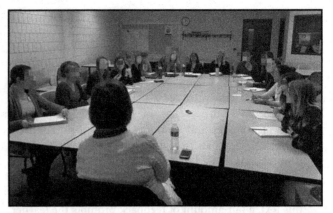

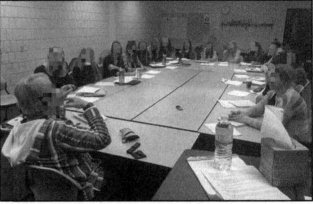

Figure 2-3a and 2-3b. Actual collaborative counseling sessions.

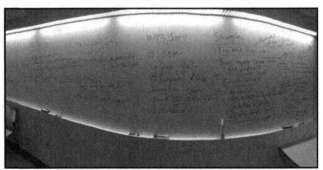

Figure 2-4. Example of white board notes by instructor.

Guided Apprenticeship

Acquiring skills in counseling is an ongoing process. Developing a counseling voice takes time, reflection, and models from others. Approaches like collaborative counseling, identified earlier, provide multiple opportunities to refine one's approach as well as multiple models of interaction to consider. One's personal counseling voice may become an amalgamation of elements from peers and mentors, which fit within one's own comfort level and style. Seeing approaches in action and trying them on for size often facilitates refinement of one's own approach. Clinical supervisors and mentors often find themselves in the position of working alongside a new or developing clinician. Whether or not the learner has previous experience in counseling, the supervisor-mentor may possess specialized skills and knowledge pertinent to a particular subset of clients they serve. Models of how to explain a concept to clients or family members, responses to difficult questions, and the mentor's interactional behaviors in a challenging counseling moment provide contextualized learning opportunities.

In situations where the mentor works alongside the learner, this is a good match for cognitive apprenticeship and situated learning. In traditional apprenticeship models, like those used in trades, the mentor demonstrates or models a technique while working alongside or in collaboration with the apprentice (Collins et al., 1991; Hautemo & Dalvit, 2016). Typically, the model is readily observable, concrete, and tangible. In cognitive apprenticeship, the mentor models their thoughts through *think alouds* or verbalizing a response. The apprentice contributes, as well. Initially, the mentor provides more models and scaf olds to support the apprentice's ability to act increasingly independently. As the apprentice's skills improve, the mentor fades those supports. Situated learning models emphasize the importance of conducting this type of collaboration in authentic contexts, with authentic tasks and consequences (opportunities for assessment; Herrington & Oliver, 2000). Like cognitive apprenticeships, situated learning fosters collaboration and reflection in the moment. Apprentices or learners see expert performance, in an authentic context and receive coaching and/or scaf olding to implement the approach in that same context. Knowing and doing are not equivalent but are also inseparable (Brown et al., 1989; Collins et al., 1989; Herrington & Oliver, 2000). Both learning (knowing and applying) and doing (executing the skill) happen within context. In speech-language pathology, our authentic context is the clinic, so training must take place in a clinical context. Learning and providing a service in an authentic context is emphasized, as it creates more realistic challenges and social relationships (Donaldson, 2015; Sheepway et al., 2011).

Peer Discussions

A natural extension of counseling practice or collaborative implementation in authentic contexts is peer discussion. Peer discussions are valuable for several reasons, including (a) providing a context for thinking through and verbalizing the rationale of one's approach, (b) providing a context for evaluating outcomes of one's approach, (c) providing an opportunity to compare one's own approach with that of peers, and (d) providing a debriefing context for dif using upsets and stressors crucial for coping and self-care of the counselor(s). This Vygotskian principle can be summed up as learners assisting other learners to advance skills through engaging in meaningful interactions. Vygotsky (1987) emphasized the importance of leveling the disparity between the expert and learner. Since authentic contexts are unpredictable, there is typically less disparity among peers. All are learners in a unique scenario, drawing upon what they know to do their best in that context.

Think aloud and verbalization of rationales for one's approach. Ongoing reflection on interactions fosters more awareness of what one is doing and why. In the realm of motivational interviewing, we often use the expression, "*saying is believing.*" That is true regarding commitment to one's own counseling approach, as well. Connecting explicit rationales to one's approach requires one to identify supporting evidence for that approach.

Evaluating outcomes of one's approach. While it falls short of empirical evidence, peer discussions begin an *n-of-one* discussion of outcomes. What worked? What failed? What requires ongoing work? Addressing these types of questions provides a starting point for refining counseling approaches with an individual and considering elements that may generalize across clients and families. Reciprocal conversations with fellow clinicians broaden that informal basis for evaluating what works and what does not. Ideally this fosters an exchange of ideas pertinent to everyday counseling moments.

Peer support and self-care. A consequence of effective counseling is engagement in more challenging counseling moments and having to process the challenges that clients bring to us. Caring for oneself is a critical element of remaining in a position to help others and preventing caregiver burnout. Practicing clinicians identify self-care and coping strategies as important to their practice but rarely addressed within counseling training (Townsend & Hoepner, 2021). Having peers who are readily available for sharing, venting, and putting things into context is a crucial element of self-care.

Self-care techniques are particularly important for disciplines that counsel others, as counseling puts those professionals in a context where they may confront strong personal emotions, human struggles, and ultimately mortality (Rosenzweig et al., 2003). Knowledge of self-care techniques is important not only in the long term but can affect counseling training learning experiences (Baker, 2003; Weiss, 2004). Mindfulness approaches are one means of proactive self-care for counselors (Christopher et al., 2006). Creative writing and journaling also show promise for promoting self-care (Warren et al., 2010).

While the importance of peer discussions has not been revisited recently, past research has identified those relationships as crucial for self-care and avoiding burnout. Specifically, increased work-group social supports were found to decrease stress among psychotherapists (Mallinckrodt, 1989). While speech-language pathologists are not professional counselors like psychotherapists, burdens of supporting clients through challenging times remain. More broadly, Robinson-Kurpius and Keim (1994) found that team building improved job satisfaction and lowered burnout among health care professionals. As such, team building workshops are recommended for graduate students to prevent stress in their future work settings (Coyne et al., 1993). Quality peer relationships provide a context for venting and dif using upset in everyday moments.

Chapter Summary

In summary, counseling is learned by doing. Engaging in counseling "practice" provides opportunities for self-assessment, practice, and self-reflection. Because every counseling moment is unique, multiple models in multiple authentic contexts are necessary. Guided apprenticeship models allow collaboration in authentic counseling moments, where the client's needs are met while the mentor and apprentice-learner hone their counseling skill sets. Self-efficacy is a strong indicator of readiness to serve as a counselor in clinical contexts. Ongoing peer discussions are useful for ongoing development of counseling skills, as well as serving as a context for self-care to cope with the potentially heavy burden of inviting others to open up to you.

Key Takeaways

- Counseling is one of the eight pillars of clinical practice, which has applications to students, clinical instructors, and course instructors.
- We learn to counsel, not just through reading about it, but by engaging in counseling practice and reflection.
- Seeing models from seasoned counselors and peers through videos and in-person interactions exposes learners to multiple ways of saying things and helps learners to develop their own unique counseling voice.
- Peer discussions help learners to recognize why techniques were implemented and to become more intentional about implementing such techniques themselves.

References

American Speech-Language-Hearing Association. (2016). *Scope of practice in speech-language pathology* [Scope of Practice]. http://www.asha.org/policy/.

Baker, E. K. (2003). *Caring for ourselves: A therapist's guide to personal and professional well-being.* American Psychological Association.

Bandura, A. (1991). Social cognitive theory of self-regulation. *Organizational Behavior and Human Decision Processes, 50*(2), 248-287. https://doi.org/10.1016/0749-5978(91)90022-L

Beutler, L. E., Machado, P. P., & Neufeldt, S. A. (1994). Therapist variables. In A. E. Bergin & S. L. Garfield (Eds.), *Handbook of Psychotherapy and Behavior Change* (pp. 229-269). John Wiley & Sons.

Borders, L. D., Brown, J. B., & Purgason, L. L. (2015). Triadic supervision with practicum and internship counseling students: A peer supervision approach. *The Clinical Supervisor, 34*(2), 232-248. https://doi.org/10.1080/07325223.2015.1027024

Bradley, C., & Fiorini, J. (1999). Evaluation of counseling practicum: National study of programs accredited by CACREP. *Counselor Education and Supervision, 39*(2), 110-119. https://doi.org/10.1002/j.1556-6978.1999.tb01222.x

Brown, J. S., Collins, A., & Duguid, P. (1989). Situated cognition and the culture of learning. *Educational Researcher, 18*(1), 32-42. https://doi.org/10.3102/0013189X018001032

Christopher, J. C., Christopher, S. E., Dunnagan, T., & Schure, M. (2006). Teaching self-care through mindfulness practices: The application of yoga, meditation, and qigong to counselor training. *Journal of Humanistic Psychology, 46*(4), 494-509. https://doi.org/10.1177/0022167806290215

Collins, A., Brown, J. S., & Holum, A. (1991). Cognitive apprenticeship: Making thinking visible. *American Educator, 15*(3), 6-11.

Collins, A., Brown, J. S., & Newman, S. E. (1989). Cognitive apprenticeship: Teaching the crafts of reading, writing, and mathematics. In L. B. Resnick (Ed.), *Knowing, learning, and instruction: Essays in honor of Robert Glaser* (pp. 453-494). Lawrence Erlbaum Associates, Inc.

Coyne, R. K., Wilson, F. R., Kline, W. B., Morran, D. K., & Ward, D. E. (1993). Training group workers: Implications for the new ASGW training standards for training and practice. *The Journal for Specialists in Group Work, 18*(1), 11-23. https://doi.org/10.1080/0193392930841 3730

Crews, J. (1999). *Counselors-in-training self-monitoring traits and counseling skills acquisition: Skills-based versus interpersonal process recall methods* [Unpublished doctoral dissertation]. University of Nevada.

Donaldson, A. L. (2015). Pre-professional training for serving children with ASD: An apprenticeship model of supervision. *Teacher Education and Special Education, 38*(1), 58-70. https://doi.org/10.1177/0888406414566995

Doud, A. K., Hoepner, J. K., & Holland, A. L. (2020). A survey of counseling curricula among accredited communication sciences and disorders graduate student programs. *American Journal of Speech-Language Pathology, 29*(2), 789-803. https://doi.org/10.1044/2020_AJSLP-19-00042

Downing, T. K., Smaby, M. H., & Maddux, C. D. (2001). A study of the transfer of group counseling skills from training to practice. *Journal for Specialists in Group Work, 26*(2), 156-167. https://doi.org/10.1080/01933920108415735

English, K., Lucks, L., Rojeski, T., & Hornak, J. (1999). Counseling in audiology, or learning to listen: Pre- and post-measures from an audiology counseling course. *American Journal of Audiology, 8*(1), 34-39. https://doi.org/10.1044/1059-0889(1999/007)

Fitch, T. J., & Marshall, J. L. (2002). Using cognitive interventions with counseling practicum students during group supervision. *Counselor Education and Supervision, 41*(4), 335-342. https://doi.org/10.1002/j.1556-6978.2002.tb01295.x

Geller, E., & Foley, G. M. (2009a). Broadening the "ports of entry" for speech-language pathologists: A relational and reflective model for clinical supervision. *American Journal of Speech-Language Pathology, 18*(1), 1-21.

Geller, E., & Foley, G. M. (2009b). Expanding the "ports of entry" for speech-language pathologists: A relational and reflective model for clinical practice. *American Journal of Speech-Language Pathology, 18*(1), 22-41.

Gottwald, S. & Parris, D. (2006). *Helping people change: Teaching counseling skills in clinical practica.* American Speech-Language-Hearing Association Annual Convention.

Hautemo, A. M., & Dalvit, L. (2016). *Situated learning: A theoretical base for online learning.* eLmL. 69.

Herrington, J., & Oliver, R. (2000). An instructional design framework for authentic learning environments. *Educational Technology Research and Development, 48*(3), 23-48.

Hill, C. E., & O'Brien, K. M. (1999). *Helping skills: Facilitating exploration, insight, and action.* American Psychological Association.

Hoepner, J. K. (2018). Course embedded practical experiences: A reflection on innovation. *The Journal for Research and Practice in College Teaching, 3*(2), 185-190.

Hoepner, J. K. & Zigler, E. (2021). *Examining the collaborative counseling approach as a course-embedded clinical training tool.* [Unpublished manuscript].

Holland, A. L., & Nelson, R. L. (2020). *Counseling in communication disorders: A wellness perspective* (3rd ed.). Plural Publishing Inc.

Kaderavek, J. N., Laux, J. M., & Mills, N. H. (2004). A counseling training module for students in speech-language pathology training programs. *Contemporary Issues in Communication Science and Disorders, 31*(Fall), 153-161.

Larson, L. M., & Daniels, J. A. (1998). Review of counseling self-efficacy literature. *The Counseling Psychologist, 26*, 179-218.

Luterman, D. (2020). On teaching counseling: Getting beyond informational counseling. *American Journal of Speech-Language Pathology, 29*(2), 903-908.

Mallinckrodt, B. (1989). Social support and the effectiveness of group therapy. *Journal of Counseling Psychology, 36*, 170-175.

Melchert, T. P., Hays, V. L., Wiljanen, L. M., & Kolocek, A. K. (1996). Testing models of counselor development with a measure of counseling self-efficacy. *Journal of Counseling & Development, 74*(6), 640-644.

Robinson-Kurpius, S. E., & Keim, J. (1994). Team building for nurses experiencing burnout and poor morale. *The Journal for Specialists in Group Work, 19*(3), 155-161.

Rosenzweig, S., Reibel, D. K., Greeson, J. M., Brainard, G. C., & Hojat, M. (2003). Mindfulness-based stress reduction lowers psychological distress in medical students. *Teaching and Learning in Medicine, 15*(2), 88-92.

Sheepway, L., Lincoln, M., & Togher, L. (2011). An international study of clinical education practices in speech-language pathology. *International Journal of Speech-Language Pathology, 13*(2), 174-185.

Simmons-Mackie, N., & Damico, J. S. (2011). Counseling and aphasia treatment. *Topics in Language Disorders, 31*(4), 336-351.

Smaby, M. H., Maddux, C. D., Torres-Rivera, E., & Zimmick, R. (1999). A study of the effects of a skills-based versus a conventional group counseling training program. *Journal for Specialists in Group Work, 24*(2), 152-163.

Terrell, P. A., & Osborne, C. (2020). Teaching Competence in Counseling: A Focus on the Supervisory Process. In *Seminars in Speech and Language* (Vol. 41, No. 04, pp. 325-336). Thieme Medical Publishers.

Townsend, A. K., & Hoepner, J. K. (2021a). *Counseling practices survey among speech-language pathologists: The state of counseling in speech-language pathology.* [Unpublished manuscript].

Townsend, A. K., & Hoepner, J. K. (2021b). *Counseling practices of speech-language pathologists serving persons with aphasia: Examining training and preparedness within clinical practice.* [Unpublished manuscript].

Urbani, S., Smith, M. R., Maddux, C. D., Smaby, M. H., Torres-Rivera, E., & Crews, J. (2002). Skills-based training and counseling self-efficacy. *Counselor Education and Supervision, 42*(2), 92-106.

Victorino, K. R., & Hinkle, M. S. (2019). The development of a self-efficacy measurement tool for counseling in speech-language pathology. *American Journal of Speech-Language Pathology, 28*(1), 108-120.

Vygotsky, L. S. (1987). *The collected works of LS Vygotsky: Vol. 1, Problems of general psychology.* (R. W. Rieber & A. S. Carton, Eds., N. Minick, trans.). Plenum Press.

Warren, J., Morgan, M. M., Morris, L. N. B., & Morris, T. M. (2010). Breathing words slowly: Creative writing and counselor self-care—the writing workout. *Journal of Creativity in Mental Health, 5*(2), 109-124.

Weiss, L. (2004). *Therapist's guide to self-care.* Routledge.

Williams, K. S. (2019). *Compassion fatigue: The cost of caring.* ASHA Leader Live. https://blog.asha.org/2019/02/20/compassion-fatigue-the-cost-of-caring/.

Zimmick, R., Smaby, M. H., & Maddux, C. (2000). Improving the use of a group counseling scale and related model to teach theory and skills integration. *Counselor Education and Supervision, 39*(4), 248-295.

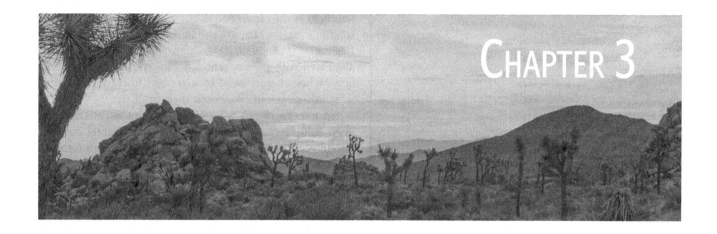

CHAPTER 3

Foundational Counseling Principles and Skills

Jerry K. Hoepner, PhD, CCC-SLP

Start where they are, not where you are. ~ Tony DiLollo

Where Counseling Fits in the WHO-ICF Framework

The World Health Organization's International Classification of Functioning, Disability and Health (WHO-ICF; 2001) is a framework for classifying health and health-related conditions (Figure 3-1). Speech-language pathologists should be familiar with this framework, as it helps contextualize an individual's activity and participation with respect to their impairment and contextual factors. While other assessment and treatment approaches within speech-language pathology address all elements, including body functions and structures (impairments), counseling primarily addresses activity, participation, and contextual factors. Activity includes what our clients want and need to do, while participation addresses their engagement in those activities. Contextual factors include barriers and facilitators to participation within the physical and partner environments.

Personal factors include internal states (e.g., fatigue, hunger, thirst, pain), feelings, beliefs, attitudes, and motivation.

Before we address specific counseling assessments or methods, there are a number of core skills and concepts to consider.

Cultural Humility and Responsiveness

The American Speech-Language-Hearing Association (ASHA, n.d.) calls for speech-language pathologists to be culturally competent. Certainly, this is an important aspirational goal and even expectation. A challenge for practicing clinicians, particularly those who work within linguistically and culturally diverse regions, is truly having knowledge of all languages and cultures. For instance, I have spoken with speech-language pathologists in California who have representation from upward of 30 languages in their region and

Hoepner, J. K. (Ed.). *Counseling and Motivational Interviewing in Speech-Language Pathology* (pp. 27-46).
© 2024 Taylor& Francis Group.

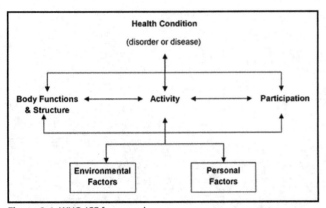

Figure 3-1. WHO-ICF framework.

caseload. Obviously, along with linguistic diversity, there is a range of cultural diversity, economic diversity, and other familial factors that make achieving "competence" less than feasible. That is not to say that speech-language pathologists in those contexts should give up but rather to recognize constraints of their human capacity to learn, instead being forthright about limits to their knowledge (cultural humility), demonstrating authentic curiosity in learning about individual client's cultures, and responsivity to their values and preferences (culturally responsive). **Cultural humility** is defined as the "ability to maintain an interpersonal stance that is **other-oriented**, in relation to aspects of cultural identity that are most important to the person" (Hook et al., 2013; p. 2). The National Institutes of Health defines cultural humility as "a lifelong process of self-reflection and self-critique whereby the individual not only learns about another's culture, but one starts with an examination of her/his own beliefs and cultural identities." Tervalon and Murray-Garcia (1998) coined the term cultural humility and identified key tenets for implementation. First, we must acknowledge that we will never know everything there is to know about a given culture or its values. This is couched as a **lifelong commitment to self-evaluation and self-critique**. We should attempt to **address power imbalances,** recognizing the inherent competence and value of all people. Thus, we need to recognize our **clients and families as the experts** on their lives. It is not enough to address our own cultural humility through self-evaluation, reflection, and addressing power imbalances in our clinical interactions. We have the responsibility to address cultural humility at a systems level. This means developing partnerships with people and groups to **advocate for others**. Think of your current or future position as a speech-language pathologist in a rehab department or school. You are surrounded by a system that needs to be culturally responsive in order for your clients to thrive. Because you are a part of the system, every action you take either adds to or reduces the cultural responsivity of the entire system. "**Cultural responsiveness** is a congruous approach to cultural competences in which the provider recognizes the importance of including the client's cultural references in all aspects of their teaching and learning. Cultural responsiveness sees

the client as the expert and engages with them to help create solutions that are effective and impactful on their treatment." (Hamilton et al., 2020, p. 3). Culturally responsive practices align well with person-centered care and most counseling approaches, characterized by a genuine interest in learning what matters to our clients and their families.

A number of resources are available from ASHA to address cultural competence (or perhaps more aptly, cultural humility). This includes structured reflection tools for personal reflection, implementation of service delivery, and system-based policies and procedures (ASHA, 2010). Note that these three tools parallel Tervalon and Murray-Garcia's (1998) tenets for implementation of cultural humility (self-evaluation/self-critique, leveling power disparities in service delivery, and system-level advocacy).

- The Cultural Competence Checklist for Personal Reflection: https://www.asha.org/siteassets/uploadedfiles/cultural-competence-checklist-personal-reflection.pdf
- The Cultural Competence Checklist for Service Delivery: https://www.asha.org/siteassets/uploadedfiles/multicultural/culturally-responsive-practice-checklist.pdf
- The Cultural Competence Checklist for Policies and Procedures: https://www.asha.org/siteassets/uploadedfiles/cultural-competence-checklist-policies-procedures.pdf

Culturally humble and responsive clinicians recognize and value their clients as experts in their own lives and use counseling skills to understand and work effectively within the culture of the clients they serve. All of the foundational skills discussed in this chapter rely upon culturally responsive, flexible implementation to meet individual cultural needs and values. Likewise, Chapter 4 addresses communicatively accessible, structured interview tools and inventories (e.g., Talking Mats, LIV Cards, Activity Card Sort, Values Inventories), which are not only rich sources of interests, wants, and needs but of cultural beliefs and values as well. This is a great starting point for authentic curiosity about clients and family members, allowing speech-language pathologists to be culturally responsive. Solutions Focused Brief Therapy (SFBT) uses the technique of **not-knowing**, as a way to authentically inquire about client's backgrounds, beliefs, and values (De Jong & Berg, 2013; Iveson & McKergow, 2015). This can serve as a tremendous asset in learning about our individual client's and family member's cultures. Indeed, over time we learn about cultural practices and preferences for groups of people (e.g., third-generation Hmong people) but also need to recognize the dangers of overgeneralizing cultural ideals to individuals. For an excellent description of implementing culturally responsive practices, see the entry by Becca Jarzynski in Chapter 8.

In the context of linguistic diversity, as with cultural competence, it is not feasible for speech-language pathologists to know all languages in their region, particularly in more diverse settings. That being said, it is our responsibility to work with interpreters to deliver assessment, intervention, and informational and personal adjustment counseling to clients in a language they comprehend effectively. While it is beyond the scope of this text to detail that process, it certainly requires a complex skill set, as delivering information or support through an intermediary unquestionably changes the dynamics of our interactions.

Foundational Principles and Skills

When We Are Uncomfortable, We Avoid

When we are uncomfortable with our role in counseling or not confident in the techniques to employ, we are more likely to avoid counseling moments (Simmons-Mackie & Damico, 2011). A lack of clarity regarding scope of practice is one element that leaves speech-language pathologists feeling uncomfortable about their role. A consequence of this lack of comfort is that we intentionally or unintentionally avoid counseling moments. Townsend and Hoepner (2021) interviewed speech-language pathologists regarding their training, current counseling practices, and confidence in responding to counseling moments. One speech-language pathologist shared that if a patient is crying, she leaves the room and tells them she will be back later when they're not upset. Lacking preparedness and confidence in implementing counseling techniques further contributes to avoidance. How do we confront this avoidance? It begins with having a clear sense of scope of practice (if you're not sure, refer back to Chapter 1). Gaining knowledge and skills in implementing counseling approaches is up next. Feeling more comfortable in really difficult situations? That takes time and a good game face. Please read the example in Box 3-1, a real-life story about one of the uncomfortable clinical, counseling moments I faced.

As clinicians, we need to summon the strength to be (i.e., appear) comfortable by preparing for difficult conversations. Many of these conversations we can prepare for or preempt with some good planning and possibly scripting (physical or mental scripting). As we develop a strong therapeutic relationship, we are better prepared to engage in difficult conversations (Hall et al., 2010; Lawton et al., 2016; Morrison & Smith, 2013; Pinto et al., 2012; Worrall et al., 2011).

Assumptions can lead to uncomfortable moments. For instance, assumptions about religious beliefs can lead you to avoid the conversation or to you making faux pas (e.g., saying, "I'll pray for you" to a person who is agnostic or simply does not share your beliefs). Often, our assumptions stem from our own culture and belief systems.

Other moments may feel taboo, depending on your culture, belief systems, and personal experiences. Those taboo topics, however, are a part of life for all of us and may be affected by the communication and physical disorders

---

Box 3-1
An Uncomfortable Conversation

One of the fringe benefits of learning how to confront difficult conversations is that your dear colleagues entrust you with those opportunities whenever they arise. In one such situation, I was working with a 16-year-old girl with a traumatic brain injury. She was still in posttraumatic amnesia, a state where she was confused and could not track new memories. My rehabilitation team and I learned from nursing staff that Chantel's 21-year-old boyfriend was making visits, with the door latched. I was selected as the therapist to have a conversation with Chantel's parents. I mentally scripted, practiced, and slammed a cup of coffee before meeting with the parents. The occupational therapist and physical therapist stood beside me for moral support. Without mincing words, I proceeded to tell Chantel's parents that her boyfriend had been having sex with her in her hospital bed with the door closed. It was one of the hardest things I have had to do, followed by an even trickier moment. Her parents said, "Yes, we're aware that they are intimate, and they have our approval. They are planning to get married." That really caught me off guard, but it set me up for an unscripted and equally difficult conversation. No judgment, I thought (although inside that was not my feeling). This was not about whether they are okay with this but educating them about the current context. "That's good that you're aware of this. Our concern right now (telepathically calling for the moral support of my colleagues) is that Chantel is still disoriented and confused, she cannot remember or process what is happening to her in the moment. Nor can she make a decision about it, even if she's already made that decision in the past." And their response reinforced why such conversations matter, "That makes sense, we didn't even think about that. We'll have a conversation with the boyfriend." Internally, I was thinking, "Oh, thank goodness!"

---

our clients experience. This can include imminent death, imminent physical and cognitive decline (e.g., dementias, amyotrophic lateral sclerosis), depression, anxiety, and other mental health concerns or sexuality and intimacy in adolescence or following brain injury, stroke, or other disease onset. An empathetic conversation about death can allow decisions to be made, loss to be processed. Talking about death doesn't bring about death nor speed its arrival. We can have a conversation about imminent cognitive decline with kindness and empathy without mincing words, which only leads to further uncertainty or even misleads our clients and their families. Such a conversation may offer the individual with dementia an opportunity to contribute to planning. Likewise, it can help partners begin to prepare and know what to expect. Depression and anxiety screeners can open the door to a conversation about mental health and potential referrals. You don't have to open a conversation about sexuality and intimacy, as that might be awkward. However, you can open the door to that conversation, inviting a conversation if they wish to have it in the future. That invitation can allow them time to mull it over and lets them know that you're not afraid of that discussion.

Finally, no one likes to deliver bad news. In the case of speech-language pathologists, we regularly have conversations about discharge, and often this is before a client and their family are ready for discharge. Whether it is due to a plateau in progress, third-party insurance payor restrictions, or a child who no longer qualifies for services, telling someone that services are ending is hard. In some cases, therapists even avoid telling clients that discharge is imminent, leaving their clients surprised and even less prepared for the transition. For a sneak peek at some discussions about having difficult conversations, please read Box 3-2.

Withholding Judgment

When we encounter people from a variety of socioeconomic, cultural, and educational backgrounds, we are likely to encounter ways of doing, ways of looking at things, and ways of living that differ from our own. Our own experiences, perspectives, beliefs, and biases can affect how we respond to others. Yes, this is another one of those *game face* situations where you have to inhibit your internal tendencies to respond to something that differs from your way of doing things. This includes both your verbal and nonverbal responses. No widening of your eyes, jaw dropping, head shaking, or even dropping your chin to avert your gaze allowed. Instead, a steady, respectful response is needed—as if it is no surprise to you, nothing unusual. Iveson and McKergow (2015) suggest that the use of not-knowing questions may help us to suspend judgment and inhibit our tendency to provide solutions and advice.

Listening Skills

Listening is a crucial element of effective counseling. Luterman (1999) emphasizes that "content-based (educational or informational) counseling cannot be successful until parents have opportunities to work through their feelings; when affect is high, cognition shuts off and parents are helped more by being listened to than by being talked at" (p. 1038). That being said, effective listening is more

---

Box 3-2
Insights About Having the Hard Conversations

If you're thinking to yourself, "What—how—tell me more about how to lean into these conversations instead of avoiding them," I invite you to take a sneak peek at some expert ideas of how to handle these tough situations. Clearly, there are many more difficult conversations than are described here, but here's a few to preview.

- Communicatively accessible depression and anxiety screening measures are discussed in Chapter 4.
- Chapter 7 includes an entry by CeCelia and Wayne Zorn about living with primary progressive aphasia (PPA) that includes a terrific focus on having the hard conversations. Included in this section are examples of questions to ask and conversations to offer.
- Also in Chapter 7, Wendy Allen shares the frustrations, struggles, and successes of raising a child with a profound cognitive impairment. Her perspectives on collaborating are a great starting point.
- In Chapter 8, social worker and death/bereavement expert Nancy Pederson (Ability KC) shares insights into having a conversation about death, dying, and bereavement.
- Robin Pollens (Western Michigan University) addresses important conversations in palliative care and end of life care in Chapter 8. Included in this discussion is information about collaborating with social workers in the palliative care context.
- Emma Power et al. (from the University of Sydney and the University of Technology Sydney) share perspectives on how to initiate and carry out conversations about sexuality and intimacy in Chapter 8. Power and her team are renowned for their work on addressing sexuality and intimacy following stroke and brain injury.
- Later in this chapter, we discuss the issue of discharge, drawing heavily on the important work of Deborah Hersh et al.

---

than sitting quietly and idly by. Active listening involves attentiveness, open-ended questions, follow-up and clarifying questions, reflecting, summarizing, and paraphrasing (Rogers & Farson, 1957). It involves truly processing and remembering what your client said, while withholding judgment. Empathetic listening involves fostering and affirming a client's emotions and feelings. To be effective in active and empathetic listening, you need to put aside your own interests and respond only to the client. This means leaving out the "I find," "I think," and "In my experience" statements.

What does it take to be attentive? Begin by placing your total focus on the client, no multitasking. Taking notes is fine, if it is for the purpose of processing and responding to what they say. Note that you need a system of key points or shorthand for this to be effective. You cannot effectively write what they say verbatim and remain engaged in the conversation. Further, while taking notes is totally acceptable in many situations, it is probably not a good choice for moments of intensely emotional disclosure.

Open-ended questions are discussed further in Chapter 5, as they are a core technique in motivational interviewing. That being said, one could argue that they are a core technique across all counseling approaches. Broadly, open-ended questions provide more flexibility for the client to control the direction of the conversation. Conversely, closed-ended questions yield a "yes" or "no" response and sometimes nothing more. Closed-ended questions put the question asker (the clinician) in control of the direction of the conversation, making your interactions clinician directed.

Follow-up questions demonstrate that you are listening and are seeking more information. Clarifications function similarly and seek verification regarding your understanding or interpretation.

Reflecting is a method for repeating and restating feeling statements. Likewise, summarization restates, paraphrases, and reiterates multiple client statements for emphasis.

Acknowledging and Revealing Competence

The concepts of *acknowledging* and *revealing competence* were not developed as counseling techniques, but I believe they have relevance to all counseling and therapeutic relationships. These principles are akin to unconditional positive regard (Rogers, 1959), which is revered by many as a core counseling approach in person-centered therapy. Kagan (1998) identified acknowledging and revealing competence as central components of supported conversation techniques for persons with aphasia. Acknowledging competence is achieved when our words and actions demonstrate that we believe our client has inherent value as a human being, has ability and intelligence, is capable and worthy of making choices about their own life, and should be treated with respect. Other actions erode acknowledgment of competence, such as talking about the person while in their presence (vs. talking to the person), making choices for them without their input, asking a partner instead of asking them, and a host of nonverbals that indicate our inner assessment of them (e.g.,

not looking at them, dismissing their ideas or attempts to communicate, failure to invest time or energy supporting them, patronizing tone). Acknowledging competence is a prerequisite to establishing rapport, alliance, and trust. Of course, there will often be situations where we second guess that competence (at least internally). They are too young to know, they're making bad decisions, or they are losing competence (e.g., a person with dementia or someone who is confused post brain injury or stroke, a child with severe intellectual impairments). Regardless of whether they're calling all of the shots, we need to acknowledge that children, people who make bad choices, people with temporary confusion, or those progressing toward further loss of orientation all have a stake in their own lives, are human, and inherently deserve our respect. Failure to do so erodes authenticity and relational trust. Internally, we may have our doubts but on the outside, we should exude confidence in their competence. See Box 3-3 for an example. If we believe that an individual has inherent value and competence, we should employ tools to reveal that competence. Simply said, revealing competence is ensuring a means of response or a means of participation. Providing alternate means of expressing their ideas or demonstrating their competence (however limited or complete it may be) is our bread and butter as speech-language pathologists. Throughout this text, we will discuss tools to reveal competence, a core element of speech-language pathology and counseling within speech-language pathology.

Working With the Experts

After 4 years of undergraduate training and 2 or more years of master's level training, it is not surprising that speech-language pathologists feel they have earned the title of expert in the domains of communication, cognition, and dysphagia. Pat yourselves on the back, you've earned it—or you soon will. Okay, now that we have that out of our system, it's time to recognize that our clients and their families are the experts on living with communication disorders. That means they must be partners in the therapy process. Partnerships require joint decision making and sharing of information (education). Stewart and Leahy (2010) suggested that we need to take a nonexpert stance, recognizing our clients (who stutter) as experts in their own lives. Ylvisaker et al. (2007), in their seminal work on project-based interventions, identified the importance of putting individuals with brain injuries in the role of expert. This can have a profound impact on confidence, self-efficacy, sense of identity, and sense of worth. Beyond acknowledging competence, acknowledging expertise helps to level the power disparity that typically occurs between a therapist and client. Think about this: We get to ask them about their family, work, past experiences, values, and struggles, but it would generally not be accepted for them to ask the same of us. In describing what it takes to level power differentials between therapist and clients/families, Tervalon and Murray-Garcia (1998)

Box 3-3
The Power of Withholding Judgment

Throughout this text, I will occasionally share experiences from my professional and personal life. One such experience is being a foster parent and family. I'm not sure that this is true of everyone who becomes a foster parent, but my family and I went into it with helping the foster children as our sole reason. It was not about helping the biological parent(s), or at least that was our initial misconception. I recall in our initial trainings, listening to the trainers talk about the role of foster parents in supporting the biological parents, but it was lost on me until I experienced it. One such lesson happened as our first set of foster siblings (the two older siblings) and their mom began the process of reunification and return to the mom's care. My wife was working the day of that team meeting with social workers, the biological mom, another family who was caring for the newborn sibling, and myself. The purpose of the meeting was to lay out all of the logistics and timeline for the transition, including dry runs, check-ins, and eventual full-time transition back to home. As the meeting got underway, the mom turned physically toward me and her very good, primary case worker and harshly away from the other foster parents (who made it clear that they did not believe that mom should ever have custody of the infant). Speaking to me she said, "You and Carol [my wife] are the only ones who didn't look down at me, treat me like a meth head, like a bad mom. You treated me with respect and believed in me." Her words hit me like a fast-moving train. I responded with an admission: "I am so glad that is what you felt, but don't put us on a shelf. We had all of those same thoughts and feelings. But you changed our minds." I felt like she needed to know at that point. Later, we talked about it further. She shared that it didn't come across that way and reiterated that it did for everyone else. I shared that we used to hold those thoughts and feelings, but that had changed. Initially, we did think she was a bad mom who didn't deserve those beautiful kids, but then we got to know her—she changed and we changed. This is not a pat on my back, on our backs (as I shared, we were no angels in our thinking). This is only to demonstrate the power of acknowledging competence. It might be one of those "fake it until you make it" moments, but we moved from holding onto what felt like microscopic evidence of value and worth initially. She's somebody's daughter, sister, friend, and *mom*. She is loved by these children, regardless of what she has done. And there was evidence of her positive influence on them (amid piles of negative influences), such as their love for reading and singing together. Identifying those little shreds of competence allowed us to put on our game faces and instill a sense of acknowledging competence and no judgment.

emphasize the importance of recognizing clients/families as the experts in their own lives and experiences of living with health conditions. Simply by living with a communication disorder, our clients and their families have knowledge, experiences, and perspectives that we do not (and typically cannot) possess. Uncovering that expertise and encouraging them to use it can empower clients to take ownership in their own development or recovery. A basic assumption of solution-focused brief therapy (see Chapter 6) is that clients are experts of their own lives, being competent and coequal to the clinician (Hanton, 2011; Jones-Smith, 2012; Lipchik et al., 2012). Likewise, in discussing the spirit of motivational interviewing, Miller and Rollnick (2013) identified the approach as collaborative, where the clinician yields their expert role in favor of a partnership and joint decision making. They go on to emphasize that this is particularly important in a counseling relationship, as the client is the only one who can enact change.

Uncovering Backstories

Ever notice that when someone you respect misses a meeting, is late, forgets to do something, or just flat out drops the ball and screws up that we are much more likely to forgive them and overlook it than we are with someone new or whom we don't know as well? When old reliable misses a meeting, you say, "Oh my gosh, no worries. That happens to all of us at times." Backstories humanize our clients and fundamentally shape the way we see their flaws and missteps. That is why seeking out those backstories is so crucial, but how or when does this happen? Learning about what the person values is a good start, including a bit of their social history. Sometimes, we learn in the moment of a meltdown or a particularly difficult moment. Let's return to your respected, reliable friend. When they do something really out of character (e.g., a big blow-up, tirade, perhaps even directed at you), sure, we might initially repel, but if that relationship is strong, you may be more likely to just check-in with a simple, "Hey, what's going on? What's wrong? This is not like you." We do this because we know it is out of character for them, and something must underlie this behavior shift. If we begin to make this assumption for our clients and suppress our human reciprocal response to react defensively or even to attack back, we can get at the backstory. McMorrow (2003) identifies two types of *reciprocity*: *reinforce-reinforce* and *attack-attack* reciprocity. When a relationship has a history of positive interactions, we tend to respond positively, setting into motion a cycle of positive interactions (reinforce-reinforce). Conversely, when there is a history of negative interactions, we bark back at anything we perceive as an attack on us, which is likely to yield a cycle of attacks. Returning to the concept of acknowledging competence, if we make the assumption that most people are good (even when there isn't an established track record), we can uncover what underlies less than positive behaviors. This may reveal the backstory of the moment or a deeper, formative backstory. It could be as simple as "I'm tired," "I'm hangry," or it could be something more catastrophic. You need to be prepared to respond to everything along that continuum. Your reaction to the revealing of something catastrophic should be understated (i.e., no jaw dropping, gasping, or "Oh my gosh, that's horrible" responses), compassionate, and affirming (e.g., "That must have been difficult"). Further, this may be one of those moments where you recognize the need for a referral to mental health professionals. Even though you know that is one of your next steps, it does not let you off the hook in the moment. You need to hold steady and remain composed, to the extent that is humanly possible—you are not a robot, so do not hold yourself to the standard of having no emotional response, but you want to have a controlled emotional response. An emotional response can convey empathy, but as soon as that response becomes the focus of that moment or interrupts your ability to respond to the client, it is problematic (e.g., sobbing profusely). You want to support their disclosure and processing. In some cases, this is an opportunity to gather some information that will be very helpful in your referral to mental health professionals (see Box 3-4 for examples).

Both simple and more substantive backstories can be helpful pieces of information that allow us to interpret future behaviors in light of that knowledge. For instance, when I'm getting a little crusty, my wife might ask, "Need something to eat?" which instantly draws my attention to my own salty behavior. With the right tone, it is not confrontational but rather an opportunity for self-assessment. For something more significant, backstories can contextualize (not necessarily excuse or condone but explain) current behaviors.

Box 3-4
Pivotal Moments

Gigantic caveat: We are *not* psychotherapists or mental health professionals and should not attempt to assume that role. That being said, we are experts in fostering communication and thus put our clients in the position to reveal things. Once revealed, we cannot simply say "Okay, I'll make a referral to Dr. Jones and she'll take care of that for you." A few simple steps can be helpful to address things in the moment.

If suicidal ideations are revealed (you now know you are firmly in referral mode), a couple of simple questions are necessary. Do you have a plan? Do you have the means to carry out that plan? Generally speaking, if there is no plan— you can have a conversation about referral to someone who is trained to handle this. If there is a plan, move more directly to an intervention (e.g., an emergency room, direct admission). If you aren't sure, better to err on the side of caution.

When a client discloses physical, emotional, or sexual abuse or assault (you are now firmly in referral mode), a couple of steps are necessary. Is there immediate or ongoing exposure or risk involved? If so, there is more urgency in addressing the issue through referral and reporting. Is the person a minor or vulnerable adult? If so, you are a mandated reporter. This means it is your responsibility to report the incident to the appropriate people within the system.

Adverse childhood experiences are traumatic experiences that are remembered into adulthood, such as physical, emotional, and/or sexual abuse; physical and/or emotional neglect; household dysfunction (e.g., incarcerated relative, divorce, witnessing parent/household substance use/ alcoholism and/or domestic violence); mental illness (CDC-Kaiser, 2019). To read more about the warning signs associated with adverse childhood experiences, see Box 3-5.

Interactional Capital

Interactional capital is the mutual positive regard and the presence of positive past shared experiences within a relationship. McMorrow (2003) refers to this idea as *interactional money in the bank*. Miller and Rollnick (2013) contended that authentic positive interaction is a crucial process for developing interactional capital in the form of recent mutual, positive experiences. Having a recent mutual, positive experience to draw upon is crucial to asking our clients to engage in challenging tasks (e.g., therapy in general). Likewise, McMorrow suggests that this capital is helpful when collaboratively facing a challenging situation or

Box 3-5
Warning Signs: Recognizing Potentially Suspicious Behavior

Caveat: Many of these signs can be present for a variety of reasons. It is not our job to investigate what underlies them but to be watchful and document what we see. This can be helpful in the case of referral.

- Anxiety can obviously be present for many reasons but it is worth noting as a potential warning sign, particularly when paired with other concerns
- Restlessness
- Detachment
- Children may wear unsuitable clothing for the temperature inside or season outdoors, such as a winter coat, long pants, or sweatshirt/long-sleeved shirt, refusing to take it off
- Self-injurious behaviors
- Universal (typically negative, hostile, or fearful) response to individuals of a particular gender
- Eating disorders
- Overly aggressive
- Extreme mood changes
- Withdrawal from social interactions

problem. Never empty the bank account! In other words, the generation of interactional capital needs to be authentic, not a fee for service sort of thing. That means, don't engage in 5 minutes of positive interaction to force or leverage participation in 5 minutes of difficult intervention time. Regardless of age or communication impairment, people can recognize inauthenticity from a mile away. Engaging in a fee-for-service, tit-for-tat type of relationship feels cheap and disingenuous. Rather, authentic positive interactions are the foundation for relationship-based care. Box 3-6 shares a clinical example relevant to McMorrow's interactional money in the bank concept.

Therapeutic Alliance

Therapeutic alliance is the extent to which a client and their family believe that a clinician has their best interests in mind and will engage them in interventions that will help them to improve. Therapeutic alliance is a combination of rapport and working alliance. Rogers (1957) described elements of **rapport** as a relationship where clients see clinicians as warm, genuine, and understanding, and the clinician's approach is congruent with the client. A **working alliance** applies to individuals with shared goals and shared responsibility for tasks involved in achieving those goals (Bordin, 1979). Bordin (1979) identified three key elements of therapeutic/working alliance: (a) client and clinician agree on the therapy tasks, (b) client and clinician agree on goals, and (c) the interpersonal bond between client and clinician. That should make it clear why this text emphasizes the importance of identifying client values/interests, collaborative goal setting, and establishing an effective therapeutic relationship. A large-scale meta-analysis of psychotherapy found that therapeutic alliance accounted for 26% or more of the variability in therapeutic outcomes (Horvath & Symonds, 1991). Pinto et al. (2012) identified communication interaction styles as crucial in their meta-analysis of therapeutic alliance (physicians and physiotherapists). This included both verbal and nonverbal communication. Facilitating, involving, and supporting patients was associated with therapeutic alliance. Specifically, listening, asking open-ended questions, and showing sensitivity to emotional concerns were identified as crucial interaction styles.

Given the crucial role of communication in relationships, therapeutic alliance is gaining interest and direction in speech-language pathology. Individuals with brain injuries identify practitioner-client relationships as having the greatest impact on perception of treatment, even more than technical experience (Darragh et al., 2001). Further, individuals involved in treatment planning feel more in control of their treatment (Darragh et al., 2001). Individuals who stutter identify therapeutic alliance and active listening as crucial ingredients for effective speech-language pathology (Plexico et al., 2010). Clients who stutter emphasize the importance of speech-language pathologists building a supportive and trusting relationship by learning about their job, hobbies, home life, in addition to their stuttering and their feelings about it. This creates a safe space for them to share and be vulnerable. Family perceptions and functioning also appear to have an important influence on therapeutic alliance, at least for individuals recovering from traumatic brain injury. Sherer et al. (2007) found that high levels of family dysfunction were associated with poor therapeutic alliance, which reduced effort during therapy. In aphasia and stroke rehabilitation, a number of elements are involved in therapeutic alliance, including "instigating readiness, recognizing personhood, sharing expectations, role delineation, encouraging goal ownership, therapeutic responsiveness, and resolving conflict" (Lawton et al., 2018a, 2018b in Lawton et al., 2019, p. 459). Five distinct viewpoints of persons with aphasia arose from a Q-sort methodology, including challenge me/direct me, acknowledge me/help me to understand, respect me/listen to me, laugh with me/help me to understand, hear me/encourage me (Lawton et al., 2019).

DiGiuseppe et al. (1996) considered factors related to developing therapeutic alliance with children and adolescents. They identify a common pitfall of focusing exclusively on development of rapport/bond and failing to address agreement on goals and tasks of therapy. DiGiuseppe et al. (1996) suggest

Box 3-6

When You Make a Large Withdrawal From Your Interactional Bank Account

Years ago, I supervised a clinical fellow who covered one of my hospital's satellite sites. Therefore, I would travel there a couple of times per week to meet and complete my observations of her development. One day, as we were discussing her caseload, she shared a concern regarding a fairly new patient she was seeing in rehabilitation. The gentleman was just a couple of weeks out from a large middle cerebral artery stroke that resulted in moderate nonfluent aphasia. In fact, I had seen this gentleman initially at my hospital, which was a regional stroke center. When he left my facility, he was fairly hopeful and positive about the road to recovery ahead of him. Like many individuals with stroke, this sense of hope and motivation was swallowed up by the onset of depression and inaction. My clinical fellow shared her concern that he might not qualify for ongoing rehabilitation if he didn't start to participate consistently in therapies. He had stopped participating in occupational, physical, and speech therapy services, refusing participation and often shutting down or pretending to sleep when people entered his room. He also stopped cooperating with nursing staff to help complete his cares and other daily routines. I asked her to tell me about the gentleman, to which she responded by sharing the results of his aphasia battery and other testing. I clarified, "What makes him tick? What does he value or like to do?" and she responded, "I don't know, he won't respond to any of my interactions." I suggested she find out by reaching out to family, having them complete a biographical sketch (Garrett & Beukelman, 1992, 2007) and return it to her. Once they provided that information, she learned he loved playing cards with his wife and friends (sheepshead, to be specific, a northern Wisconsin card game). She learned he was a retired farmer who loved to travel, used to go hunting out west for elk and mule deer, and take fishing trips with his sons and brothers to Canada each year, along with several other details about his culture and values. She immediately began to authentically connect with the gentleman, building participation on the low-linguistic and high-salience of the sheepshead game. Initially sharing that she had never played the game, she set out to learn it with his help. Little by little he opened up, engaging more and more. Eventually, this resulted in his return to participation in occupational and physical therapy and cooperation with nursing to complete his cares. Things weren't perfect, but he was back on track. Observing their sessions, you could see the synergy and alliance between them. And then one day, several days after beginning the card playing and conversational interactions, she laid down the law, "It's time to get to work [on real therapy, she implied]." I wondered, so what you were doing wasn't "real therapy"? The interactions that drew him out of his inaction and fostered his return to participation in therapies wasn't "real therapy"? Nonetheless, she drew a line in the sand, pushed for more. He leaned back (and I held my breath) and then leaned back in and got to work. You see, there was plenty of capital, and although her ask was difficult, he trusted her.

Fast forward a couple of months, I was doing my regular check ins. She shared about another gentleman, so similar to the first. She no longer asked for my advice, she knew what to do. She found out about his interests and engaged with him right away. Her quick action and new-found skills helped her to pull him out of his funk much more quickly than the other gentleman. A couple of days and he was back on track and then, she did it—she made the same type of big ask but without the necessary capital. He shut down and retracted into himself. Within a week, he was discharged and transferred to long-term care, as he was no longer qualifying for rehab. It is much harder to undo this sense of betrayal or being used. Authenticity matters.

that clinicians need to acknowledge that children are not self-referred. As such, goals and therapeutic tasks are often imposed on them as well. This places them in an ambiguous and precontemplative stage of readiness to change. In fact, children may have goals that differ from or strongly oppose parent and/or clinician goals. Children in family-oriented approaches are more likely aware of the therapist goals, as they are more likely to be discussed. DiGiuseppe et al. (1996) acknowledged the challenges associated with helping younger children to understand goals. They emphasize approaches that foster collaboration, choice, and connections between

what is being addressed in therapy and what they want to do. Green et al. (2001) demonstrated that clinician alliance with parent and child do not always correlate. Further, alliance with the child is more predictive of outcomes than alliance with parents (Green, 2006). That is not to say we don't need to nurture alliance with parents or other partners, rather we need to nurture both client and family relationships.

Teletherapy contexts are no exception, when it comes to the importance of therapeutic alliance. Box 3-7 addresses some tools that can help you establish and maintain therapeutic alliance in virtual contexts.

Box 3-7
Teletherapy Contexts

With the rapid shift to teletherapy in 2020-2021, largely due to the COVID-19 pandemic, speech-language pathologists were challenged to establish and maintain therapeutic alliance in a context foreign to many of them and their clients. This context certainly brings new challenges and opportunities. The inability to provide concrete, physical supports or directly interact in play certainly poses a challenge. This creates an opportunity to engage *e-helpers* (e.g., parents, partners, siblings, aids, other disciplines) to deliver those physical supports with your guidance (Walker, 2020). Certainly, an e-helper, although likely necessary to deliver communicatively accessible counseling tools, is likely to alter the counseling context. That is something we need to navigate on an individual basis with our clients and their families. On a positive note, we gain the opportunity to engage with clients in their home environments, allowing connections with family, pets, hobbies, and other activities we would not typically engage with during in-person therapy. Harnessing those opportunities involves collaborative goal development, utilizing client-identified therapy tasks within the home, and establishing rapport/bond. This means either creating digital access to sorting tools or creative use of webcams and document cameras. Walker (2020) also recommended sending a physical tool kit for clients and e-helpers to access at home. A recent interdisciplinary investigation addressed parent engagement and therapeutic alliance with a psychologist, speech pathologist, and occupational therapist (Fairweather et al., 2021). Qualitative analyses identified factors that parents described as affecting their engagement and alliance, including the importance of initial engagement, collaboration, and rapport. Specifically, parents evaluated therapist efforts in communicating (with a desire for clear and frequent communication), truly partnering with them (discussing their ideas), and building rapport with them and the child (using parent observations of nonverbal communication to support engagement).

Freckmann et al. (2017) examined therapeutic alliance using the Therapeutic Alliance Scales for Children—Revised, finding that there was no significant difference between alliance for teletherapy vs. in-person therapy. The authors also suggest that the Therapeutic Alliance Scales for Children—Revised appears to have good potential for examining therapeutic alliance in speech-language pathology. Of course, not all clients are good candidates for teletherapy contexts. The Telepractice Technology Checklist (Walker, 2015) is a measure of communication candidacy and addresses necessary technology access. As a discipline, we have much to learn about therapy and relationships in the teletherapy context, but we can begin to build on knowledge of what supports alliance within face-to-face contexts.

Even Data Collection Can Be a Counseling Moment

Developing interactional capital and establishing therapeutic alliance depends on mutual direction, trust, and authentic interactions. This extends to how we collect session data. I have seen clinicians who try to hide their clipboard, as if their clients are not allowed to see what they are writing. Nothing says trust and collaboration like hiding stuff! Rather, it only serves to broaden the power differential in the clinical relationship. Lori Tufte, a wise externship supervisor in the schools (a setting I only worked during my externship), shared her system for collecting data and this rationale. Every production receives a +, there are no negatives. Of course, everyone makes errors but her point was this: all of our clients are going to get it right, it is just a matter of whether they get it right on their own or whether they need our help to do it. When they get it right independently, they receive a +. If they require our support, they receive a ⊕. This is a simple but effective way to tally productions in an errorless framework.

Noticing Small Steps and Incremental Change

Wheeler (2001) described the basic assumptions of SFBT, noting that "Small steps can change a vicious cycle of problem maintenance to a virtuous cycle of problem resolution" (p. 294). Likewise, Jones-Smith (2012) stated that SFBT therapists assume that small changes are constantly occurring and that small change can lead to a ripple effect, whereby larger changes begin to take place. Likewise, motivational interviewing assumes that even small changes are good changes (Miller & Rollnick, 2013). Affirming those changes moves clients toward bigger changes. My wife, Carol, is a nurse who serves as a complex care coordinator, serving patients with complex needs and high recidivism (e.g., frequent hospitalization and reactive care, rather than proactive prevention). She is a master at motivational interviewing, particularly skilled in withholding judgment and recognizing the value of incremental change. For instance, when she asks a patient with diabetes if they have been checking their blood sugars and what those levels are, they might respond,

"Yes, sometimes, but I can't do it every day. My typical numbers are around 350," she doesn't bat an eye. They are used to a negative response and may even be fishing for one but she responds, "That's great, you weren't checking them at all last week when we started, and your numbers were in the 400 to 500s then. You're already on the right track." While it would be easy to say that 350 is still unacceptable, expecting a blood sugar of 110 isn't realistic. Typically, this success breeds success, and in this case, numbers continued to plumate. In speech-language pathology, this could translate to hydration, dropping from four cups of coffee per day to two and increasing water intake from one to two glasses. We can get there by saying, "I love coffee too, and I'm not always good about drinking water either. What is a reasonable starting point?" Maybe for parents, this is reading to their toddler two nights every week instead of none. We can get there by saying, "I know you're very busy, so reading every night isn't an option. What would you be willing to try?" All too often we identify some end goal that seems unachievable. The funny thing is, when we prescribe unrealistic goals (particularly when we set the goal, not our clients), we don't move the needle, but when we allow clients to identify goals, they just keep blowing past their own increments, often surprising us and themselves in the process.

Finding Your Counseling Voice

"It feels uncomfortable, unnatural, it's just not me, it sounds patronizing, it feels stilted, I just can't say it that way . . ." These are common responses, as people initially attempt to employ counseling skills. They are not saying, "It sounds weird when Stephen Rollnick uses a specific technique or approach." Rather, it sounds fine when he does it and weird when I do. It is a matter of being comfortable and confident with our own counseling voice, which takes time and practice to develop. If saying, "How does that make you feel?" makes you feel like a bad actor portraying a psychoanalyst in a movie, then don't ask that question that way. *Finding your counseling voice* takes time, practice, trial and error, and seeing multiple models. The best way to learn counseling is by practicing actually implementing the approaches. You will likely make many missteps and have many awkward moments. That is a part of the development process. Try on different counseling voices for size. This includes wording/word choice, tone of voice, and where you comfortably fall on a continuum of indirect to direct statements. Viewing multiple models is a good starting point. It is helpful to see models that are a bit indirect, "So, it sounds like you feel frustrated with the situation. Is that right?" and others that are more direct, "You are frustrated with the situation." And perhaps everything in between. When using specific techniques, like reflection, it may feel okay to simply repeat exactly what the person says for emphasis, or you may want to paraphrase and/or emphasize a key element (e.g., C: "I think what they did is stupid." Y: "You feel that what they did is stupid." vs. C: "I put a lot of time and effort into this project." Y: "That was a lot of time and effort on your part." C = client, Y = you). What feels comfortable and works well for one person can feel awkward and uncomfortable for another. If you feel confident and comfortable, that is the message you will convey to your clients. Conversely, if you feel uncertain, patronizing, uncomfortable, or stilted, that is the tentative message you will convey to your clients. That is not to say that every client requires the same approach, but rather, make sure the approach you use fits you. Viewing others in action helps people to become an amalgam of features, drawn from what one sees as the best parts of those models. For instance, my counseling voice is part Stephen Rollnick, part Audrey Holland, part Carol Hoepner (my wife), part Mary Beth Clark (my clinical mentor), pieces of many talented students, and of course part Jerry Hoepner (and a hodgepodge of many other colleagues and friends). Box 3-8 shares a real-life story of a student who was searching to find her counseling voice.

A key caveat for your counseling voice—what feels comfortable to you still needs to convey professionalism. Our ability to code switch between casual and a bit more formal is important. This means we need to strike a balance by communicating in language that feels approachable to our clients but credible as a professional. Of course, all of our clients are unique, so we need to be flexible enough to modify our language to fit our clients. This takes time to develop, so you'll need to self-assess and reflect upon this throughout your career. This same set of skills helps us translate information about the anatomy and pathophysiology of disorders, along with purpose and methods for clinical assessment and interventions, into client and family-friendly education.

Educational and Informational Counseling

Speech-language pathologists typically feel more comfortable with educational-informational counseling than personal adjustment counseling (Townsend & Hoepner, 2021). Likewise, Luterman (2020) contended that most students and clinicians who have counseling coursework focus on informational counseling rather than personal adjustment counseling. That being said, effective educational counseling is not a simple skill set. For the purpose of this discussion, we'll use the concepts of health literacy as synonymous with literacy for educational materials provided within the schools. Health literacy is "the capacity to obtain, process, and understand basic health information and services needed to make appropriate decisions" (Institute of Medicine, 2004). Did you know that 90 million adults in the United States have basic or below basic health literacy skills? The Joint Commission for health care (2010) describes the importance of patient-centered communication as the "successful joint

Box 3-8
That's Not Your Counseling Voice

Several years back, before I began to actively discuss counseling voice with students in my counseling course, I had a graduate student in my counseling course who came from a small rural community a few hours away from my university. Her everyday language was often pretty informal, characterized by some regional slang and idiosyncratic wordings. She was very bright and very capable. Somehow, she got the impression that to counsel well, she needed to adopt the language of a somewhat prototypical counseling voice (if there is such a thing). As I viewed her practice counseling videos, I immediately got the impression that it did not fit her and that she felt very uncomfortable and tentative in her newly adopted counseling voice. It was so stark that I asked her to meet with me to chat about her video. After asking about her comfort level and confidence, she disclosed that she felt very stilted and unnatural. I explained that she should develop a counseling voice that fit her and the individuals she served. She planned to return to work in her home region after graduation. I suggested that perhaps her greatest strength was her unique ability to speak in a counseling voice that matched the tone and wording that people from that area share with her. It was the voice of "her people" (so to speak) and one that made her an insider—a respected insider with a master's degree. She seemed quite relieved that she didn't have to masquerade in a professional/expert façade that didn't reflect who she was.

establishment of meaning wherein patients and healthcare providers exchange information, enabling patients to participate actively in their care and ensuring that the responsibilities of both patients and providers are understood. To be truly effective, communication requires a two-way process in which messages are negotiated until the information is correctly understood by both parties" (p. 1). Effective education is thus collaborative and reciprocal in nature—we cannot simply dispense information. Evidence-based health literacy practices are designed to foster accessible health information that prepares patients to be informed collaborators in their care. This applies to both families and the client themselves. "Patient-centered protocols and strategies to minimize the negative consequences of low or limited health literacy" (Barrett et al., 2008). We accomplish this by speaking to clients and families on their level—the unspoken/unwritten

piece of this imperative is that we need to know what "their level" is. The CDC (n.d.) suggests, "using familiar concepts, words, numbers, and images, presented in ways that make sense to the people who need the information" (https://www.cdc.gov/healthliteracy/learn/). This is our charge future and current speech-language pathologists! Effective educational counseling is more than simply providing information, for real-life examples of the missteps and assumptions we can all encounter, please read Box 3-9.

Twelve factors to consider related to educational/informational counseling:

1. **Timing:** There are two ways to consider timing of educational counseling: one in light of learning readiness and the second in light of continuous education. As you will learn, there are points in time where clients, parents, partners, and families are in a better position to listen and learn. That being said, we cannot afford to simply wait until those moments arise. It is important, however, to recognize which type of moment it is (i.e., ready for learning or not ready). That will relate to how much information you share, in what formats, and how you document needs for ongoing education in the future. For instance, if a learner is not ready (perhaps they're staring through the walls), it is even more important than ever not to share too much at that point, to assure that they have a tangible (likely written) form of information to take away and refer to later, and that you make a note about returning to the information later.

2. **Learning readiness and comprehension issues:** For parents who just received a new diagnosis for their child or those who care for a child with special needs, they may already have a lot on their plates or be overwhelmed with new diagnoses or challenges. Likewise, clients and families confronted with a life-changing trauma or impairment may struggle to learn in their current context. Knowing that there are times when learners are not ready for information or simply struggle to comprehend what you share, it is important to distribute information, rather than providing everything at once. Further, include a tangible resource that they can review later, when they are better positioned to learn.

3. **Instruction format(s):** We certainly know that verbal explanations alone are not enough to foster sustainable learning. Those words often evaporate into space once they have left our tongues, regardless of how eloquently they were presented. There are a wide variety of modalities for instruction, including verbal, paper (e.g., booklets, brochures, flyers, handouts, posters), electronic, videos, audio, and social media. All of these can be modified to make them more communicatively accessible. Video explanations and demos can be a terrific way to make our intangible words tangible and reviewable. This can include creating screencasts that use images to help explain pertinent anatomy and function (check out screencast-o-matic.com and www.educreations.com for easy-to-use screen casting

---

Box 3-9
Pat Yourself on the Back . . . or No?

Early in my clinical career, I was working in a subacute rehabilitation facility. A new patient with global aphasia, Al, was admitted and I was thrilled to share the knowledge I had gained in my training program, through my work with aphasia groups, and mentorship. A standard part of our rehabilitation program was weekly rehab meetings with patients and their families. So, when it came around to my time to share about this gentleman's status, I discussed his aphasia and the approaches that helped him to comprehend and express himself. His wife asked, "What is aphasia?" and I was stunned, as that was obviously a prominent impairment, along with paresis and difficulties with self-cares. I proceeded to eloquently share (at least in my mind, it was eloquent) what aphasia was and what aphasia was not; what worked and what did not work; and how we could collaborate to help. His family said, "Wow, I cannot believe no one else told us any of this. We've never heard the word aphasia and certainly hadn't heard what it means for Al." As I left the meeting, my rehab director said, "Great job, I'm so glad to have you on the team. That was an awesome explanation of aphasia." I walked with a serious bounce in my step back to my office, thinking to myself, wow, I'm really terrific! And I thought, wow—I cannot believe no one at that hospital told them about aphasia, shame on them. It didn't take me too long to fall off of this delusional ego high. I thought to myself, there is *no* way that someone from the acute care hospital, a well-respected facility, did not tell them about aphasia and what it means. I started to recognize, in my mind, that they almost certainly had been told about aphasia and many more things. Part of me also knew that somewhere down the road, someone would educate them about something I had already taught them, and they'd say, "Jerry never shared that with us." Of course, they're adjusting to this life changing event, Al's stroke, and they don't have past knowledge about communication, language, neuroanatomy, etc. to relate to all of this new information. Education is more than telling people something. Timing, readiness, competing demands, past knowledge, and many more factors affect learning and retention.

A few years later, one day in aphasia group, this lesson was reinforced again. I was sitting next to a first-timer and her partner while a colleague was making opening comments for the day and explaining what we were going to do for the session. The first-timer was currently an outpatient with another colleague. Five minutes into the session, her partner turned and asked, "What is this aphasia thing that they keep talking about?" Oh boy, it's just the reason you're here and clearly, my colleague had mentioned it in their sessions and perhaps when he invited them to the *aphasia* group. Learning is hard when you are thrust into a life-changing context with new demands, emotions, and adjustments to make.

---

tools). There are also a lot of great videos and social media resources already available online. Note that we also have a role in either curating or helping clients and families to vet the accuracy of online or social media content, particularly when it is produced by others.

4. **Balancing the need for more with less:** People with aphasia and their partners identified the need for more information (Draper & Hill, 1995; McKenna et al., 2003). Conversely, they identified the importance of not overwhelming the reader with too much complex information (Parr et al., 1997). Even though it may sound like these two points contradict each other, in reality they do not. People desire ongoing education in manageable bites. This allows them to acquire more information but not all at once, in a way that is less overwhelming.

5. **Communicatively accessible content:** See Figure 3-2 for the anatomy of an accessible education document. See Box 3-10 for strategies for creating accessible written information and Box 3-11 for creating accessible electronic information.

6. **Types of education documents:** (a) Basic information about a disorder, (b) information about how to support a person with a communication disorder, or (c) a combination of information and supports.

7. **Prior knowledge:** What is the client's and family's current knowledge about the information? How do they prefer to receive information? Our previous exposure to information affects our ability to learn more about it. Certainly, an ENT admitted to the hospital with an ear-nose-throat disorder would have different learning needs than someone with no medical background. Learning about a client's or family member's prior knowledge is important, as it helps us to adjust our messages to fit them. A word of caution, however: Even if we know a person has prior knowledge, it is important not to assume they understand everything. We cannot simply hand them a stack of medical journal articles and call it good. We still need to check comprehension. See Box 3-12 for examples.

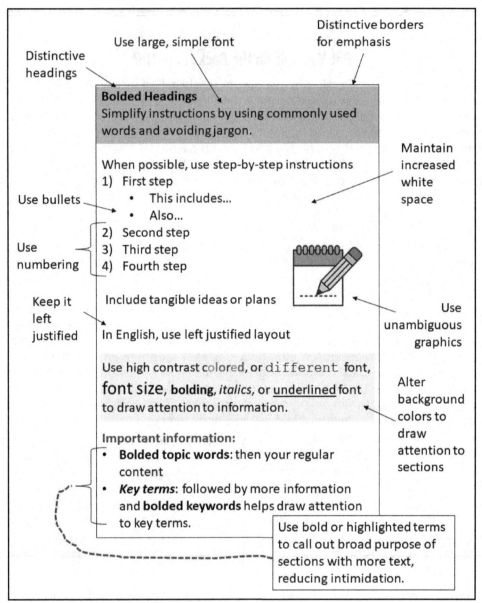

Figure 3-2. Anatomy of an accessible document.

8. **Sensitivity to cultural learning variables:** You cannot know everything about learning preferences with every culture. That being said, it is feasible to learn what each of your clients prefers. No doubt, over time you'll be able to generalize some of that knowledge, but the best approach is to learn directly about your client's and family's preferences. In this case, it is better to ask than to assume. This can begin with a simple, "How do you prefer to learn?" and "Is there anything specific I should know about your culture that affects your preferences?" which can be shortened to "cultural preferences?"

9. **Return demonstrations and return explanations:** How do we know if our clients and families understand what we've taught them? *Return demonstrations* are used when we teach clients and families a skill (e.g., how to use supported conversation techniques).

This is also known as the ***Teach-Back Method*** (Aazh, 2016; Schillinger et al., 2003). Along with explaining, modeling, and practicing the techniques, in a return demonstration, we ask them to demonstrate the trained skill independently to assess their learning. *Return explanations* are similar. After we teach clients or families about specific content knowledge, we ask them to explain it back to us in their own words. Instead of asking, "Do you understand how to use written choice?" or "Do you get how to do the supraglottic swallow?" you would say, "I want to make sure you know how to use written choice. Try asking me a question" or "Let's make sure you understand how to do the supraglottic swallow and why. Show me how you would do it . . . Now, explain to me in your own words why it is important to use it."

Box 3-10

Creating Accessible Written Information

Egan et al. (2004, p. 269) summarized evidence and recommendations to create accessible text design for people with language impairments. Their 10 suggestions include:

1. Simplify written instructions into short phrases and sentences.
2. Use commonly occurring words with the emphasis on simplicity.
3. Use large font (size 14 to 18 pt.).
4. Use simplified font styles (e.g., Times New Roman, Comic Sans MS, Arial, Verdana).
5. Format with bulleting and numbering to set out points clearly rather than embedding points in paragraphs of running prose.
6. Break down instructions or less into clearly defined steps and then order these steps in a logical sequence from simple to more complex.
7. Use generous spacing between lines of text to maximize the effect on white paper.
8. Use unambiguous graphics (e.g., clipart, photos) to support the meaning of the text rather than replace text altogether.
9. Align text where possible from left margin to simplify page layout presentation.
10. Use different formatting techniques to make headings and important points stand out (e.g., a change in font size, font style, color, or the use of borders around a text selection).

Check out this toolbox for more Teach-Back ideas and video demonstrations: www.teachbacktraining.org.

10. **Community-resources:** It may be useful to develop a repository of contacts and resources for the types of clientele you serve in your workplace. This includes community support groups, online groups, and a variety of community resources (e.g., respite care, long-term care facilities). It may include a list of potential providers for referrals (e.g., mental health counselors with experience supporting individuals with communication disorders, neurologists, otolaryngologists). To some extent, we may have to do some vetting of those third-party resources, as a client's or family's experience with those connections will likely reflect on us.

11. **Contingencies and how to reconnect:** Given factors like learning readiness, coupled with constraints of the health care and education settings, sometimes our

Box 3-11

Creating Communicatively and Cognitively Accessible Electronic and Internet Materials

In addition to the communication impairments that have potential to affect the accessibility of electronic, internet, and social media content for our clients, many of our clients have sensory, cognitive, or motoric impairments that further limit access. Gao et al. (2012) eloquently summarized modifications to sensory, cognitive, and motoric adaptations necessary to support access to our clients. Certainly, if you are developing digital resources for your clients and their families, these are important ingredients. Similarly, as you seek out digital resources to share with your clients and their families, these are important considerations.

Sensory (visual and auditory adaptations)

- Larger font, icons, and buttons
- Use simple font, such as sans serif type
- Increase spacing and white space
- Place important information at screen-center
- Color and contrast considerations—generally speaking we want high contrast
- Audio outputs should be in the low to middle frequency ranges
- Reauditorization of speech and closed captioning is useful

Cognitive

- Reduce demands on working memory by
  - Simplifying text
  - Decreasing number of successive operations to access functions
  - Simplifying menu hierarchies, this also improves navigation performance
- Avoid moving or expandable menus
- Minimize irrelevant information, redundant information, or design complexity
- Avoid interface that requires a lot of scanning

Motor

- Avoid moving targets
- Eliminate demands for rapid and repetitive movements
- Minimize use of scrollbars

Box 3-12
Prior Knowledge

In Chapter 7, CeCelia and Wayne Zorn share a story about the moment when Wayne was diagnosed with PPA. CeCelia has a PhD in nursing and had many years of practice-based knowledge to draw upon. Knowing this, the neurologist attempted to adjust the information provided to fit her knowledge, sharing journal articles about PPA. Unfortunately, what he did was a serious overshoot. Handing her a stack of jargon-filled medical journal articles without any interpretation or explanations was a big miss on his part. He didn't share an overview or check her comprehension with a return explanation. Rather, he handed the articles to her on the way out of the office.

Full disclosure, I have lived with a rare spinal disorder for the past 18 years. That disorder has occasionally landed me in a well-known teaching hospital, where my regular physician and his large group of residents would assess and treat me. One day in morning rounds, a new batch of residents came in to do their daily assessment and status check. After doing their assessment, they began reporting my status to me in simple terms, perhaps too simple. "The spinal cord is a group of nerves that…" It was aimed at about the sixth-grade level. My physician, who had reached a point of age and wisdom, just allowed them to teach me. When they were done with their education, my physician stepped in and said, "Okay, this is Dr. Hoepner, he is a professor from Wisconsin who teaches neuroanatomy and physiology…" and the residents' collective jaws fell to the floor. You could see the embarrassment on their faces, knowing that they had seriously undershot with their teaching. Taking advantage of every teaching moment, my physician said, "See why it's important to learn about the patient's background?"—a lesson that I'm sure those residents will never forget.

clients and their families exit the system with learning and work yet to be done. Establishing a means for them to reconnect with the system is crucial.

12. **Health information accessibility and readability:** Accessible health information can reduce anxiety, encourage clients to become more involved in their own interventions, increase compliance, increase sense of control, increase client's understanding of their condition, and improve the relationship between client and therapist (Rose et al., 2003). Access to health information can improve understanding of health issues and improve coping. Clients want more such information and are often dissatisfied with the information they receive. Modifications are necessary to ensure accessibility of content provided. Deciding the best way to provide health information is complex. Possibilities include verbal, written brochures, posters, audio recordings, videos, and the internet among others (Rose et al., 2003). In spite of the possibilities (which are all potentially great options), patients often prefer printed educational materials (Draper & Hill, 1995). Of course, this may change as technology becomes increasingly ubiquitous. Printed educational materials (PEMs) are printed booklets, pamphlets, handouts, or brochures used to provide health-related information. They supplement and reinforce verbal information, are cost-effective, allow self-paced learning, and can be referred to for reminders and clarification (Rose et al., 2003). Please complete the PEM assignment within Box 3-13.

Key Timepoints for Counseling

Counseling moments can arise at any time throughout therapy. For some clients, it is nearly a daily event. That being said, for many other clients, it seems to cluster around specific landmarks: initial meetings, transitions, and discharges. These are key time points for both educational counseling and personal adjustment counseling. Providing educational counseling at these beginnings, transitions, and endings is one way to distribute content and knowledge.

For new beginnings, there is a need to provide information about disorders, prognoses/what to expect, and first steps for supporting a client with a communication disorders. A common pitfall here is providing too much or too complicated materials. Depending on the situation, the client and their family may be spending all of their energies processing what just happened or the loss of the dreams they had planned. Either way, seeing you is new and likely brings new information and challenges to address.

Transitions happen as clients shift from one setting to another. This could include elementary school to middle school, acute care to rehabilitation, rehabilitation to home, or assisted living to skilled nursing care. Likewise, it could include return to school or return to work transitions. Obviously, there are far more permutations than those listed previously but you get the idea. Several of those transitions are marked by an increase in demands, while a few are marked by new restrictions in activity level or the need for extra supports. Whatever the case, this is a time when information about the upcoming changes can reduce anxiety and stress, and help set clear expectations. Creating a communicatively accessible support document can be very useful (e.g., ideas for returning home, activity ideas, ideas for returning to school, how to help Johnny to be successful at home, tips for communicating with Agnes). Often, these tools can serve multiple purposes, in that they help partners/families know what to expect, help the client by providing specific information or supports, and help staff at the next facility to know a bit about the new person and how to help them.

Discharges are inevitable for most of our clients. Certainly, in a case where someone meets all of their goals, is "fixed," or is graduating the program, this is a very positive experience. Some discharges also represent a transition to another program or next step, which is sometimes a very positive thing and other times can seem like a step backward. Unfortunately, some of our discharges happen because the client is no longer making progress or due to limitations in insurance coverage or because a student no longer meets criteria for services. In these cases, clients and family members can feel very disappointed. Hersh (2009) examined perceptions of individuals with aphasia and their partners regarding discharge. Clients and their partners were often unsure of why they were being discharged. Their assumptions were that it was either client-related, therapist-related, or externally imposed. **Client-related** reasons are somewhat shocking and speak to our need to provide a clear reasoning and plan for discharge. Reasons included:

> *improving and no longer needing therapy, no longer improving, therapy was not enjoyable, therapy was not doing them any good, refused group therapy as stigmatizing, did not like the setting, put off by transport issues, responsibility to move on so that others could have a chance at therapy, responsibility not to waste the therapist's time, and they had not worked hard enough to deserve more therapy. (p. 342)*

This begs the question, exactly what kind of a message are we sending to our clients? Are we giving them the impression that they are a burden or not living up to our expectations? When clients assumed it was a **therapist-related** decision, they identified the following reasons:

> *the therapist had done everything possible, the therapist believes the client doesn't need any more intervention, the therapist is too busy and needs to move people off of the books, the therapist has other priorities, and the therapist no longer knows what to do. (p. 342)*

Again, we are not sending a clear message about the discharge plan or instilling confidence about our competence in carrying out our job. **Externally imposed** reasons included:

> *imposed time restrictions on the therapist, imposed financial restrictions on the therapist, and limited service options to refer to for further therapy. (p. 343)*

Patients with stroke discharged from physiotherapy (physical therapy in the United States) were often surprised by termination of therapy, as they did not think they had reached their expectations for recovery (Wiles et al., 2004).

Box 3-13

Design Your Own Communicatively Accessible Paper Education Material

Drawing upon the principles for accessible written information, develop PEM for one of your current clients/their family members.

Remember, this may include (a) basic information about a disorder, (b) information about how to support a person with a communication disorder, or (c) a combination of information and supports.

Read on to learn about key timepoints and transitions, where PEMs are particularly helpful (e.g., return to school, return to work, returning home, tips for communicating, activity ideas, safe swallowing).

In this case, while their therapists judged that they had reached a plateau, they did not feel comfortable explaining this to patients, so they avoided telling them. Avoiding the conversation limits our ability to collaborate on a plan and to fully understand one's current situation.

Regardless of the reasons for discharge, clients and family members need to be involved in the process. A qualitative review of discharge from the hospital following brain injuries found that most studies reported that families and caregivers were not involved in discharge arrangements (Piccenna et al., 2016). As a result, those patients and family members did not feel adequately prepared at the time of discharge to transition to home. Similarly, only 4 of 21 interviewees in Hersh's (2009) study were involved in decision making about their discharge. Manskow et al. (2018) also identified problems with discharge, noting that family members reported not receiving information about long-term consequences and dependency level following brain injury. Further, this transition has been identified as a time of increased family burden, distress, anxiety, and depression (Gouick & Gentleman, 2004). This leaves family members feeling underprepared for supporting loved ones following discharge (Gouick & Gentleman, 2004; Manskow et al., 2018; Piccenna et al., 2016; Turner et al., 2008). Hersh (2009) identified inconsistency in timing, noting that discharge was sprung suddenly on some families, while others had more time to prepare. Further, offers for follow-ups were inequitable, with some families receiving clear instructions for follow-ups and others not receiving these opportunities.

Hersh and Cruice (2010) suggested that we need to have a clear plan for addressing discharge. They note the subtleties of discharges that serve as a transition from one site to another are quite different than final discharges from therapy.

As such, speech-language pathologists need to consider the sociopolitical, geographic, cultural, clinical, and relational contexts of discharge. Sociopolitical factors relate to the reimbursement systems. Geographic factors include availability of services, including low or no cost services at universities or community-based programs. Certainly, cultural contexts alter expectations for services. Likewise, clinical contexts relate to a speech-language pathologist's adherence to evidence-based practices but may also be influenced by the therapy model being followed. Relationships with partners, parents, and other caregivers are also crucial. Establishing home programs and follow-ups can help them to feel more prepared to carry out supports and ongoing interventions. Along with understanding these contextual factors, speech-language pathologists need a clear idea of how to discharge and hands-on experience, models, and scaffolding to carry it out.

Key Points for Discharge

- **Communicate:** Establish explicit communication about the discharge process. Don't avoid this communication. Knowing what to expect, even if it isn't ideal, is better than not knowing what comes next.
- **Timing:** Don't wait until the last minute to inform clients about discharge.
- **Collaborate:** Work with clients and their families on discharge planning.
- **Why:** Make it clear why a client is being discharged.
- **What to expect:** Provide families with clear information about the long-term consequences and level of support needed for a client.
- **Put it on paper:** Create an accessible document with a plan for the transition, supports needed at home, and next steps.
- **Plan:** Establish a follow-up plan and contacts.
- **Resources:** If this is the "final" discharge, connect the client and their family with other community resources such as support groups, university services, respite, and other community-based options.

Complete the exercise in Box 3-14, using the information about effective discharge planning to create a client-/family-friendly discharge plan.

Chapter Summary

Within the WHO-ICF framework (2001), counseling primarily addresses activity, participation, and contextual factors. In particular, feelings, beliefs, attitudes, and motivation are often addressed in the context of a client's current and desired participation in personally relevant activities. In our role as counselors, we will encounter topics and situations that are very uncomfortable to discuss. We need to be prepared to lean into those difficult conversations, as they

---

> ## Box 3-14
> ### Discharge Plan
>
> Consider one of your current or past clients. Develop a communicatively accessible and clear discharge plan for the client and their family.

---

are a necessary part of moving forward. A number of foundational counseling skills help prepare us for these conversations. Listening skills are crucial to all counseling methods and listening means more than simply sitting back quietly. Active and empathetic listening includes demonstrating that we are attentively listening through our affirmations, reflections, follow-up questions, and nonverbals. Our words and actions also demonstrate when we acknowledge a client's inherent competence and personhood. Using communication supports to ensure a means of response helps us to reveal that competence. After all, our clients and their families are the experts in living with a communication disorder and have earned a collaborative voice at the table to express their priorities and make choices about the direction of therapy. Uncovering our client's backstories allows us to see their inherent personhood and cut them a bit of slack when things don't go perfectly. Developing authentic interactional money in the bank is necessary, as we ask our clients to do difficult things every day in therapy. Establishing therapeutic alliance allows our clients and families to feel a sense of trust that what we do in therapy will help them move toward meeting their therapy goals. Finding and owning our counseling voice allows us to be confident and authentic in the words we use to support our clients. This takes time to develop and becomes unique to each of us.

One of the first foundational counseling tools we employ is educational counseling. This is more complex than simply giving our clients and their families information about the communication disorders they experience. Knowing how much information to provide and when varies by individual situation, thus we need to be responsive to client's learning readiness and prior knowledge. For persons with communication disorder, providing the information in a communicatively accessible format allows them to understand the content. Having such information can reduce anxiety, improve their follow through, and provide a sense of partnership in therapy. Both educational counseling and personal adjustment counseling can happen at any moment but both also cluster around key time points, including initial meetings, transitions, and discharge. We need to be prepared to address those moments head on, as clients and families often report that these time points can be frustrating and confusing.

Key Takeaways

- Counseling addresses feelings, beliefs, attitudes, and motivation to engage in personally relevant activities.
- As speech-language pathologists, you will encounter uncomfortable counseling moments. Preparation is the antidote to avoidance.
- Affirming, reflecting, and summarizing demonstrate that we are actively listening.
- There are tools for making communicatively accessible education documents.
- Return demonstrations and return explanations are techniques for evaluating the effectiveness of our client's learning in response to our education.
- Initial sessions, transitions, and discharges are often key opportunities for educational and personal adjustment counseling.
- Along with presenting education, expectations, and establishing a transition/discharge plan verbally, communicatively accessible printed materials can help clients and families feel better about transitions and discharges.

References

American Speech-Language-Hearing Association. (n.d.). *Cultural Competence*. (Practice Portal). http://www.asha.org/Practice-Portal/Professional-Issues/Cultural-Competence/.

American Speech-Language-Hearing Association. (2010). *Cultural competence checklist: Personal reflection*. http://www.asha.org/uploadedFiles/Cultural-Competence-Checklist-Personal-Reflection.pdf.

Aazh, H. (2016). Feasibility of conducting a randomized controlled trial to evaluate the effect of motivational interviewing on hearing-aid use. *International Journal of Audiology, 55*(3), 149-156.

Bordin, E. S. (1979). The generalizability of the psychodynamic concept of the working alliance. *Psychotherapy: Theory, Research, and Practice, 16*, 252-260.

Centers for Disease Control and Prevention. (n.d.). *Talking points about health literacy*. https://www.cdc.gov/healthliteracy/shareinteract/Tell Others.html

Centers for Disease Control and Prevention. (2016). *About the CDC-Kaiser ACE study*. Centers for Disease Control and Prevention, 8.

Centers for Disease Control and Prevention, Kaiser Permanente. (2016). *The ACE study survey data* [Unpublished data]. U.S. Department of Health and Human Services, Centers for Disease Control and Prevention.

CDC-Kaiser, A. C. E. (2019). *Study (2019)*. Adverse Childhood Experiences (ACEs).

Darragh, A. R., Sample, P. L., & Krieger, S. R. (2001). "Tears in my eyes cause somebody finally understood": Client perceptions of practitioners following brain injury. *American Journal of Occupational Therapy, 55*(2), 191-199.

De Jong, P., & Berg, I. K. (2013). *Interviewing or solutions* (4th ed.). Thomson Brooks/Cole

DiGiuseppe, R., Linscott, J., & Jilton, R. (1996). Developing the therapeutic alliance in child—adolescent psychotherapy. *Applied and Preventive Psychology, 5*(2), 85-100.

Draper, M., & Hill, S. (1995). *The role of patient satisfaction surveys in a national approach to hospital quality management*. AGPS.

Egan, J., Worrall, L., & Oxenham, D. (2004). Accessible internet training package helps people with aphasia cross the digital divide. *Aphasiology, 18*(3), 265-280.

Fairweather, G. C., Lincoln, M., Ramsden, R., & Bulkeley, K. (2021). Parent engagement and therapeutic alliance in allied health teletherapy programs. *Health & Social Care in the Community, 30*(2), e504-e513.

Freckmann, A., Hines, M., & Lincoln, M. (2017). Clinicians' perspectives of therapeutic alliance in face-to-face and telepractice speech-language pathology sessions. *International Journal of Speech Language Pathology, 19*(3), 287-296. https://doi.org/10.1080/17549507.2017.1292547

Gao, Q., Ebert, D., Chen, X., & Ding, Y. (2012). Design of a mobile social community platform for older Chinese people in urban areas. *Human Factors and Ergonomics in Manufacturing & Service Industries, 25*(1), 66-89. https://doi.org/10.1002/hfm.20523

Gouick, J., & Gentleman, D. (2004). The emotional and behavioural consequences of traumatic brain injury. *Trauma, 6*(4), 285-292.

Green, J. (2006). Annotation: The therapeutic alliance—a significant but neglected variable in child mental health treatment studies. *Journal of Child Psychology and Psychiatry, 47*(5), 425-435.

Green, J., Kroll, L., Imre, D., Frances, F. M., Begum, K., Gannon, L., & Anson, R. (2001). Health gain and predictors of outcome in inpatient and day patient child psychiatry treatment. *Journal of the American Academy of Child and Adolescent Psychiatry, 40*, 325-332.

Hall, A. M., Ferreira, P. H., Maher, C. G., Latimer, J. & Ferreira, M. L. (2010). The influence of the therapist-patient relationship on treatment outcome in physical rehabilitation: A systematic review. *Physical Therapy, 90*, 1099-1110.

Hamilton, A. F., Ramos-Pizarro, J. F., Rivera Peréz, J. González, W., & Beverly-Ducker, K. L. (2020). *Exploring cultural responsiveness: Guided scenarios for communication sciences and disorders (CSD) professionals*. ASHA Press.

Hanton, P. (2011). *Skills in solution focused brief counselling and psychotherapy*. Sage.

Hersh, D. (2009). How do people with aphasia view their discharge from therapy? *Aphasiology, 23*(3), 331-350.

Hersh, D., & Cruice, M. (2010). Beginning to teach the end: The importance of including discharge from aphasia therapy in the curriculum. *International Journal of Language & Communication Disorders, 45*(3), 263-274.

Hook, J. N., Davis, D. E., Owen, J. W., & Worthington, E. L. E., & Utsey, S. (2013). Cultural humility, measuring openness to culturally diverse clients. *Journal of Counseling Psychology, 60*(3), 353.

Horvath, A. O., & Symonds, B. D. (1991). Relation between working alliance and outcome in psychotherapy: A meta-analysis. *Journal of Counseling Psychology, 38*(2), 139.

Institute of Medicine (US) Committee on Health Literacy. (2004). Health literacy: A prescription to end confusion. Nielsen-Bohlman, L., Panzer, A. M., Kindig, D. A. (Eds.). National Academies Press (US); 2004. PMID: 25009856.

Iveson, C., & McKergow, M. (2015). Brief therapy: Focused description development. *Journal of Solution-Focused Brief Therapy, 2*(1), 1-17.

Joint Commission. (2010) *Advancing effective communication, cultural competence, and patient- and family-centered care: A roadmap for hospitals*. The Joint Commission.

Jones-Smith, E. (2012). *Theories of counselling & psychotherapy: An integrative approach*. Sage.

Kagan, A. (1998). Supported conversation for adults with aphasia: Methods and resources for training conversation partners. *Aphasiology, 12*(9), 816-830.

Lawton, H. M., Haddock, G., Conroy, P. & Sage, K. (2016). Therapeutic alliances in stroke rehabilitation: A metaethnography. *Archives of Physical Medicine and Rehabilitation, 97*, 1979-1993.

Lawton, M., Conroy, P., Sage, K., & Haddock, G. (2019). Aphasia and stroke therapeutic alliance measure (A-STAM): Development and preliminary psychometric evaluation. *International Journal of Speech-Language Pathology, 21*(5), 459-469.

Lawton, M., Haddock, G., Conroy, P., Serrant, L., & Sage, K. (2018a). People with aphasia's perception of the therapeutic alliance in aphasia rehabilitation post stroke: A thematic analysis. *Aphasiology, 32*(12), 1397-1417. https://doi.org/10.1080/02687038.2018.1441365

Lawton, M., Haddock, G., Conroy, P., Serrant, L., & Sage, K. (2020). People with aphasia's perspectives of the therapeutic alliance during speech-language intervention: A Q methodological approach. *International Journal of Speech-Language Pathology, 22*(1), 59-69.

Lawton, M., Sage, K., Haddock, G., Conroy, P., & Serrant, L. (2018b). Speech and language therapists' perspectives of therapeutic alliance construction and maintenance in aphasia rehabilitation post-stroke. *International Journal of Language & Communication Disorders, 53*(3), 550-563. https://doi.org/10.1111/1460-6984.12368

Lipchik, E., Derks, J., Lacourt, M., & Nunnally, E. (2012). The evolution of solution-focused brief therapy. In C. Franklin, T. Trepper, W. Gingerich, & E. McCollum (Eds.), *Solution-focused brief therapy: A handbook of evidence-based practice* (pp. 3-19). Oxford University Press.

Luterman, D. (1999). Counseling families with a hearing-impaired child. *Otolaryngologic Clinics of North America, 32*(6), 1037-1050.

Luterman, D. (2020). On teaching counseling: Getting beyond informational counseling. *American Journal of Speech-Language Pathology, 29*(2), 903-908.

Manskow, U. S., Arntzen, C., Damsgård, E., Braine, M., Sigurdardottir, S., Andelic, N., . . . Anke, A. (2018). Family members' experience with in-hospital health care after severe traumatic brain injury: A national multicentre study. *BMC Health Services Research, 18*(1), 951. https://doi.org/10.1186/s12913-018-3773-7

McMorrow, M. J. (2003). *Getting ready to help: A Primer on interacting in human service.* Paul H. Brookes Publishing.

Morrison, T. L. Smith, J. D. (2013). Working alliance development in occupational therapy: A cross-case analysis. *Australian Occupational Therapy Journal, 60*, 326-333.

Parr, S. Byng, S., Gilpin, S., & Ireland, C. (1997). *Talking about aphasia: Living with loss of language after stroke.* McGraw-Hill Education.

Piccenna, L., Lannin, N. A., Gruen, R., Pattuwage, L., & Bragge, P. (2016). The experience of discharge for patients with an acquired brain injury from the inpatient to the community setting: A qualitative review. *Brain Injury, 30*(3), 241-251.

Pinto, R. Z., Ferreira, M. L., Oliveira, V. C., Franco, M. R., Adams, R., Maher, C. G., & Ferreira, P. H. (2012). Patient-centered communication is associated with positive therapeutic alliance: A systematic review. *Journal of Physiotherapy, 58*(2), 77-87. https://doi.org/10.1016/S1836-9553(12)70087-5

Plexico, L. W., Manning, W. H., & DiLollo, A. (2010). Client perceptions of effective and ineffective therapeutic alliances during treatment for stuttering. *Journal of Fluency Disorders, 35*(4), 333-354.

Rogers, C. R. (1957). The necessary and sufficient conditions of therapeutic personality change. *Journal of Consulting Psychology, 21*(2), 95.

Rogers, C. R. (1959). Client-centered therapy. *American Handbook of Psychiatry, 3*, 183-200.

Rogers, C. R., & Farson, R. E. (1957). *Active listening* (p. 84).

Rose, T., Worrall, L., & McKenna, K. (2003). The effectiveness of aphasia-friendly principles for printed health education materials for people with aphasia following stroke. *Aphasiology, 17*(10), 947-963.

Rose, T. A., Worrall, L. E., Hickson, L. M., & Hoffmann, T. C. (2011). Aphasia friendly written health information: Content and design characteristics. *International Journal of Speech-Language Pathology, 13*(4), 335-347.

Schillinger, D., Piette, J., Grumbach, K., Wang, F., Wilson, C., Daher, C., . . . & Bindman, A. B. (2003). Closing the loop: physician communication with diabetic patients who have low health literacy. *Archives of Internal Medicine, 163*(1), 83-90.

Sherer, M., Evans, C. C., Leverenz, J., Stouter, J., Irby Jr, J. W., Eun Lee, J., & Yablon, S. A. (2007). Therapeutic alliance in post-acute brain injury rehabilitation: predictors of strength of alliance and impact of alliance on outcome. *Brain Injury, 21*(7), 663-672.

Simmons-Mackie, N., & Damico, J. S. (2011). Counseling and Aphasia Treatment. *Topics in Language Disorders, 31*(4), 336-351. https://doi.org/10.1097/tld.0b013e318234ea9f

Stewart, T., & Leahy, M. M. (2010). Uniqueness and individuality in stuttering therapy. In A. Weiss (Ed.), *Perspectives on individual differences affecting therapeutic change in communication disorders* (pp. 205-220). Psychology Press.

Teach-Back Training. (2017). Always use Teach-Back! Training toolkit. http://www.teachbacktraining.org/

Tervalon, M., & Murray-Garcia, J. (1998). Cultural humility versus cultural competence: A critical distinction in defining physician training outcomes in multicultural education. *Journal of Health Care for the Poor and Underserved, 9*(2), 117-125.

Townsend, A. K., & Hoepner, J. K. (2021a). Counseling practices of speech-language pathologists serving persons with aphasia: Examining training and preparedness within clinical practice. [Unpublished manuscript].

Townsend, A. K., & Hoepner, J. K. (2021b). Counseling practices survey among speech-language pathologists: The state of counseling in speech-language pathology. [Unpublished manuscript].

Turner, B. J., Fleming, J. M., Ownsworth, T. L., & Cornwell, P. L. (2008). The transition from hospital to home for individuals with acquired brain injury: A literature review and research recommendations. *Disability and Rehabilitation, 30*(16), 1153-1176.

Walker, J. P. (2015). *University of Maine, Speech Therapy Terapractice and Technology Program manual.* University of Maine Faculty Monographs, Book 220. http://digitalcommons.library.umaine.edu/fac_monographs/220

Walker, J. P. (2020). In Hall, N., Juengling-Sudkamp, J., Gutmann, M. L., & Cohn, E. R. (Eds.), *Tele-AAC: Augmentative and Alternative Communication Through Telepractice.* Plural Publishing.

Wheeler, J. (2001). A helping hand: Solution-focused brief therapy and child and adolescent mental health. *Clinical Child Psychology and Psychiatry, 6*(2), 293-306.

Wiles, R., Ashburn, A., Payne, S., & Murphy, C. (2004). Discharge from physiotherapy following stroke: the management of disappointment. *Social Science & Medicine, 59*(6), 1263-1273.

World Health Organization. (2001). ICF: International Classification of Functioning, Disability and Health.

Worrall, L., Sherratt, S., Rogers, P., Howe, T., Hersh, D., Ferguson, A., & Davidson, B. (2011). What people with aphasia want: Their goals according to the ICF. *Aphasiology, 25*(3), 309-322.

Ylvisaker, M., Feeney, T., & Capo, M. (2007). Long-term community supports for individuals with co-occurring disabilities after traumatic brain injury: Cost effectiveness and project-based intervention. *Brain Impairment, 8*(3), 276.

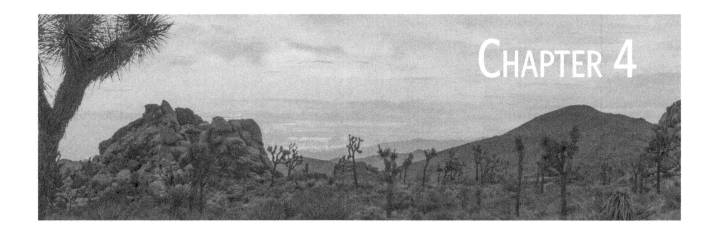

CHAPTER 4

Assessment and Interviewing

Jerry K. Hoepner, PhD, CCC-SLP

Everybody is a genius. But if you judge a fish by its ability to climb a tree, it will live its whole life believing that it is stupid. ~ Albert Einstein

It's not what you have that matters but what you do with what you have that matters. ~ Mark Ylvisaker

Assessment in Counseling?

You might be wondering, is there really assessment in counseling? Just like assessment throughout the profession of speech-language pathology, counseling assessment guides our intervention. Further, it doesn't just happen at the outset of treatment or the end. Effective assessment in counseling needs to be ongoing. Miller and Rollnick (2013) refer to this as ***routine assessment*** and caution about the impracticality and consequences of beginning a therapeutic relationship with a barrage of questions in your initial meeting. They note that a lengthy initial assessment is unlikely to promote engagement and sometimes results in making clients more passive or not returning. If this is true for individuals without communication disorders, it is likely amplified for those with communication disorders. Thus, our initial interactions

need to be focused on promoting engagement and any information-seeking interviews or assessments need to be highly collaborative, and perhaps limited in scale or length. Multiple investigations report that motivational interviewing improves client retention (see Miller & Rollnick, 2013 for the complete list), so using the motivational interviewing framework within the initial session may be worthwhile. Preceding any initial interview with 10 minutes of engaging and focusing is recommended. For some individuals, 20 to 30 minutes is necessary (Miller & Rollnick, 2013). In either case, much of the needed information is often identified during the more conversational engaging and focusing time, reducing the need for more formal interviewing.

So, what does this assessment look like for persons with communication disorders? This includes our exploration of values, needs, and goals. Framing your initial interview with Maslow's hierarchy of needs in mind is helpful in developing a counseling approach that fits the individual you are

Hoepner, J. K. (Ed.). *Counseling and Motivational Interviewing in Speech-Language Pathology* (pp. 47-68).

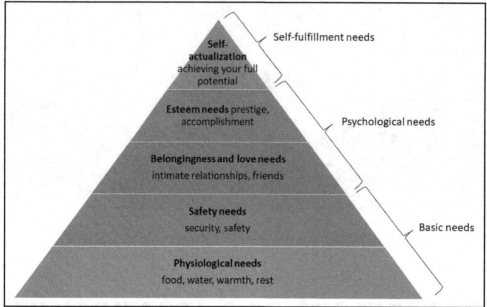

Figure 4-1. Maslow's hierarchy of needs.

working with (Figure 4-1). The hierarchy was not developed specifically for individuals who experienced a developmental or acquired disorder. Rather, it was an early attempt to understand what motivates people. Generally speaking, basic needs must be met before one can address psychological needs. We are not motivated or in a position to consider higher-level needs until we have met those more basic needs. Likewise, self-actualization cannot be addressed until basic and psychological needs have been addressed. So, we need to get a sense of the person's physical needs, social-emotional context, and living situation. See Box 4-1 for an application of Maslow's hierarchy.

Once we have completed an interview, sharing our findings is an important part of the process. Our clients need to know why we're asking for specific information and how we plan to use it. In this case, we need to let them know that learning about their needs, values, and goals or any perceived barriers and concerns is central to setting goals together and selecting personally relevant therapy tasks. It also demonstrates our commitment to building an authentic relationship by learning about them as individuals. Collectively, this information is crucial for enhancing their engagement and motivation. Before we dive head over heels into assessing needs, values, and goals, let's revisit a concept that undergirds the importance of these assessments, ***therapeutic alliance***. Recall that Bordin (1979) identified three key elements of therapeutic/working alliance: (1) client and clinician agree on the therapy tasks, (2) client and clinician agree on goals, and (3) the interpersonal bond between client and clinician. Therefore, assessment of counseling should address these three elements along with mood states that are likely to affect motivation and participation.

Eliciting Person-Centered Goals and Interests (Bordin's Principle of Shared Therapy Goals and Tasks)

Effective counseling is person-centered. As such, eliciting information about an individual's values, interests, and goals is a crucial step. Regardless of the presence or severity of a communication impairment, collecting that much information is a lot to ask, particularly in an interview that is exclusively verbal. Establishing tangible and reviewable interviews is the first step in making the conversation accessible. A number of tools and frameworks exist that can help you to elicit this information, which will be discussed in the upcoming sections. Acknowledging competence and the personhood of an individual with a communication disorder is a critical first step. The concept of "personhood" acknowledges all people as valuable and deserving of respect and a voice in their own care (DiLollo & Favreau, 2010; Kitwood, 1997). Personhood shifts away from an emphasis on impairments toward understanding how their experience is shaped by those around them (Davies, 2020). It's easy to assume that this only applies to some of our clients. For instance, you wouldn't ask a toddler what goals they have for their speech; likewise, you wouldn't ask a person with moderate to severe dementia about their swallowing priorities. True, you wouldn't ask in that manner, but those impairment-based elements are just part of goals. Giving those individuals a voice/choice in what they do does matter. This may be conducted through proxy interviews ("What does your child like to do?" or "What kinds of food does your mum

---

Box 4-1

Insights From the Other Side, "Survival Mode"

As a foster parent, I gained the unique perspective of seeing children come from an environment where physiological and safety needs were not being met. Coupled with conflicting messages from parents about belonging and love, the children my family and I encountered needed to experience a sense of consistency and trust in meeting those needs. Some of the things we encountered may relate to the challenges that children or adults you encounter in clinical contexts.

- Every child that entered our home hoarded food for at least 2 weeks to a month, not confident of when their next meal would come. We would regularly find boxes of food squirreled away in their bedrooms. Once they experienced consistency and trust, this behavior ceased.

- Many of the children we encountered had impoverished language environments, thus their reaction to books or even oral stories took some time to develop.

- None of the children that entered our home had a sense of routine or regularity for what happens on a weekday or weekend. Establishing a routine takes at least a month, and thus it takes at least a month to see the positive behaviors that follow the consistency of a regular routine.

- Sense of safety and trust is also an important factor early on. One 9-year-old boy who we fostered wore jeans and a sweatshirt for the first month with us—even though it was July and very hot! Once he began to feel safe and gain trust, he was willing to wear short-sleeved shirts and shorts, a preference that he now carries into Wisconsin winters as well.

- Most of the children did not receive empathetic concern for their physical or emotional well-being. At minimum, that empathy was highly inconsistent and unpredictable. As such, they did not attempt to convey or communicate about pain. In one instance, a child entered our home with lots of behavioral outbursts and what some may call obstinate or oppositional behaviors. As a 4-year-old, her communication was actually pretty close to what I expected for a typical 4-year-old. At some point I noticed what I thought was lip reading, prompted by the fact that she spoke loudly and didn't seem to listen when she wasn't looking at me. I shudder to say this was 2 weeks after she had been in our home when I made the realization. I grabbed an otoscope from my office and checked her ears that evening. To my horror, I found a fully perforated tympanic membrane and prominent evidence of scar tissue on the other side. In a visit with our ENT, it nearly brought him to tears. He remarked that he had been a medic/physician in the Gulf War and this sweet girl's pain tolerance was comparable to the soldiers he treated. Two weeks . . . and no outward complaints about any pain. Sadly, she did not expect anyone to respond to this basic physiological need.

---

like?"), but given communication supports, it's best to elicit as much of the interest, values, and activity-participation oriented information from the person themselves as possible.

Autobiographical/Biographical Sketches and Inventories

Garrett and Beukelman (1992, 2007) developed an Inventory of Topics and Biographical Information Sketch for individuals with severe communication impairments such as global aphasia. This tool has value far beyond that narrow scope, as a way to efficiently collect personal background, interests, and values. Whether completed directly by the individual with a communication disorder or a partner/family member, having this information positions the speech-language pathologist well to probe even more deeply about

those interest areas. As a caveat, it may be helpful and culturally sensitive to inform clients and family that they may skip items that they are not comfortable including in a response. As much as I value this tool, it's important to note that you can make your own homegrown versions too that may get at age- and culture-specific content that you hope to explore.

Tangible Sorts and Multimodal Structured Interview Tools

Personal Values Card Sort

Values sorts are an important piece of interviewing and assessment in counseling. Central to motivational interviewing, values sorts are a way to map agendas and set goals. One such tool, the *Personal Values Card Sort*, is a set of terms and descriptors of personal values (Miller et al., 2011), which is downloadable at https://motivationalinterviewing. org/personal-values-card-sort. There are five sorting headers, including **most important**, **very important**, **important**, **somewhat important**, and **not important**. Miller et al. (2011) emphasize the flexibility to add other values and to move beyond the initial sort to evoke more specific information from the clients. For instance, once the initial sort is made, have them rank order the top five most important values. A core value of motivational interviewing is to make this as conversational as possible, rather than a transaction. The end goal is not to compile a list but to get a deeper sense of values. While this tangible sort is a good starting point for interviewing, it remains linguistically complex. For instance, the tool includes 100 values to sort, which would be overwhelming for most of our clients. Individualized modifications would be necessary to make this communicatively accessible. A number of communication-friendly and accessible tools exist that can further support this exploration of values and goals.

Q Sort

Another tool to consider for rank ordering value and interest is the Q sort (Rogers, 1954; Stephenson, 1953). While conceptualized as a research tool to help identify most important items to include in scaled assessments (e.g., A-STAM; Lawton et al., 2019) and interview sorts (e.g., Activity Card Sort; Baum & Edwards, 2001), it can also be used as a clinical assessment tool. This method can be used to elicit rankings for things like **how relevant**, **how valuable**, **how important**, or **how interesting** a topic is to an individual. You may have encountered a scenario where an individual identifies everything as important, which makes prioritizing and goal setting challenging. The framework somewhat forces the issue of getting to most valued items or ideas by only allowing one or two spaces for those top priorities. The traditional Q sort asks clients to sort statements and resort them until they are happy with the results (see Figures 4-2a for a visual representation of the sort and 4-2b for the sorting grid layout). A communication-friendly, accessible version may use images and perhaps limited accompanying text. In the context of supporting individuals with communication disorders, we are less concerned with the numbers on the sorting grid and more concerned with the prioritization and ranking it achieves. Nevertheless, the numbers associated with each card can be used to indicate priorities. Further, a smaller grid with fewer items to sort may be more appropriate for individuals with communication and cognitive impairments. Nevertheless, the framework is an important consideration as we consider communication-friendly tools like Talking Mats, Activity Card Sort, Life Interest and Value Cards (LIV Cards), or homegrown values and goal setting sorts. Lawton et al. (2020) used the Q sort methodology to elicit subjective

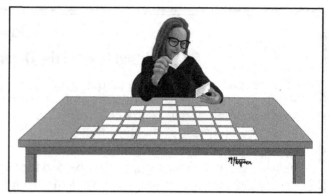

Figure 4-2a. Q sort.

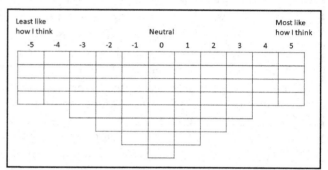

Figure 4-2b. Sorting grid for Q sort.

perceptions of individuals with aphasia about therapeutic alliance with their speech-language therapists. Questions explored included: "I trust my therapist," "My therapist is interested in me as a person," and "My therapist shares things about their life." This illustrates the ability of the Q sort to address complex, abstract concepts with individuals with aphasia. The method was effective in eliciting perceptions of individuals with communication impairments.

Multimodal card sorts and structured interview tools, such as Talking Mats (https://www.talkingmats.com/), Activity Card Sort (Baum & Edwards, 2008), and LIV Cards (Haley et al., 2010) can be very useful in scaffolding communication when conducting values inventories and goal setting. The pairing of iconic visuals and limited text scaffolds comprehension and expression, while reducing demands on memory. Sometimes seeing the visuals and keywords enables the client to share other related information verbally as well. Two points of caution, as you prepare to use a picture-based, structured interview tool: (1) make sure your clients or families know the purpose of the interview, and (2) address the potential for the images and/or process of sorting cards to feel patronizing. I often use the disclaimer that some cards may feel a little hokey but the process helps us to gain a lot of information about their values, interests, and goals. One more caveat—the use of tangible, structured interviews to gather information about values, interests, and goals fits primarily into the World Health Organization (WHO-ICF, 2001) domains of activity and participation assessment. That being said, such tools are not only an assessment but a counseling tool and communication support.

Talking Mats

Talking mats is an icon-based sorting tool that can be used for interviewing, goal setting, and as a communication support. The framework aligns with the WHO-ICF framework (2001) for goal setting and intervention planning (Bornman & Murphy, 2006). It comes in an original, mat-based format and in a digital, app-based format. There are sets for *education*, for consulting children and young people; *health care*, for consulting adults and children in medical settings; *social work*, focused on assessment of needs in home-health/wellness-community contexts; and *residential care*, focused on communication (particularly social) and involvement of residents in their own care. All of these versions have relevance to speech-language pathologists and cross contextual bounds (i.e., residential care version is useful in home and medical settings, social work version is useful for speech-language pathology assessments).

Talking Mats uses a three-point visual analog scale (top-scale symbols), ranging from thumbs down to thumbs up, unsure is at the midpoint (Figures 4-3a and 4-3b). In the traditional, mat-based format (see Figure 4-3a), the speech-language pathologist lays these icon-based cards across the top of the mat. They simply appear at the top of the app-based version (see Figure 4-3b). A central topic symbol (e.g., leisure) is placed at the bottom center of the mat to identify the parameter for the sort (or selected in the app-based version). You may want to add a resorting topic at the top as well (i.e., "Which leisure activities do you enjoy?", "Which leisure activities do you get to do?", "Which leisure activities would you like to return to?"). Without this visual support, clients may forget the parameters for a given sort and/or revert back to/perseverate on a previous sorting parameter. A set of icon-based cards (option symbols) are associated with each topic. Depending upon the linguistic and cognitive level of the client, you can hand the small stack of cards to the client and allow them to place them or hand them to the client one by one. In the app-based version, the icons simply populate the screen based upon the topic area, which works well for some clients but can be challenging for others. In either case, allowing the client to place the cards in the appropriate area is important (i.e., don't simply place them for the client by asking them to point, if avoidable).

Like more linguistically laden values sorts discussed previously, the end goal is not to make a list but to foster flexible, ongoing communication that is more like a conversation than an interrogation. As such, effective use moves from one topic sort to another. For instance, in a sort of recreation cards, one may begin with sorting, "Which ones do you enjoy the most?" followed by, "How often do you get to do them?" and perhaps a third round of, "Of those that you enjoy but don't get to do as often as you would like, which ones would you like to do more?" The key here is not simply conducting a sort for the sake of sorting but rather to move you further along, into a better understanding of the person's values, goals, and priorities. By capturing images of

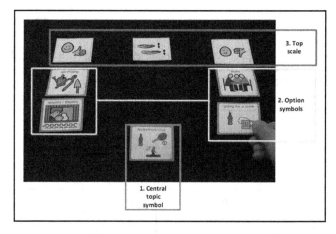

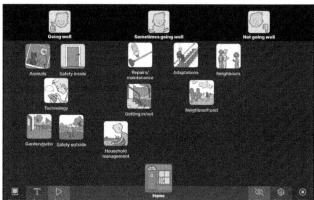

Figure 4-3a and 4-3b. Talking Mats.

each sort, you also create a photographic record of the client's values, goals, and priorities that can be useful as you explore goal planning and discrepancies between values and behaviors (see Chapter 5). Murphy and Oliver (2013) found that Talking Mats helped people to feel more involved in decision making and more satisfied with outcomes of those decisions. Evidence exists across the lifespan and contexts about the value of Talking Mats (Table 4-1).

Activity Card Sort

The *Activity Card Sort* (ACS) is a tool for identifying a client's participation in a range of activities (Baum & Edwards, 2001, 2008). See Figure 4-4 for an example. It includes a set of 89 photographs of individuals engaged in various activities. Since it was developed for occupational therapists, it focuses on social, instrumental activities of daily living, and leisure activities. There are three versions, including the *Community Living* version for community-dwelling adults; *Institutional* version for adults in a hospital, skilled nursing, or rehabilitation context; and the *Recovery* version for adults recovering from disease or injury. All versions use the same photographs but sorting suggestions are different (see Table 4-2 for sorting parameters for each version). Simply prompt clients to "sort these cards into each of these piles [pointing to parameter

TABLE 4-1*
Evidence for Talking Mats Across Lifespan and Contexts

IMPAIRMENT OR CONTEXT	CITATIONS
Dementias	Murphy et al., 2007, 2010; Murphy & Oliver, 2013; Oliver et al., 2010; Reitz & Dalemans, 2016
Long-term care	Murphy & Boa, 2012
Frail elderly	Murphy et al., 2005
Huntington's disease	Ferm et al., 2010, 2012; Hallberg et al., 2013
Learning disabilities	Bell & Cameron, 2008; Brewster, 2004; Bunning & Steel, 2007; Cameron & Murphy, 2002; Germain, 2004
Anxiety (children)	Nilsson et al., 2012
Children and adults with profound, complex learning impairments	Gridley et al., 2014; Whitehurst, 2007
AAC users (children)	Midtlin et al., 2015
Aphasia	Gillespie et al., 2010; Pettit et al., 2017

*While this table is not exhaustive, it provides a sense for the scope of evidence regarding Talking Mats.

cards] according to your level of participation." Modify language as necessary to support comprehension. Clients view each of the photographs and sort them into piles (per version) to indicate their level of participation in each activity. Further sorts can be useful to determine barriers to activity and to prioritize most valued activities, particularly in relation to restricted participation in those valued activities. This can be used to prioritize activity-focused intervention goals. It comes with a helpful scoring sheet, but scoring is not always necessary to document status. Depending upon level of communication impairments, there is also a 55-item checklist version (Everard et al., 2000). Multiple versions now exist across languages (English, Hebrew, Spanish, Korean, Chinese, and Dutch).

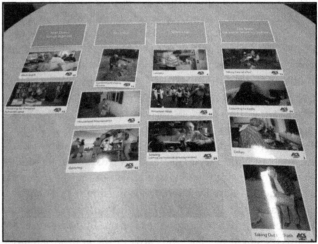

Figure 4-4. Activity Card Sort.

Infant Toddler Activity Card Sort

The **Infant Toddler Activity Card Sort** (ITACS) was developed to identify infant-toddler activity and participation, in order to set appropriate family-centered goals (Hoyt et al., 2020). Based upon the ACS (Baum & Edwards, 2001), it follows the WHO-ICF (2001) framework. Parents are asked to respond to a set 40 photographs of infants and toddlers engaged in various activities. While developed for occupational therapists, the ITACS includes a number of activities relevant to speech-language pathologists (Table 4-3). For each photograph, parents are asked, "Does your child participate in this activity?" Depending on their responses, "yes" or "no",

follow-up questions probe for the underlying reasons (e.g., haven't tried yet, tries but not yet successful).

Preschool Activity Card Sort

The **Preschool Activity Card Sort** (PACS) is intended to address 3-6-year-old children's activity and participation profile through parent interview (Berg & LaVesser, 2006). Like the ITACS, this tool was based upon the ACS (Baum & Edwards, 2001). The World Health Organization International Classification of Functioning, Disability, and Health (WHO-ICF, 2001) identifies activity and participation

TABLE 4-2

Sorting Parameters by Activity Card Sort Version

HEALTHY ADULT VERSION	INSTITUTIONAL VERSION	RECOVERING VERSION
Never done	Done prior to illness	Not done before illness/injury
Not done as an adult	Not done	Continued to do after illness/injury
Doing now		Doing less after illness/injury
Doing less		Gave up due to illness/injury
Given up		Beginning to do again

TABLE 4-3

Validated List of 40 Activities Included in the Infant Toddler Activity Card Sort

Reading books	Playing with blocks	Sleeping	Running errands
Going to school	Tummy time/floor play	Changing diaper	Going for walks
Listening to music	Crawling	Breastfeeding	Playing outside
Watching television	Swinging	Bottle feeding	Playing with children
Pretend play	Walking	Spoon feeding	Playing with adults
Social interaction	Running	Finger feeding	Playing with pets
Tablet	Taking a bath	Using a cup	Meal preparation
Drawing	Toilet learning	Brushing teeth	Going to a restaurant
Puzzles	Getting dressed	Riding in a car	Crying
Playing	Climbing on playground equipment	Going to religious services	Smiling

Reproduced with permission from Hoyt, C. R., Fernandez, J. D., Varughese, T. E., Grandgeorge, E., Manis, H. E., O'Connor, K. E., ...& King, A. A. (2020). The infant toddler activity card sort: A caregiver report measure of children's occupational engagement in family activities and routines. *OTJR: Occupation, Participation and Health, 40*(1), 36-41.

domains (i.e., learning and applying knowledge, general tasks and demands, communication, ***domestic life***, ***self-care***, ***education***, ***interpersonal interactions and relationships***, and ***community-social-civic-leisure activities***). The PACS includes six of those nine domains, which preschoolers engage in (domestic chores, self-care, community mobility, education, social interaction, leisure/play). Like the ACS, the PACS was developed for occupational therapists. As such, it does not directly address communication but does address interpersonal interactions and relationships. It uses photographs of preschoolers engaged in typical activities to elicit parent responses about their child's participation. It can also be useful in determining barriers to participation, such as child (is the child physically able, have they tried an activity, are they interested, is the activity age-appropriate), family (has the parent tried to support them), or environmental factors (do they have access to the activity). Parents are asked to respond to 73 photographs of children engaged in activities. For each photograph, parents are asked, "Does your child participate in this activity?" Parent responses could include, "Yes, my

child participates", "Yes, with adult assistance (beyond that necessary for a typical preschooler)", or "No, my child does not participate." Note, if the answer given is simply, "Yes", you may have to probe to see if extra assistance is necessary. If the response is "No", follow-up questions explore potential barriers/reasons (child, parent, environment). If a parent indicates that they have tried in the past, follow-up questions can begin to focus more on child and environmental barriers. There are also Spanish (Stoffel & Berg, 2008), Japanese (Igarashi et al., 2020), and Arabic (Malkawi et al., 2017) versions of the PACS.

Adolescent and Young Adult Activity Card Sort

Because the transition to adulthood includes a shift toward employment, higher education, and domestic life, an activity-participation assessment must address these and other changing activities. The **Adolescent and Young Adult Activity Card Sort** includes chores, leisure, social, health and fitness, work, education, and parenting domains (Berg et al., 2015). Like the PACS, it is developed based upon the framework of the ACS (Baum & Edwards, 2001). The Adolescent and Young Adult Activity Card Sort includes 67 photographs of young adults engaged in activities and 67 matching line drawings. Responses are elicited directly from the adolescent/young adult, "Do you participate in this activity?" Again, follow-up questions are prompted depending on the individual's responses to explore the nature of the barriers.

Life Interest and Value Cards

LIV Cards are a counseling tool to help clients identify what activities they wish to address in therapy (Haley et al., 2010, 2013). LIV Cards offer individuals the opportunity to make their own choices about activities for home, community, physical exercise, social events, and hobbies or entertainment. This is central to person-centered and participation-based goal setting. While LIV Cards were designed for individuals with aphasia, there appears to be potential to support individuals with a variety of communication disorders using this tool. Individuals with aphasia showed that they are consistent over time, identifying the same goals 78% of the time (Haley, Womack et al., 2019). Family members and friends were less accurate in predicting the individual's goals, highlighting why it is so important for individuals to make their own choices.

You can begin your interview with composite cards (Figure 4-5), which include the topics of home and community activities, relaxing and creative activities, physical activities, and social activities. You may ask, "Which one do you want to discuss first?" which doesn't require a verbal response. Selecting a **composite card** allows the client to choose the direction of the discussion. Each composite card has a set of topic cards associated with it. If yes/no is consistent, you can offer dichotomous choices that can be answered verbally or through gesture. A simple decision tree of "Do you currently do this?" leads to "Yes" and then "Would you like to do it more?" or "No" followed by, "Would you like to start doing it?" Or you may simply have the client sort into "yes" (green ☑) and "no" (red ☒) piles. Following the first sort, you can follow up with previously suggested resorts. Depending on level of verbal or written expression, you may ask more open-ended questions about each card. Like Talking Mats, the point isn't to get through the sorts as quickly as possible but rather to make it conversational and express authentic interest. You can access the LIV Cards Activity Score sheet online (https://www.med.unc.edu/ahs/sphs/card/resources/liv-cards/score-sheets/), as well as the LIV Cards Questionnaire for Friends and Family Members.

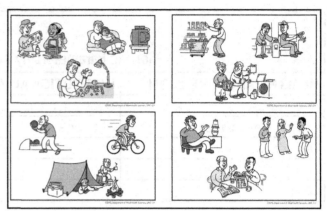

Figure 4-5. LIV Cards.

Obligatory Versus Nonobligatory Interview

I've long since lost the source for this tool that was shared with me several decades ago by my clinical mentors. I've continued to use it, modifying it to reduce linguistic demands on individuals with communication impairments. The **obligatory vs. nonobligatory interview** framework is simple, just ask your client and their partners to sort by two parameters, "Put those things you do because you have to in the obligatory pile and those things you do because you want to in the nonobligatory pile." For individuals who have sustained a stroke or brain injury, it can be a helpful conversation for goal planning and to gain insights into the spouse/partner's demands. Ask both individuals (client and their partner) to sort as they would have **before stroke/brain injury** and as they would **after stoke/brain injury**. Frequently, you see a profound shift in both individuals' lists with partners adding several obligations and engaging in fewer activities just because they want to. Likewise, individuals with stroke/brain injury often have reductions in both categories; in some cases, they have no obligations, which has implications for sense of worth and contribution. Modifications to the traditional form include using images from other card sorts rather than writing the list down. See Table 4-4 for the framework. Like the card sorts discussed previously, the obligatory vs. non-obligatory interview can be useful in goal setting. For instance, in viewing a partner's sort, a client may say, "My wife has been making coffee every morning but that's something I could do." In this way, tangible tasks can be added back onto their obligatory list. While making coffee may not feel like a speech and language goal, success in non- to low-linguistic tasks fosters confidence to engage in more activity. This includes contexts for contextualized interactions.

TABLE 4-4			
Obligatory Versus Nonobligatory Interview			
BEFORE INJURY/ILLNESS		**AFTER INJURY/ILLNESS**	
Do because you have to	Do because you want to	Do because you have to	Do because you want to

Homegrown Sorts

While there is tremendous value in these package tools, there is room for development of homegrown, personalized tools. The Aphasia Institute has a number of free, online resources available in their Participics repository (https://www.aphasia.ca/participics/) that can be used to generate your personalized, homegrown tangible interview. Likewise, Boardmaker and Talking Mats have online tools for personalized visual supports and interview development, noting that there is a cost associated with both of those programs. Alternately, capturing your own photos or simple image searches can be useful in finding the right images for an idea or choice. You can draw upon the rich source of frameworks discussed previously to facilitate a communication-friendly means of response.

Delivering Communicatively Accessible Interviews

Beyond providing scaffolding through tangible values sorts, speech-language pathologists need to open up their full communication toolbox to support counseling assessments. Adapting a framework from Kagan (1998) for supported conversation is a great place to start when considering communication accessibility. This includes providing supports for *getting the message in* (supporting comprehension) and for *getting the message out* (supporting expression). Approaches for getting the message in include use of short, syntactically simple sentences, augmented by gestures, pictures, and keywords. The intent is not to dumb-down the message but rather, to make it accessible given an individual's communication status. Approaches to getting the message out include providing a preferred modality of response (e.g., written or object choices, gestures, augmentative and alternative communication [AAC], pictures, drawings), asking one thing at a time, and allowing time for formulating a response. For those of us working in the adult, neurogenic world, that means implementation of written choice, rating scales, drawing, keywords, self-generated photographs, and AAC. In the pediatric or school-based world, that means providing tangible choices (e.g., "Do you want to play with this toy or this toy?") and multimodal communication (i.e., speech, gestures, sign language, AAC/speech-generating devices, picture exchange communication systems). For some minitutorials regarding these communication supports, see Box 4-2.

While such communication supports and ramps are an important element of communicatively accessible interactions, a word of caution is warranted. There are definitely times when scaffolding responses through choices and other modalities is necessary. Likewise, there are times when we risk inadvertently compromising a client's message through our intended supports. Leaman and Archer (2022) advocated waiting for and promoting self-repair on the part of individuals with aphasia. Their article, aptly titled, "If you just stay with me and wait . . . you'll get an idea of what I'm saying," addresses the concern that sometimes scaffolding constrains or changes a client's message (Leaman & Archer, 2022). Supports like written choice may favor progressivity over autonomy, sacrificing the client's intended message. While progressivity, or moving the conversation along, is advantageous and certainly more comfortable for the communication partner, it may not always be the right choice when we hope to let the client take the lead. Sometimes we may want to foster progressivity but other times we need to wait. It may be an overgeneralization, but lighthearted conversations may benefit from progressivity, particularly when there is a history of therapeutic alliance and joint knowledge of topics. In other situations, where our primary intent is to empower the client's autonomy, we need to be patient through the struggle. This really parallels what we know about counseling in general, clinicians (human beings) are often uncomfortable with waiting and listening, so they try to scaffold client responses. This can limit their ability to really reveal the client's voice and foster agency.

Box 4-2

Just-in-Time Minitutorials on Communication Supports

Written choice uses a syntactically simple written sentence paired with a verbal sentence (sometimes slightly more elaborated), followed by three or four simple choices and an "other" or "something else" choice. Typically, begin with broader questions and work toward narrower, more specific questions.

Example: What kinds of activities do you like? *(Verbalized: "What kinds of recreation activities or hobbies do you like?")*

- Outdoor
- Indoor
- Both
- Something else

A person makes their choice, you circle it, and verify that it is correct. If they select "something else" you generate a new list of options.

Rating scales provide an alternative to asking "Do you like x?" by offering a continuum of how much they like or dislike something. Whenever you want a qualitative evaluation (i.e., how important), rating scales are a good choice. Prompt with a simple written question, paired with a slightly expanded verbal question.

Example: Reading? *(Verbalized: "How important is working on reading?")*

←——————————————————————————————————————→

Not important   Somewhat important   Very important

A person may point or make a hatch mark. In either case, you should circle and verify their mark placement.

Jotting down **keywords** can support comprehension and serve as an artifact that can be used to support expression.

Example: When brainstorming goals with the client, I might take note of key ideas they shared verbally and ideas I've shared. The visual shows the client that I'm listening, creates a sense of collaboration, and an artifact to reference as they formulate ideas or goals.

Concerns/struggles? Goals? Potential solutions?

Work

Friends

Organizing my planner

Remembering

Self-generated photographs are a way to express things that are difficult to express verbally, either because they are intangible or ambiguous, or because expressing things in general is difficult. This can include photographs taken in the moment to capture a feeling or idea, or images selected to represent a feeling or idea (e.g., an internet image search). Initial use of self-generated photography was typically for the former, helping people to express complex, intangible ideas through a visual representation. Miller and Happell (2006) used this to help individuals with schizophrenia express their emotions. For instance, an image of a tree with no leaves is a powerful response to a question about how one feels in the present moment. Imagine verbalizing "I feel like a tree that has lost its leaves." That image carries a lot of emotional significance, right? Given the eloquence of captured or found photographs to represent feelings or complex thoughts, the method has been extended to helping individuals with communication disorders like aphasia and learning disabilities to express themselves (Baier et al., 2017; Brown et al., 2010; Germain, 2004; Hoepner et al., 2017). As a tool to support expression of thoughts that are hard to verbalize or share, this is a helpful tool in a counseling toolbox when working with individuals with communication disorders.

Drawing to communicate serves many of the same functions as self-generated photographs, namely the ability to express ideas that are difficult to express verbally. In the context of emotional expression, I am drawn to this example by a person with aphasia: (insert animated drawing by person with aphasia and apple with tears streaming down his face).

		TABLE 4-5
		Self-Selected Goal Attainment Scale Framework

		Goal: This goal should be framed in the client/family's words or words they agree upon and understand.
+2	5	Dream a little—if you woke up tomorrow morning and everything was great, this is what it would look like (equidistant from Better Than Expected)
+1	4	Better Than Expected—equal increment from Expected Outcome level
0	3	Expected Outcome—equal increment above Baseline
-1	2	Baseline—this is how you're performing at the outset
-2	1	Worsened—equidistant increment below Baseline

Collaborative Goal Setting (Bordin's Principle of Shared Goals)

Collaborative goal setting is the process of empowering clients and their family members/partners to select end-goals that fit their values, needs, and priorities. Clinicians often default to identifying goal areas based upon deficits rather than client values and needs, which creates a potential break in therapeutic alliance and trust. Client goals tend to be activity- and participation-based, if we consider elements of the WHO-ICF (2001). As such, their goals are about things like participating in conversations, playing games with friends, or even playing a team sport effectively. Of course, all of those activity- and participation-based goals are dependent on communication. That is where we fit in. Eliciting activity and participation elements of goals begins with an inventory and prioritization or ranking of their values, interests, and needs. The good news is that we can build upon communication-accessible values sorts discussed previously (e.g., Talking Mats, Activity Card Sorts, LIV Cards). The process involves eliciting interests and then moving toward prioritization of activity- and participation-based goals. Then, it is a matter of mapping our interventions onto those goals. This addresses how those goals will be achieved (i.e., the type and level of support to be provided and/or the skill/ability developed through the intervention). Collaborative goal setting is an essential precursor to ensuring salience and motivation, which are a crucial element of effective counseling. Prescott et al. (2019) identified the importance of involving clients in goal setting as crucial to developing a person-centered approach. When involved in cooperative treatment planning and goal setting, individuals feel more in control (Darragh et al., 2001). Hersh et al. (2012) eloquently identify a framework for aligning person-centered, collaborative goals with objective standards of SMART goals, which is discussed further in Chapter 5, as goal setting straddles assessment and intervention. This framework is intended to facilitate ongoing shared decision-making regarding goals.

Goal Attainment Scales

The way that we elicit, measure, and monitor intervention goals should align with the principles of collaborative goal setting. This includes (1) self-selected goal targets, (2) self-assessed performance outcomes, and (3) review of concrete evidence to elicit self-confrontation. Goal attainment scales (GAS) have been shown to increase goal achievement (Hoepner et al., 2021; Malec, 1999; Turner-Stokes, 2009). Table 4-5 provides a generic framework for setting and measuring goals through GAS. Overarching goals and levels are set by the client with the help of the clinician. Typically, the baseline level is established first, in the client's words. Next, the end goal or ceiling criteria is set, which is what the client ultimately hopes to accomplish. The clinician can work backward to establish the "expected" and "better than expected" levels, so that there are equal increments between criteria levels. Then set the regression below baseline last, following the equal intervals from the already established levels. The process for measuring and continuous monitoring of goals should also be consistent with underlying theoretical principles of collaborative goal setting. Ask the client to recall their goals, in their own words, at the outset of each session. Before the close of the session, have them rate their performance according to their own criteria. Ask questions to corroborate and validate their assessment (e.g., "What makes your performance a 2?" or "Explain to me why you think it is a 2."). If you believe the rating is inaccurate, reviewing the criteria for each level can be helpful. There should not be any confrontation or dispute on your part, simply self-confrontation prompted when you ask them to review the criteria and explain their rating. Often, this leads them to adjust their ratings to match the criteria.

<table>
<tr><th colspan="2" align="center">TABLE 4-6</th></tr>
<tr><th colspan="2" align="center">Mapping FOURC Onto Steps of Motivational Interviewing</th></tr>
<tr><th>FOURC ELEMENT</th><th>MOTIVATIONAL INTERVIEWING STEP</th></tr>
<tr><td>Pre-FOURC</td><td>Engaging: positive, nondirectional conversation that precedes assessment</td></tr>
<tr><td>Choosing a communication goal</td><td>Focusing: identifying an area to work on</td></tr>
<tr><td>Creating client solutions</td><td>Evoking: eliciting client solutions</td></tr>
<tr><td>Collaborating on a plan and Completing/continuing the plan</td><td>Planning: making an actionable plan with clear steps and indicators for success</td></tr>
</table>

Box 4-3

LIV Cards and FOURC

Check out this great podcast conversation on Aphasia Access Conversations Podcast Episode #25 with Dr. Katarina Haley. She discusses LIV Cards and the FOURC model.

https://aphasiaaccess.libsyn.com/25-aphasia-access-conversations-katarina-haley

---

FOURC

Haley et al. (2019) developed the FOURC model as a way to systematically address counseling and treatment planning. Note that FOURC is not an acronym but rather addresses four Cs: (1) choosing a communication goal, (2) creating client solutions, (3) collaborating on a plan, and (4) completing/continuing the plan. In this way, the model aligns with the steps of motivational interviewing with the exception of engaging, which Haley refers to as pre-FOURC (Table 4-6). The FOURC model is a method for approaching goal setting and therapy planning, which focuses on considering possibilities and setting priorities, rather than addressing impairments (Haley, Cunningham et al., 2019). As such, it is strengths based and life participation focused. Instead of asking about problems, the FOURC model asks, "Who are your communication partners? What is important to you? How can you grow? What resources can you pull from?" (Haley et al., 2019, p. 3). The four prongs of FOURC address the elements of any treatment approach, including skills and abilities, intentional strategies, environmental supports, and confidence and motivation. The four prongs are addressed explicitly with the clients, so they can see how their therapy approaches map onto their communication goals. As such, Haley et al. (2019) have color coded those elements to match parts of the treatment plan. In this way, a client can use the four prongs as a framework for addressing their goals: (1) I'm working on expressing myself clearly, (2) I have strategies like self-cuing, (3) I use context-specific scripts to say what I want to say, (4) I want to be confident to engage in social settings (e.g., coffee with friends). For an engaging conversation about the FOURC model and LIV Cards, see Box 4-3.

COM-B and Goal Mapping

Hart et al. (2018), in their description of the Rehabilitation Treatment Specification System model, identified three basic constructs, **ingredients** (what the therapist does or selects), **mechanisms of action** (how the treatment is expected to work), and **targets** (aspect of functioning directly targeted for change). Within this construct, there are only three types of treatment targets across all types of rehabilitation, **organ functions** (e.g., repair or augment a body part—hearing aid, prosthetic), **skills and habits** (i.e., improve ability to perform), and **representations** (i.e., how you think and feel, attitudes, motivation). Counseling assessment approaches like motivational interviewing fit within representation. Addressing **representations** is where collaborative goal setting and attitudes/motivation collide. Hart et al. (2018) refer to the COM-B framework (Michie et al., 2011) as a mechanism for addressing this construct. In this model, volitional behavior (**B**) is a function of three elements, **C**apability, **O**pportunity, and **M**otivation. To assess capability, we consider, "Does my client have the ability to do a task, and do they know how to do it?" Regarding opportunity, "Does my client have the time, space, and access (e.g., transportation, proximity to activities) to engage in a task?" To address motivation, "Is my client motivated to complete the task or goal?" Once we've addressed these questions, we can begin to collaborate on addressing their treatment targets. Sometimes we conflate treatment targets (what we're working on during a session) with aims (which typically take multiple targets to achieve). Things like returning to work, dating again, and successfully returning to social settings are **aims**, as they require multiple treatment targets. Conceptualizing the path from target, to target, to aim (participation-based goal) is nebulous for our clients. Lyn Turkstra (2021), in her discussion of the Rehabilitation Treatment Specification

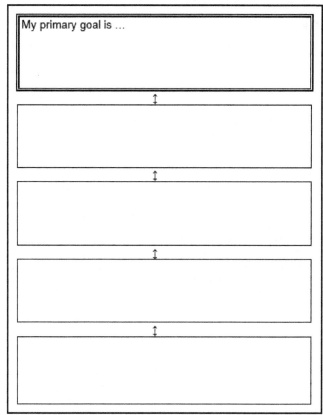

Figure 4-6. Goal Map. (Reproduced with permission from Lyn Turkstra and Spain Rehabilitation Speech Pathologists.)

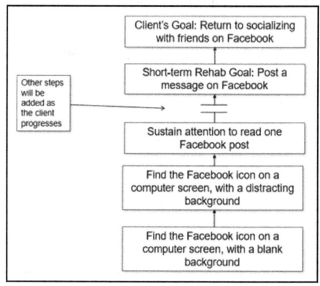

Figure 4-7. Example Goal Map for social media. (Note: See that the progression begins at the bottom and culminates at the top. Reproduced with permission from Lyn Turkstra and Spain Rehabilitation Speech Pathologists.)

System, noted that she uses a goal mapping process to help explicitly connect what we do in therapy with a client's aim (participation-based goal). This is especially important when working toward an aim, as it helps clients to connect the work we're doing on each target task to their ultimate goal. See Figure 4-6 for a template and Figure 4-7 for an example of a goal map from Lyn Turkstra.

Collaborative goal setting is also emphasized in developmental contexts, although the collaborator is typically a parent, rather than the child (Crais et al., 2006; Forsingdal et al., 2014). Darrah et al. (2012) identified active collaboration as central to family-centered practices. Parents value goals that are concrete, observable, contextualized, and written down (Øien et al., 2010). Collaborating in the process allows parents to focus on meaningful activity and repetition of practice in the child's everyday environment, increasing their participation (Bexelius et al., 2018). Parents who are involved in treatment planning take an active role both within and outside intervention sessions (Davies et al., 2017; Forsingdal et al., 2014). As was mentioned previously, this collaborative goal setting conversation is not a simple one and done. Goals continuously evolve and some "potential" goals arise in the moment and thus constitute an opportunity for returning to collaborative goal setting mode. See Box 4-4 for a few examples of collaborative goal setting exchanges.

Formulations

Formulations are a mechanism for mapping out information about a client's background, ability, needs, identity, and goals. More than a diagram, formulations create a comprehensive description of our clients' strengths, challenges, and interests (Wilson et al., 2009). Formulations collect and integrate information acquired through assessment, including psychological, biological, and systemic factors (British Psychological Society Division of Clinical Psychology [BPS-DCP], 2011). It should draw upon theory and research to create a framework that represents a client's needs and challenges. Formulations draw upon elements of the WHO-ICF (2001) to capture the influence of impairments, environment, and interests on participation in personally identified activities. This creates a shared narrative that relates to personal meaning of the events and experiences of the client (Harper & Spellman, 2006). This can help us, as speech language pathologists, to have a clear, holistic picture of our clients and identify gaps in our knowledge about the client. It can also help to prioritize issues and problems, support goal setting, build therapeutic alliance, normalize problems, and increase a client's sense of agency (BPS-DCP, 2011). Clinicians identify the value of identifying a team approach, helping team and client/family to work together, building consensus, and sense of balanced collaboration through use of formulations (BPS-DCP, 2011). Johnstone and Dallos (2006) note that formulations should summarize a client's core impairments, suggest relationships between difficulties, lead to intervention plans, be iterative and evolving, and be used as a tool to share information/discuss goals with clients and families. See Figure 4-8 for a formulation template and the chapter Appendix for a worksheet to use with your clients. As you

Box 4-4
Collaborative Goal Setting Examples

C = client, Y = you, P = parent/partner

Scenario #1:

C: Nika is frustrated because no one will play or talk with her during recess. The flip side of that problem is, she wants to be able to play and talk with other kids during recess, which is the end goal/"why" in this collaboration. Her "activity- or participation-based" part of the goal is playing and talking with kids during recess. You might elicit this during a values inventory OR you might encounter the sadness, frustration, anger, and other emotions when a counseling moment arises in the moment. Either way, this is a counseling moment, a moment for assessment of client values and behaviors and a moment primed for a counseling response (which we will get to in upcoming chapters). Hopefully, the counseling response will evoke her ideas, potential solutions, and reasons to address this activity/ participation concern.

Y: As a speech-language pathologist, you may have immediate thoughts about social communication interventions and supports. That is your part of the goal. That is the "how" in this collaboration. Addressing this part of the goal without consultation/collaboration with the client is where breakdown can occur—not that it isn't a good thing to work on but that it does not necessarily connect to the client's end goal.

Scenario #2:

C: Clayton just got fired from his job as a laborer and concrete apprentice. At the root of the issue is Clayton's struggle to code switch between front office and back room talk. Profanity and obscenities are a fairly acceptable part of the exchange between Clayton and his coworkers or even his foreman. That being said, this language has become a common element in his communication since his brain injury. Concerns arise when customers are present, as his coworkers alter their language accordingly, but Clayton does not. Clayton has received several stern warnings from his foreman, and he knows he is on thin ice. While you may elicit this concern during a goal setting discussion, it is perhaps more likely that it will arise when you ask how work is going. In either case, this is definitely a counseling and goal setting moment (to be discussed in upcoming chapters). Hopefully, the counseling response will elicit his self-confrontation, awareness, and motivation to self-regulate a bit more effectively. Clayton's end goal/participation-based part of that goal will be to use context-appropriate language in order to keep his job.

Y: As a speech-language pathologist, you probably have many thoughts about social communication and self-regulatory interventions for this *and* related social situations regarding Clayton. Social communication and self-regulatory interventions are the "how" in this collaboration. Self-confrontation and awareness are key to making this collaboration work, highlighting why he needs to be in on this goal.

Scenario #3:

P: Carla is Kennedy's mom. Kennedy is a 4-year-old girl with severe impairments to articulation and expressive language. Carla wants her two other children, Colton (age 6 years) and Caeden (age 7 years) to be able to understand Kennedy. Carla is really close to her own siblings but tends to ask Colton and Caeden to keep Kennedy out of the room when she's visiting with her own siblings. What used to be cute is now bordering on embarrassing. Carla acknowledges that she knows she does this, and she didn't do it with the other kids. If you ask Carla what her goal is for Kennedy, she would tearfully say, "I just want Ken to be normal." Um, that's Carla's participation-based goal. She wants you to fix that, "help her to talk normal."

(continued)

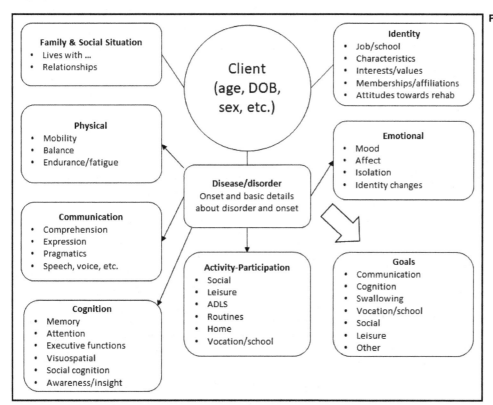

Figure 4-8. Formulation template.

collect information about the client's interests, values, family, and status (physical, communication, cognition, and emotional status) you can summarize it in the formulation. This is meant to be an iterative and evolving document that is updated as the client changes.

This section has discussed several tools to support collaborative goal setting (FOURC, goal mapping, formulations). Additionally, the SMARTER collaborative goal setting tool is described in Chapter 5. Using one of these formats, create your own tangible collaborative goal setting "formulation" to complete the assignment in Box 4-5.

Therapeutic Alliance (Bordin's Principle of Client-Clinician Bond)

Measures of therapeutic alliance in speech-language pathology are relatively new. In terms of the WHO-ICF model (2001), assessment of therapeutic alliance primarily falls within personal factors. Freckmann et al. (2017) examined therapeutic alliance using the Therapeutic Alliance Scales for Children—Revised (TASC-r) and suggest that the

TASC-r appears to have good potential for examining therapeutic alliance in pediatric speech-language pathology. The TASC-r (Creed & Kendall, 2005) is a 12-item scale that addresses therapy tasks, goals, and bond. Questions are rated on a 4-point scale (from "not at all like my client" to "very much like my client") and examples include "The child considers you an ally" and "The child feels that you spend too much time focusing on his or her problems." While further psychometric testing of the TASC-r is still necessary for use in speech-language pathology, it appears to be an appropriate tool. The Aphasia and Stroke Therapeutic Alliance Scale (A-STAM) includes clinician and client versions, both of which have strong internal consistency and test-retest reliability (Lawton et al., 2019a). Both forms are highly correlated with existing measures of therapeutic alliance with strong psychometric properties. Items from the client A-STAM are rated on a 5-point scale from "never" to "all of the time" and include "my therapist really listens to me," "my therapist is interested in me as a person," "we get on well," "my therapist is honest with me," "my therapist recognizes that I am still a capable person," "my therapist and I want different things from therapy," "my therapist gives me the choice to involve my family," and "we work on things that are important to me." While further psychometric testing is still needed for the A-STAM, it appears to be a promising measure. While numerous measures of therapeutic alliance exist outside of speech-language pathology, clearly there is a need for validation of more communicatively accessible measures across the lifespan and disorders.

Other Constructs That Underlie Motivation

DARN and COM-B

Because the assessment of DARN (desire, ability, reasons, and need) is a part of the motivational interviewing framework (Miller & Rollnick, 2013), they are discussed further in Chapter 5. That being said, these basic precursors to motivation have relevance to other counseling approaches as well. Note the parallels to the COM-B framework (Michie

et al., 2011). The ability to engage in a target behavior depends upon capability, opportunity, and motivation. Assessment of these constructs is informal but an important part of your initial and ongoing assessment.

Agenda Mapping

Agenda mapping is a part of the motivational interviewing framework as well, so it is discussed further in Chapter 5. Again, it has relevance across a range of counseling approaches. Conceptually, agenda mapping is finding out what our client wants to do and prioritizing those goals. It should be conducted in a highly collaborative manner, where the clinician draws out the client's own agenda and reasons for change. Further, it can include a process for addressing discrepancies between their agenda (goals) and their actions. Tools like the readiness ruler offer a communication-friendly way to assess self-perceived motivation. Further, such tools create a context for a tangible discussion about change. Questions like, "So, you rated × a 2/10, why not a 1?" and "What would it take to move you from a 2 to a 3?" can elicit valuable information about barriers and facilitators to change.

Assessing Mood and Related Constructs

Depression, anxiety, and other mental health concerns are common among individuals with communication disorders, particularly adolescents and adults. Adults who stutter are twice as likely to meet criteria for a mood disorder than matched controls (Iverach et al., 2010). Depending upon the scale used, individuals with aphasia have a prevalence of anxiety ranging from 16% to 44% (Morris et al., 2017). Prevalence of clinical depression in chronic aphasia is over 19% and subthreshold depression is 22% (Ashaie et al., 2019). Rates for depression at 3- and 12-months post-onset are even higher (70% and 62% at 3 and 12 months respectively; Kauhanen et al., 2000). Nearly 25% of deaf adults self-report depression or anxiety, as compared to about 21% of hearing adults (Kushalnagar et al., 2019). In a meta-analysis of depression in autism, pooled prevalence was about 14% with studies that used a clinical interview to assess depression having the highest reported rates, at nearly 29% (Hudson et al., 2019).

For some of these individuals, assessment through traditional, linguistically laden measures is not feasible or validated. While in-depth assessment of mood falls outside of our scope of practice, screening for and reporting mood to other disciplines is a part of our role. This is particularly important as we are experts in scaffolding communication and using adapted scales to elicit client perceptions of mood. For the purposes of the counseling context, this section addresses measures of direct client report, excluding other measures of proxy reporting or observation—as there are too many to report and not all are relevant to individuals with communication disorders. Note that assessing mood and related constructs addresses personal factors within the WHO-ICF model (2001). Screening partner mood, particularly for those who serve as caregivers for individuals with communication disorders, is also an important element of holistic environmental assessment.

Adult Measures

The ***Hospital Anxiety and Depression Scale*** (HADS) was initially developed in 1983 (Zigmond & Snaith, 1983). It is widely accepted as an effective bedside measure, which takes an efficient 2 to 5 minutes to complete for persons without communication or cognitive impairments. While responses are on a 4-point scale, from 0 to 3, the scale items change from question to question. Further, questions and scale items are linguistically complex. Similarly, the ***Beck Depression Scale*** (Beck et al., 1961) is also widely used but is presented verbally and is not accessible to individuals with cognitive and language impairments. There are also a wide variety of visual scales for anxiety and depression but not all are designed specifically with communication and cognition impairments in mind. Let's consider some that are intended to be communicatively accessible.

The ***Visual Analog Mood Scales*** (VAMS; Stern, 1997; Stern et al., 1997) were designed specifically for individuals with neurological impairments, including aphasia. It includes normative data from persons with and without neurological impairments from ages 18 to 94 years. The VAMS assesses eight mood states, including sad, happy, tense, afraid, tired, energetic, confused, and angry. Each 100-mm vertical scale has a neutral line-drawn face at the bottom of the scale with a line extending up to one of the eight mood state line-drawn faces and accompanying word (e.g., neutral ☺ to sad ☹, neutral ☺ to happy 😊, etc.). In order to validate the ability of individuals with aphasia to report mood states through the VAMS, Haley et al. (2019) compared ratings of mood on VAMS scale items (happy, sad, angry, tense) to four mood cards from the LIV Cards (happy, sad, angry, and worried). There were moderate to strong correlations across these four items.

Visual Analog Self-Esteem Scale (VASES; Brumfitt & Sheeran, 1999a; 1999b) includes 10 pairs of polar opposite, simple line drawings that anchor each end of the continuum. The intent was to reduce linguistic complexity as much as possible so that individuals with severe language impairments could respond. Each line drawing indicates one pole, including cheerful/not cheerful, trapped/free, optimistic/pessimistic, confident/unconfident, frustrated/not frustrated, confused/not confused, misunderstood/understood, outgoing/not outgoing, intelligent/stupid, and angry/calm. Participants identify whether the picture is "very true of me" by pointing to ++ or "true of me" by pointing to +, or provide a neutral response by pointing to 0. Note that ++ and + were used on both ends of the scale but you can think of the (++) on the negative end of the scale as a (− −) and a (+) as (−). For instance, someone who identifies themselves as

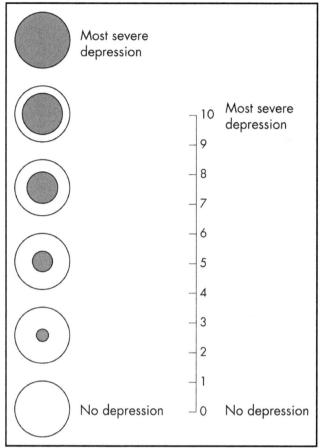

Figure 4-9. DISCs visual. (Reproduced with permission from Turner-Stokes, L., Kalmus, M., Hirani, D., & Clegg, F. (2005). The Depression Intensity Scale Circles (DISCs): A first evaluation of a simple assessment tool for depression in the context of brain injury. *Journal of Neurology, Neurosurgery & Psychiatry, 76*(9), 1273-1278.)

very pessimistic would indicate by pointing to (++) under the pessimistic line drawing, equivalent to a (− −), whereas someone who identifies themselves as very optimistic would point to (++). The higher the score, the more positive the view of the self. The VASES has good psychometric properties with individuals with aphasia and matched controls.

The ***Depression Intensity Scale Circles*** (DISCs; Turner-Stokes et al., 2005) is a vertical, 5-point Likert scale that uses black dots of increasing size to represent intensity of mood (e.g., darker/larger representing more intensity at the top of the scale, empty circle at the bottom: ○ ● ⬤ see Figure 4-9). A version with pictorial anchors is also available. Yes/No reliability must be established before asking clients to make a rating. The client is oriented to the scale, to make sure that they can see it. Instruction also includes these brief statements, accompanied by pointing: "This is a scale for measuring sadness or depression. The grey circles show how sad or depressed you feel. The bottom circle [point] shows no sadness or depression. The top scale [point] shows sadness or depression as bad as it can be. As you go from the bottom to the top circle [gesture] you can see that sadness or depression is becoming more and more severe" (Turner-Stokes

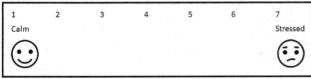

Figure 4-10. 7-point analog scale. (Adapted from Laures-Gore, J., & Rice, K. G. [2019]. The simple aphasia stress scale. *Journal of Speech, Language, and Hearing Research, 62*[8], 2855-2859.)

Box 4-6

Stress and Depression Scales for People With Aphasia

Check out this episode of the SLP Minded podcast with Dr. Jacqueline Laures-Gore as she discusses the SASS.

https://www.podbean.com/ew/pb-4mtjq-9ea7d0

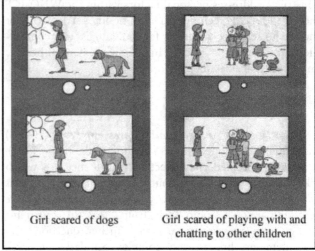

Girl scared of dogs   Girl scared of playing with and chatting to other children

Figure 4-11. Sample PAT items. (Reproduced with permission from Dubi, K., & Schneider, S. [2009]. The Picture Anxiety Test (PAT): A new pictorial assessment of anxiety symptoms in young children. *Journal of Anxiety Disorders, 23*[8], 1148-1157.)

---

et al., 2005; pp. 1274-1275). Then, the clinician asks the Yale question, "Do you often feel sad or depressed?" or "Which of these circles shows best how sad or depressed you feel today?" The DISCs have acceptable convergent validity and reliability for screening depression in clients with complex neurological impairments following brain injury. Further investigation is needed for persons with more profound language and cognitive impairments.

The ***Simple Aphasia Stress Scale*** (SASS; Laures-Gore & Rice, 2019) is a single-item scale, which has good absolute and relative stability. Across three studies, the authors compared 5- and 7-point scales and prompts. While either scale was appropriate, offering more choices offers more ability to detect subtle change, so the authors recommend the 7-point scale (Figure 4-10). This 7-point visual analog scale from not at all to very asks clients to "Please describe your stress level in the last hour." Further validation of the scale is necessary and currently underway. The authors also suggest that returning to the anchors of calm to very stressed may be a better option.

For a nice discussion of the SASS with Dr. Jacqueline Laures-Gore, please follow the link in Box 4-6.

Pediatric Measures

Many of the pediatric measures of anxiety, depression, and mood rely on clinician and parent report. Even those with a child report version are complex and lengthy, including as many as 44 items that are linguistically complex. Existing tools intended to reduce linguistic burden are limited and not specific to children with communication disorders.

The ***Picture Anxiety Test*** (PAT; Dubi & Schneider, 2009) is a tool for screening/assessing anxiety and avoidance in children. There are 17 items, each including paired pictures,

one illustrating a symptom of anxiety/avoidance (e.g., child is afraid) and a neutral image with no symptoms of anxiety/avoidance (Figure 4-11). Children are prompted to point to the picture that looks most like them. Semistructured interviews are suggested to follow-up on each symptom identified. Eleven of the items include a specific phobia (e.g., scared of dogs), two with social phobia situations, two with generalized anxiety, and two with separation anxiety. It is a psychometrically sound measure for assessing anxiety and avoidance in young children.

The ***Pictorial Instrument for Children and Adolescents—Revised*** (PICA-R; Ernst et al., 2000) is a tool for examining depression in children from ages 6 to 16 years. Like the PAT, a line-drawing picture is presented to the child and the child is asked, "How much are you like him/her?", which is paired with a 5-point visual analog scale to rate degree of severity (Figure 4-12). Other questions include "Do you get like him/her? How much? Do you feel sad the way he/she does? Do people tell you that you look sad? How much? What about crying? How much does it happen to you?" The tool appears promising, as it has good internal consistency, discriminative power, and specificity. The authors recommend only using this tool if you have psychiatric training.

Chapter Summary

Assessment is a crucial and ongoing element of counseling. Conversational engaging should precede information-seeking interviews or assessments. Those initial information-seeking interactions should feel collaborative and be limited in duration. Effective assessment addresses Bordin's (1979) principles of therapeutic alliance, fostering choice about therapy tasks, collaborative goal setting, and establishing a bond between client and clinician. A variety of communicatively accessible tools exist to elicit information about a client's values, interests, and needs across the lifespan. Those same structured interview sorts are crucial in eliciting client-centered goals that address individualized activity and participation wants and needs. A collaborative process for goal setting and mapping therapy tasks toward goal achievement can help make the intangible process more tangible and accessible. Individuals with communication disorders are often at a higher risk for mood disorders, including depression and anxiety. A small but growing list of communicatively accessible tools exist for screening and assessing mood, across the lifespan. While deep assessment and intervention of mood disorders is outside of our scope of practice, our expertise in eliciting client feelings, socioemotional status, and psychological states put us in a position to learn valuable information to share with professional counselors and to shape our interventions.

Key Takeaways

- Begin initial meetings with time dedicated for simply engaging with the client before moving into interview and assessment mode.
- Do your best to make counseling assessment and interviews feel conversational and collaborative.
- Learn about the client's social and living situation to identify whether basic physical needs are being met prior to moving toward higher level psychological needs.
- Proxy interviews and inventories can provide good information about your clients and allow you to take a slower, more methodical approach to directly eliciting their interests and values.
- Structured interview tools and sorts can elicit interests, values, and goals directly from our clients. A variety of tools exist that are designed to fit specific age groups and disorders. That being said, learning about frameworks in general will enable you to deliver an age-appropriate sort to your clients.
- Formulations can help clinicians to visualizes their clients' interests, values, and challenges, which is helpful to developing a collaborative treatment plan.
- Collaborative goal setting helps our clients and their partners to feel more in control. It is just as important for children as adults.
- Goal mapping can help clients see the therapy tasks and steps involved in achieving their goals/aims.
- Parents value goals that are concrete, observable, contextualized, and written down.
- Our discipline still has some work to do regarding assessment of mood across the lifespan. Nevertheless, several communicatively accessible tools exist that can provide some basic information to guide our interventions, referrals, and interactions with other disciplines.

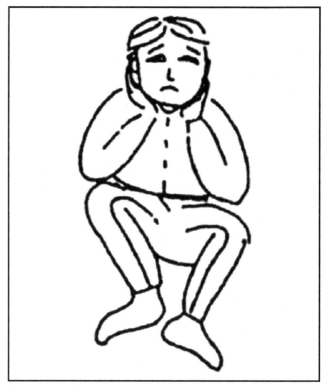

Figure 4-12. PICA-R stimuli.

References

Ashaie, S. A., Hurwitz, R., & Cherney, L. R. (2019). Depression and subthreshold depression in stroke-related aphasia. *Archives of Physical Medicine and Rehabilitation, 100*(7), 1294-1299.

Baier, C. K., Hoepner, J. K., & Sather, T. W. (2017). Exploring Snapchat as a dynamic capture tool for social exchange among individuals with aphasia. *Aphasiology, 32*(11), 1336-1359. https://doi.org/10.1080/02687038.2017.1409870

Baum, C., & Edwards, D. (2001). *ACS: Activity Card Sort.* American Occupational Therapy Association, Incorporated (AOTA Press).

Baum, C., & Edwards D. F. (2008). *Activity Card Sort* (2nd ed.). American Occupational Therapy Association (AOTA Press).

Beck, A. T., Ward, C. H., Mendelson, M., Mock, J., & Erbaugh, J. (1961). An inventory for measuring depression. *Archives of General Psychiatry, 4*(6), 561-571.

Bell, D. M., & Cameron, L. (2008). From Dare I say . . . ? to I dare say: A case example illustrating the extension of the use of Talking Mats to people with learning disabilities who are able to speak well but unwilling to do so. *British Journal of Learning Disabilities, 36*(2), 122-127.

Berg, C., & LaVesser, P. (2006). The preschool activity card sort. *OTJR: Occupation, Participation and Health, 26*(4), 143-151.

Berg, C., McCollum, M., Cho, E., & Jason, D. (2015). Development of the adolescent and young adult activity card sort. *OTJR: Occupation, Participation and Health, 35*(4), 221-231.

Bexelius, A., Carlberg, E. B., & Löwing, K. (2018). Quality of goal setting in pediatric rehabilitation—A SMART approach. *Child: Care, Health and Development, 44*(6), 850-856.

Bordin, E. S. (1979). The generalizability of the psychoanalytic concept of the working alliance. *Psychotherapy: Theory, Research and Practice, 16*(3), 252-260.

Bornman, J., & Murphy, J. (2006). Using the ICF in goal setting: Clinical application using Talking Mats. *Disability and Rehabilitation: Assistive Technology, 1*(3), 145-154.

Brewster, S. J. (2004). Putting words into their mouths? Interviewing people with learning disabilities and little/no speech. *British Journal of Learning Disabilities*, 32(4), 166-169.

British Psychological Society—Division of Clinical Psychology (BPS-DCP). (2011). Good Practice Guidelines on the use of psychological formulation. http://www.sisdca.it/public/pdf/DCP-Guidelines-for-Formulation-2011.pdf

Brown, K., Worrall, L., Davidson, B., & Howe, T. (2010). Snapshots of success: An insider perspective on living successfully with aphasia. *Aphasiology*, 24(10), 1267-1295.

Brumfitt, S. M., & Sheeran, P. (1999a). The development and validation of the visual analogue Self-Esteem scale (VASES) 1. *British Journal of Clinical Psychology*, 38(4), 387-400.

Brumfitt, S. M., & Sheeran, P. (1999b). *VASES: visual analogue self-esteem scale*. Winslow Press Ltd.

Bunning, K., & Steel, G. (2007). Self-concept in young adults with a learning disability from the Jewish community. *British Journal of Learning Disabilities*, 35(1), 43-49.

Cameron, L., & Murphy, J. (2002). Enabling young people with a learning disability to make choices at a time of transition. *British Journal of Learning Disabilities*, 30(3), 105-112.

Crais, E. R., Roy, V. P., & Free, K. (2006). Parents' and professionals' perceptions of the implementation of family-centered practices in child assessments. *American Journal of Speech-Language Pathology*, 15, 365-377.

Creed, T. A., & Kendall, P. C. (2005). Therapist alliance-building behavior within a cognitive-behavioral treatment for anxiety in youth. *Journal of Consulting and Clinical Psychology*, 73(3), 498.

Darragh, A. R., Sample, P. L., & Krieger, S. R. (2001). "Tears in my eyes' cause somebody finally understood": Client perceptions of practitioners following brain injury. *American Journal of Occupational Therapy*, 55(2), 191-199.

Darrah, J., Wiart, L., Magill-Evans, J., Ray, L., & Andersen, J. (2012). Are family-centred principles, functional goal setting and transition planning evident in therapy services for children with cerebral palsy?. *Child: Care, Health and Development*, 38(1), 41-47.

Davies, K. (2020). Conceptualizing participation and communication disorder in dementia research. *Perspectives of the ASHA Special Interest Groups*, 1(5), 256-260.

Davies, K. E., Marshall, J., Brown, L. J., & Goldbart, J. (2017). Co-working: Parents' conception of roles in supporting their children's speech and language development. *Child Language Teaching and Therapy*, 33(2), 171-185.

DiLollo, A., & Favreau, C. (2010). Person-centered care and speech and language therapy. *Seminars in Speech and Language*, 31(2), 90-97.

Dubi, K., & Schneider, S. (2009). The Picture Anxiety Test (PAT): A new pictorial assessment of anxiety symptoms in young children. *Journal of Anxiety Disorders*, 23(8), 1148-1157.

Ernst, M., Cookus, B. A., & Moravec, B. C. (2000). Pictorial instrument for children and adolescents (PICA-III-R). *Journal of the American Academy of Child & Adolescent Psychiatry*, 39(1), 94-99.

Everard, K. M., Lach, H. W., Fisher, E. B., & Baum, M. C. (2000). Relationship of activity and social support to the functional health of older adults. *Journal of Gerontology: Social Sciences*, 55(4), S208-S212.

Ferm, U., Gelfgren, E., Hartelius, L., & Wallfur, P. E. (2012). *Communication between Huntington's Disease patients, their support persons and the dental hygienist using Talking Mats*. INTECH Open Access Publisher.

Ferm, U., Sahlin, A., Sundin, L., & Hartelius, L. (2010). Using Talking Mats to support communication in persons with Huntington's disease. *International Journal of Language & Communication Disorders*, 45(5), 523-536.

Fish, J., McIntosh, J., Lack, V., & Betteridge, S. (2021). *Seeing the wood and the trees: Social cognition, social communication, and cognitive communication after brain injury*. Cognitive Communication Symposium.

Forsingdal, S., St John, W., Miller, V., Harvey, A., & Wearne, P. (2014). Goal setting with mothers in child development services. *Child: Care Health and Development*, 40(4), 587-596. https://doi.org/10.1111/cch.12075

Freckmann, A., Hines, M., & Lincoln, M. (2017). Clinicians' perspectives of therapeutic alliance in face-to-face and telepractice speech-language pathology sessions. *International Journal of Speech Language Pathology*, 19(3), 287-296. https://doi.org/10.1080/17549507.2017.1292547

Garrett, K. L., & Beukelman, D. R. (2007). In D. R., Beukelman, K. L., Garrett, & K. M., Yorkston, K. M. (Eds.), *Augmentative communication strategies for adults with acute or chronic medical conditions*. Paul H. Brookes Publishing Company.

Germain, R. (2004). An exploratory study using cameras and Talking Mats to access the views of young people with learning disabilities on their out-of-school activities. *British Journal of Learning Disabilities*, 32(4), 170-174.

Gillespie, A., Murphy, J., & Place, M. (2010). Divergences of perspective between people with aphasia and their family caregivers. *Aphasiology*, 24(12), 1559-1575.

Gridley, K., Brooks, J., & Glendinning, C. (2014). Good practice in social care: the views of people with severe and complex needs and those who support them. *Health & Social Care in the Community*, 22(6), 588-597.

Haley, K. L., Cunningham, K. T., Barry, J., & de Riesthal, M. (2019). Collaborative goals for communicative life participation in aphasia: The FOURC model. *American Journal of Speech-Language Pathology*, 28(1), 1-13.

Haley, K. L., Womack, J. L., Harmon, T. G., McCulloch, K. L., & Faldowski, R. A. (2019). Life activity choices by people with aphasia: repeated interviews and proxy agreement. *Aphasiology*, 33(6), 710-730.

Haley, K. L., Womack, J. L., Helm-Estabrooks, N., Caignon, D., & McCulloch, K. L. (2010). *The Life Interest and Values Cards*. University of North Carolina, Department of Allied Health Sciences.

Haley, K. L., Womack, J., Helm-Estabrooks, N., Lovette, B., & Goff, R. (2013). Supporting autonomy for people with aphasia: Use of the Life Interests and Values (LIV) Cards. *Topics in Stroke Rehabilitation*, 20(1), 22-35.

Hallberg, L., Mellgren, E., Hartelius, L., & Ferm, U. (2013). Talking Mats in a discussion group for people with Huntington's disease. *Disability and Rehabilitation: Assistive Technology*, 8(1), 67-76.

Harper, D. & Spellman, D. (2006). Social constructionist formulation: Telling a different story. In L. Johnstone & R. Dallos (Eds.), *Formulation in psychology and psychotherapy: Making sense of people's problems* (pp. 98-125). Routledge.

Hart, T., Whyte, J., Dijkers, M., Packel, A., Turkstra, L., Zanca, J., Ferraro, M., Chen, C., & Van Stan, J. (2018). *Manual of rehabilitation treatment specification*. http://mrri.org/innovations/manual-for-rehabilitation-treatment-specification

Hersh, D., Worrall, L., Howe, T., Sherratt, S., & Davidson, B. (2012). SMARTER goal setting in aphasia rehabilitation. *Aphasiology*, 26(2), 220-233. https://doi.org/10.1080/02687038.2011.640392

Hoepner, J.K., Baier, C.K., Sather, T.W., & Clark, M.B. (2017). A pilot exploration of Snapchat as an aphasia-friendly social exchange technology at an aphasia camp. *Clinical Archives of Communication Disorders*. 1(1). 1-13. http://dx.doi.org/10.21849/cacd.2016.00087

Hoyt, C. R., Fernandez, J. D., Varughese, T. E., Grandgeorge, E., Manis, H. E., O'Connor, K. E., . . . & King, A. A. (2020). The infant toddler activity card sort: A caregiver report measure of children's occupational engagement in family activities and routines. *OTJR: Occupation, Participation and Health*, 40(1), 36-41.

Hudson, C. C., Hall, L., & Harkness, K. L. (2019). Prevalence of depressive disorders in individuals with autism spectrum disorder: A meta-analysis. *Journal of Abnormal Child Psychology*, 47(1), 165-175.

Igarashi, G., Karashima, C., & Uemura, J. I. (2020). Items selection for the Japanese version of the preschool activity card sort. *OTJR: Occupation, Participation and Health*, 40(3), 166-174.

Iverach, L., Jones, M., O'Brian, S., Block, S., Lincoln, M., Harrison, E., . . . & Onslow, M. (2010). Mood and substance use disorders among adults seeking speech treatment for stuttering. *Journal of Speech, Language, and Hearing Research*, *53*(5), 1178-1190.

Johnstone, L., & Dallos, R. (Eds.). (2006). *Formulation in psychology and psychotherapy: Making sense of people's problems*. Routledge.

Kagan, A. (1998). Supported conversation for adults with aphasia: Methods and resources for training conversation partners. *Aphasiology*, *12*(9), 816-830.

Kauhanen, M. L., Korpelainen, J. T., Hiltunen, P., Määttä, R., Mononen, H., Brusin, E., . . . & Myllylä, V. V. (2000). Aphasia, depression, and non-verbal cognitive impairment in ischaemic stroke. *Cerebrovascular Diseases*, *10*(6), 455-461.

Kitwood, T. (1997). *Dementia reconsidered: The person comes first*. Open University Press.

Kushalnagar, P., Reesman, J., Holcomb, T., & Ryan, C. (2019). Prevalence of anxiety or depression diagnosis in deaf adults. *The Journal of Deaf Studies and Deaf Education*, *24*(4), 378-385.

Laures-Gore, J., & Rice, K. G. (2019). The simple aphasia stress scale. *Journal of Speech, Language, and Hearing Research*, *62*(8), 2855-2859.

Lawton, M., Haddock, G., Conroy, P., Serrant, L., & Sage, K. (2020). People with aphasia's perspectives of the therapeutic alliance during speech-language intervention: A Q methodological approach. *International Journal of Speech-Language Pathology*, *22*(1), 59-69.

Lawton, M., Conroy, P., Sage, K., & Haddock, G. (2019). Aphasia and stroke therapeutic alliance measure (A-STAM): Development and preliminary psychometric evaluation. *International Journal of Speech-Language Pathology*, *21*(5), 459-469.

Malkawi, S. H., Abu-Dahab, S., Amro, A. F., & Almasri, N. A. (2017). The psychometric properties of the Arabic preschool activity card sort. *Occupational Therapy International*, *2017*.

Michie, S., van Stralen, M. M., & West, R. (2011). The behaviour change wheel: A new method for characterising and designing behaviour change interventions. *Implementation Science*, *6*, 42.

Midtlin, H. S., Næss, K. A. B., Taxt, T., & Karlsen, A. V. (2015). What communication strategies do AAC users want their communication partners to use? A preliminary study. *Disability and Rehabilitation*, *37*(14), 1260-1267.

Miller, G., & Happell, B. (2006). Talking about hope: The use of participant photography. *Issues in Mental Health Nursing*, *27*(10), 1051-1065. https://doi.org/10.1080/01612840600943697

Miller, W. R., C'de Baca, J., Matthews, D. B., & Wilbourne, P. L. (2001). *Personal values card sort*. University of New Mexico.

Miller, W. R., & Rollnick, S. (2013). *Motivational interviewing: Helping people change*. Guilford Press.

Morris, R., Eccles, A., Ryan, B., & Kneebone, I. I. (2017). Prevalence of anxiety in people with aphasia after stroke. *Aphasiology*, *31*(12), 1410-1415.

Murphy, J., & Boa, S. (2012). Using the WHO-ICF with Talking Mats to enable adults with long-term communication difficulties to participate in goal setting. *Augmentative and Alternative Communication*, *28*(1), 52-60.

Murphy, J., Gray, C. M., & Cox, S. (2007). Using "Talking Mats" to help people with dementia to communicate. *JRF Findings*. https://www.jrf.org.uk

Murphy, J., Gray, C. M., van Achterberg, T., Wyke, S., & Cox, S. (2010). The effectiveness of the Talking Mats framework in helping people with dementia to express their views on well-being. *Dementia*, *9*(4), 454-472.

Murphy, J., & Oliver, T. (2013). The use of Talking Mats to support people with dementia and their carers to make decisions together. *Health & Social Care in the Community*, *21*(2), 171-180.

Murphy, J., Tester, S., Hubbard, G., Downs, M., & MacDonald, C. (2005). Enabling frail older people with a communication difficulty to express their views: the use of Talking Mats as an interview tool. *Health & Social Care in the Community*, *13*(2), 95-107.

Nilsson, S., Buchholz, M., & Thunberg, G. (2012). Assessing children's anxiety using the modified short state-trait anxiety inventory and talking mats: A pilot study. *Nursing Research and Practice*, *2012*, 932570.

Øien, I., Fallang, B., & Østensjø, S. (2010). Goal-setting in paediatric rehabilitation: Perceptions of parents and professional. *Child: Care, Health and Development*, *36*(4), 558-565.

Oliver, T., Murphy, J., & Cox, S. (2010). 'She can see how much I actually do!' Talking Mats: helping people with dementia and family carers to discuss managing daily living. *Housing, Care and Support*, *13*(3), 27-35.

Pettit, L. K., Tönsing, K. M., & Dada, S. (2017). The perspectives of adults with aphasia and their team members regarding the importance of nine life areas for rehabilitation: A pilot investigation. *Topics in Stroke Rehabilitation*, *24*(2), 99-106.

Prescott, S., Fleming, J., & Doig, E. (2019). Refining a clinical practice framework to engage clients with brain injury in goal setting. *Australian Occupational Therapy Journal*, *66*(3), 313-325.

Reitz, C., & Dalemans, R. (2016). The use of "talking mats" by persons with Alzheimer in the Netherlands: Increasing shared decision-making by using a low-tech communication aid. *Journal of Social Inclusion*, *7*(2), 35-47.

Stephenson, W. (1953). *The study of behavior; Q-technique and its methodology*. University of Chicago Press.

Stern, R. A. (1997). *Visual analog mood scales professional manual*. Psychological Assessment Resources Inc.

Stern, R. A., Arruda, J. E., Hooper, C. R., Wolfner, G. D. & Morey, C. E. (1997). Visual analogue mood scales to measure internal mood state in neurologically impaired patients: Description and initial validity evidence. *Aphasiology*, *11*(1), 59-71. https://doi.org/10.1080/026870 39708248455

Stoffel, A., & Berg, C. (2008). Spanish translation and validation of the preschool activity card sort. *Physical & Occupational Therapy in Pediatrics*, *28*(2), 171-189.

Turner-Stokes, L., Kalmus, M., Hirani, D., & Clegg, F. (2005). The Depression Intensity Scale Circles (DISCs): A first evaluation of a simple assessment tool for depression in the context of brain injury. *Journal of Neurology, Neurosurgery & Psychiatry*, *76*(9), 1273-1278.

Whitehurst, T. (2007). Liberating silent voices—perspectives of children with profound & complex learning needs on inclusion. *British Journal of Learning Disabilities*, *35*(1), 55-61.

Wilson, B. A., Gracey, F., Evans, J. J., & Bateman, A. (2009). *Neuropsychological rehabilitation: Theory, models, therapy and outcome*. Cambridge University Press.

World Health Organization. (2001). International classification of functioning. Disability and Health (WHO-ICF), 28-66.

Zigmond, A. S., & Snaith, R. P. (1983). The hospital anxiety and depression scale. *Acta Psychiatrica Scandinavia*, *67*(6), 361-370. https://doi.org/10.1111/j.1600-0447.1983.tb09716.x

Appendix: Formulation Template		
Emotional Status (mood, affect, isolation, identity changes, etc.)	**Disease/Disorder** (onset and basic details about disorder and onset)	**Identity** (job/school, characteristics, memberships, affiliations, attitudes toward rehab)
Physical Status (mobility, balance, endurance/fatigue, ADLs, etc.)	**Client Name** (age, DOB, sex, etc.)	**Family & Social Situation** (lives with . . . , relationships)
Communication Status (comprehension, expression, pragmatics, speech, voice, etc.)	**Activity-Participation** (social, leisure, routines, home, vocation, school)	**Goals** (communication, cognition, swallowing, vocation, school, social, leisure, other)
Cognition Status (memory, attention, executive functions, visuospatial, social cognition, awareness/insight, etc.)		

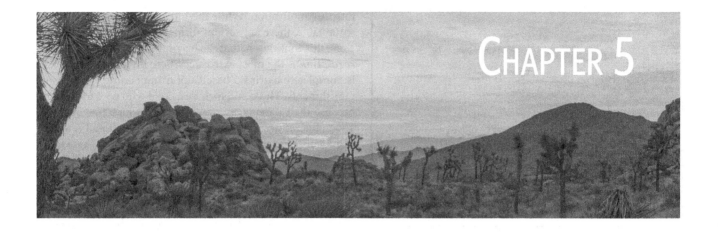

Motivational Interviewing in Speech-Language Pathology

Jerry K. Hoepner, PhD, CCC-SLP

Confidence is contagious. So is lack of confidence. ~ Vince Lombardi

If you act like you've got fifteen minutes, it will take all day. Act like you've got all day, it will take fifteen minutes.
~ Monty Roberts, horse trainer

The Roots of Motivational Interviewing

Motivational interviewing has its roots in the ***transtheoretical model of intentional human behavior change***, also known as the ***stages of change model*** (Prochaska & DiClemente, 2005). In the context of speech-language pathology, it helps to think of "change" as a desire to work on improving skills in a given area (e.g., improving clarity of speech, improving ability to express ideas, improving ability to write clearly). Central to this model is the cyclical progression from precontemplation to maintenance and/or goal completion (see Figure 5-1 and definitions of each stage). Precontemplation is marked by a lack of desire to change or even a recognition of any need to change. Prochaska and

DiClemente (2005) suggested using ***consciousness raising techniques*** to help people move from precontemplation to contemplation. This could include self-assessments or reflections on performance and/or review of videos (e.g., self-observations, video self-modeling). ***Ambivalence***, a lack of interest in change, is likely present during the transition from precontemplation to contemplation and perhaps throughout the contemplation stage. It is a normal stage in the change process. Ambivalence marks a potential tipping point, where the person is not actively resistant to change but is not actively seeking change. As such, the person is persuadable if they can contemplate their own reasons for making a change/working to improve their skills in a given area. Once reasons to change are identified and an actionable plan is developed, moving toward action is more likely. The intent is for that action to lead to goal completion or a maintenance stage. Sometimes this model includes "relapse" following action or maintenance. While speech-language pathology clients don't

Hoepner, J. K. (Ed.). *Counseling and Motivational Interviewing in Speech–Language Pathology* (pp. 69-93).
© 2024 Taylor & Francis Group.

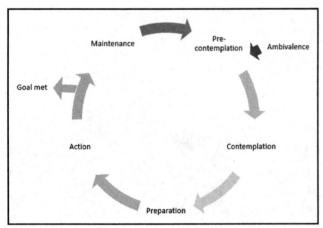

Figure 5-1. Stages of change.

really "relapse" when they stop working toward communication or swallowing goals, they may experience a "backslide" where they perhaps lose focus on the reasons for practicing, implementing strategies, or putting effort into improving a specific skill area. At that point, like those experiencing a relapse, they need to be redirected to contemplation and action. Our hope, of course, is that consistent positive behaviors result in routine or habitual behaviors that are somewhat self-maintaining. The five stages of changes include:

1. *Precontemplation* is the initial stage, where a person is unaware of a need to change and is not ready to make a change.

2. *Contemplation* is a period of considering change and may include attempts to seek out further information and potential supports.

3. *Preparation* involves making a plan to make changes.

4. *Action* includes actual steps toward change.

5. *Maintenance* is the process of making the change a routine and sticking to it. Ideally, maintenance moves the person toward goal attainment.

Motivational interviewing also has connections to self-determination theory (Ginsberg et al., 2002; Markland et al., 2005). Self-determination theory was developed to identify how to promote intrinsic motivation, particularly in the context of conflicting external pressures (Deci & Ryan, 2012; Ryan & Deci, 2000). Self-determination theory places an emphasis on autonomy, choice, and human relationships. Autonomy is enhanced through choices and personal responsibility for one's actions. It is undermined by external pressures such as rewards, punishments, deadlines, and outside judgments. Therefore, it is crucial to establish choice, yield control to the client, and facilitate a collaborative partnership to foster intrinsic motivation that is self-determined.

Ryan and Deci (2000) describe motivation on a continuum, with amotivation on one end and autonomous motivation on the other end. *Amotivation* occurs when clients do not believe they are capable of change (e.g., addressing an intervention goal, getting better at a specific skill). The remaining continuum of change goes from highly extrinsic to highly intrinsic motivation. While the intrinsic motivation is more sustainable, there are several forms of extrinsic motivation, along this continuum, that can become internalized. *External regulation* is the most extrinsic, where the motivating force is completely extrinsic based upon impending rewards or punishments. This could include a child who goes to therapy because their parents are making them, which may include a tangible reward system (e.g., stickers), emotional rewards (e.g., praise, hugs), or punishments (e.g., no video game time if you don't participate in therapy). An adult in rehabilitation may be motivated by the fear of not qualifying for rehab and the threat of discharge from services. *Introjected regulation* remains extrinsic but is controlled by consequences that a client sets for themselves, such as feeling obligated to succeed or wasteful for failing (i.e., "I'm making the most of this opportunity" or "I'm wasting this opportunity"). Identified and integrated regulation are extrinsic but moving toward more internalized. In general, clients with identified and integrated regulation are willing participants who self-identify the need for therapy. *Identified regulation* occurs when a client understands the rationale or purpose of an intervention. This helps them to recognize its value and actively engage in it, working toward a specific goal. *Integrated regulation* occurs when a client integrates the values of an approach into their everyday routines. For an example, a voice client may make stretching and warm-up exercises a part of their morning routine, prior to beginning their day as a physical education teacher. Intrinsically motivated clients do things because they want to, because they enjoy doing things for the sake of doing them. In reality, we all operate on a continuum of doing things because we should do them to those we want to do because we enjoy them.

Cook and Artino (2016) examined five prominent motivation theories (expectancy-value, attribution, social-cognitive, goal orientation, and self-determination) and identified four recurring themes: *competence*, *value*, *attributions*, and *social and cognitive elements*. For an excellent summary of all five theories, you are encouraged to read the full synthesis. *Competence* relates to expectancy for success, self-efficacy, confidence, and self-concept. *Value* is placed on successful achievement of the learning or goal. *Attributions* of success are crucial; when people perceive that the change is in their control, they are more likely to persist against challenges. *Social and cognitive elements* involve mental processes and involve interactions between individuals and the broader social context. *Cognitive evaluation theory*, an adjunct to self-determination theory, suggests that intrinsic motivation is achieved by meeting three basic psychosocial needs: *autonomy*, *competence*, and *relatedness* (see Figure 5-2). *Autonomy* includes choice and control of one's own actions. Note in the Figure 5-2 that autonomy is compromised by rewards and punishments. I think this is a trap many of us fall into, the *reward-punishment trap*. Returning to Figure 5-3, we see that rewards and punishments are external/extrinsic, which leads them to be less sustainable. It only works if someone is filling the meter, so to speak,

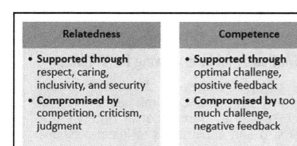

Figure 5-2. Cognitive evaluation theory.

Relatedness	Competence	Autonomy
• **Supported through** respect, caring, inclusivity, and security • **Compromised by** competition, criticism, judgment	• **Supported through** optimal challenge, positive feedback • **Compromised by** too much challenge, negative feedback	• **Supported by** choice, explanations/rationales, acknowledging feelings • **Compromised by** tangible rewards, threats, deadlines, goals imposed by others

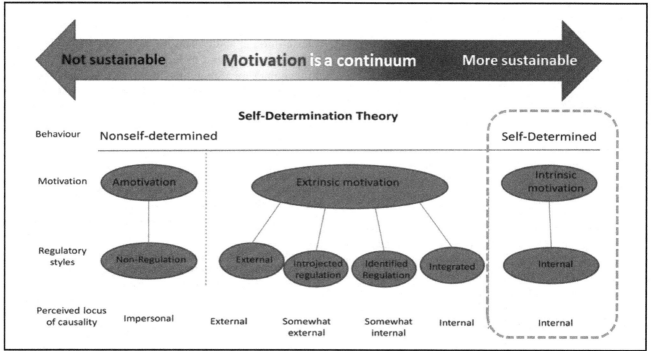

Figure 5-3. Self-determination theory.

creating dependency on those outside individuals rather than the independence and autonomy we desire for our clients. *Competence*, as described previously relates to one's self-efficacy. It is best fostered by optimum level of challenge, thus speech-language pathologists need to match level of task difficulty with client ability. Too much challenge results in frustration and poor self-efficacy. Likewise, too little challenge is boring and patronizing. *Relatedness* is an affiliation and connectedness to others (and closely relates to therapeutic alliance). It may help to think of these elements as feeding into the self-determination figure. Listen to Dr. Michael Biel discuss motivation and engagement in aphasia (see Box 5-1 for the podcast link).

Miller and Rollnick (2013) describe the "spirit of motivational interviewing" as the intersection between collaboration, acceptance, evocation, and compassion (Figure 5-4). *Collaboration* retains a sense of autonomy and sense of control, while achieving relatedness and affiliation between the counselor and client. This is a partnership but the client should do most of the talking. Speech-language pathologists should monitor the balance of talk time to ensure that

---

Box 5-1

Motivation and Engagement in Aphasia

Check out this great podcast conversation on Aphasia Access Conversations Podcast Episode #69 with Dr. Michael Biel, as he discusses motivation and engagement in aphasia.

https://aphasiaaccess.libsyn.com/motivation-and-engagement-in-aphasia-rehabilitation-in-conversation-with-michael-biel

---

it leans strongly in favor of the client. Multimodality communication is necessary to achieve this balance in interactions with individuals with communication disorders. Hersh et al. (2018) demonstrated that even individuals with severe aphasia and with little actual "talk" can benefit. *Acceptance* helps foster self-awareness and self-efficacy, which is crucial to the shift from precontemplation and ambivalence toward

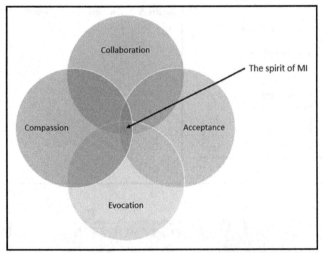

Figure 5-4. The spirit of motivational interviewing. (Adapted from Miller, W. R., & Rollnick, S. [2013]. *Motivational interviewing: Helping people change.* Guilford Press.).

contemplation and preparation to change. To achieve this, speech-language pathologists must acknowledge competence by recognizing the client's worth, ensuring a means of response, affirming their thoughts and efforts, and demonstrating empathy. Miller and Rollnick (2013) emphasize that acceptance "recognizes and supports the person's irrevocable autonomy to choose his own way" (p. 19). **Evocation** is the process of eliciting one's own reasons for change and potential solutions; valuing choice and autonomy. To accomplish this, speech-language pathologists seek to understand a client's goals, values, and abilities, rather than their impairments. **Compassion** is the merger of perceived competence and humanity with relatedness and affiliation. Authentic compassion builds trust and therapeutic alliance. See Box 5-2 for a podcast conversation with Dr. Deborah Hersh about motivational interviewing for wellness.

Motivational Interviewing

Why Is Motivational Interviewing a Fit for Speech-Language Pathology?

Motivational interviewing is not simply about fostering motivation or change. Rather, motivational interviewing is about empowering people to make their own choices, their own decisions, and finding the commitment to address them. In many cases, it is about helping them to find clarity within their own thoughts, beliefs, and priorities. Knowing what they should do is different than doing it. Actually following through requires motivation, commitment, ability, and resources. The acronym DARN (Miller & Rollnick, 2013) is a helpful way of capturing what it takes to make

Box 5-2

Motivational Interviewing for Wellness

Check out this episode of the SLP Minded podcast with Dr. Deborah Hersh as she discusses the motivational interviewing approach and applications to interprofessional wellness interventions.

https://theslpmindedpodcast.podbean.com/

change—desire, ability, reasons, and need. Our role is not to fix or prescribe but to facilitate the process of thinking through one's own situation. Once DARN is established, we can collaborate with clients on establishing commitment, activation, and taking some initial steps (CAT), referred to as **mobilizing change talk**. It may help you to follow the acronym, DARN-CAT.

Talk therapy (of which motivational interviewing is a type) works by getting people to think through and verbalize their ideas, situations, solutions, and challenges. It works best when the counselor creates a safe place for that brainstorming and releasing a stream of thoughts, as the counselor draws out the person's own perspectives, values, and potential solutions. Restating and reflecting what that person says in a less than cohesive stream of consciousness and returning it to them in the form of a cohesive, actionable plan is the powerful piece of this synergistic relationship. In the context of serving people with communication disorders, the role of scaffolding communication and cognition is brought even further to the forefront (Figure 5-5). On one end of the continuum, we may need to pull together a few thoughts that are not well described (e.g., an adult with nonfluent aphasia or a child with an expressive language delay). On the opposite end of the continuum, we may have to sift through volumes of incohesive thoughts into something meaningful (e.g., an individual with a traumatic brain injury with discourse impairments). That being said, the same basic elements remain: creating a safe therapeutic environment and alliance, eliciting the person's own ideas-frustrations-potential solutions, and then reassembling their own ideas in a cohesive or complete manner, thus creating a more actionable response. In order to do this well, we must think about the balance of **talk time**. This balance should lean firmly in the direction of the client (or family member). Johnson et al. (2018) provides a comparison of clinician-centered vs. client-centered exchanges in auditory rehabilitation. In clinician-centered exchanges, clinicians make 20% of statements, ask 70% of questions, and only respond 10% of the time vs. clients, who make none of the statements, ask 10% of questions, and are in a responding role 90% of the time. There is a marked difference in client-centered exchanges, where clinicians only make 45% of statements, ask 30% of questions, and respond 25% of time. Conversely, clients make 50% of statements, ask

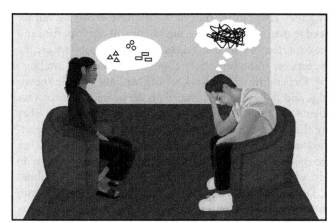

Figure 5-5. Combining incohesive or incomplete thoughts into clear affirmations, reflections, and summaries.

20% of questions, and are in a responding role 30% of the time. Obviously, there is no magic formula and percentages differ by client and type of exchange. The point is, we should be talking less and listening more and *talk time* is an indicator of balance in participation. See Box 5-3 for a disciplinary application of accessible "talk" therapy.

Interprofessional collaboration and referrals are another key application of motivational interviewing to speech-language pathology. Individuals with communication disorders are often systematically eliminated from opportunities to engage in talk therapy, including motivational interviewing, because professional counselors either lack the skills to support communication that are necessary to deliver the approach effectively, or they incorrectly believe those individuals are incapable of utilizing the approach. Part of our role is to train and collaborate with mental health professionals and counselors in order to achieve access to motivational interviewing (and other counseling approaches for that matter). Beyond the potential positive effects of accessible provision of counseling on psychosocial and mental health challenges (e.g., depression, anxiety), those trained professional counselors can now address other lifestyle and wellness goals such as diet, exercise, smoking and alcohol cessation, and the like.

Common Pitfalls (for Human Beings)

To err is human . . . This is an important admission for anyone who seeks to help another. As a speech-language pathologist, you educate yourself in order to know the answers, have the solutions, and inform your clients. Part of our human nature, particularly for "helpers" who are drawn to professions like speech-language pathology, is to prescribe, correct, and dictate, so as to put our clients on the path we believe is best for them. It takes an explicit commitment to going against our own human tendencies to inhibit our righting reflex. A "*righting reflex*," as Miller and Rollnick coined it, is our tendency to provide solutions, correct people when they are wrong or even incomplete, and it results in a fixing mentality. We quickly fall into the trap of throwing

solutions at clients but fail to recognize that they are our solutions, not theirs. Righting reflexes erode therapeutic alliance and trust, which makes them incongruent with our own goals of working successfully with our clients and fostering their independence. *Pushback* (another human response) is a common response to unsolicited advice and a common response when we fail to inhibit our righting reflex. It is human to push back when we disagree with that unsolicited advice and sometimes, we even push back when we agree with the advice (simply because the power of self-determination has been taken away from us). To see minicase examples of what the righting reflex looks like, see Box 5-4.

The Expert Trap

The expert trap is when "counselors" provide advice to clients instead of helping the client to identify their own goals, direction, and plans. When we give advice, we make the arguments for change, which puts our clients in the position of arguing against change (Miller & Rollnick, 2013). Our overall goal as speech-language pathologists is to help people

Box 5-4
Righting Reflexes

Minicase: Townes is a 25-year-old man with a traumatic brain injury who is early in his recovery, has moderate memory problems, and executive dysfunction. He is currently an outpatient and living under his parents' roof, semi-independently. He says, "I want to go back to work next week." Righting reflex response: "Are you kidding, you are not even close to ready to go back to work, I don't know if you ever will." (By the way, it is human to be thinking this type of response, internally.) A more appropriate response would be, "I can understand that you want to get back to work. What will you need to do in order to get to that goal?" Of course, there will need to be many scaffolded conversations to get Townes to actually evaluate and identify barriers and limitations in his endurance-memory-attention, etc. The point is that you turn your response from telling him what to do/not to do toward self-exploration (with lots of guidance and scaffolding).

Minicase: Nadia is a 12-year-old girl who stutters. One day in therapy, she says, "I don't see the purpose in this. It is totally unfair that I have to come here. It's not my idea, I don't care about my stutter. It's not like it's gonna get any better." Righting reflex response: "Of course it matters. Everything we do in therapy is to make it better. Besides, it is not your decision, it's your parents' decision." A more appropriate response would be to affirm her feelings. "You think it is unfair that you have to come to therapy, like you don't have a say in it, and you aren't sure how it will help anyway."

Exercise: Be honest with yourself, how would you respond (either internally or externally) to these types of scenarios? Even if you know you wouldn't outwardly say it in the way you're thinking of it, what is your righting reflex in these situations?

---

move toward more independent communication, thinking, and swallowing. Deciding what to do (based on assumptions or deficit areas from an assessment) places us in the expert role and places our clients in the dependent role (which is incongruent with our overall goal of fostering independence). It is human to believe that 4 years in undergraduate and 2 additional years in a graduate program have endowed you with a level of expertise and knowledge when it comes to communication and swallowing disorders. It might follow, therefore, that it is our role to dictate our client's goals because that is

why they come to us. Indeed, we do have expertise, but we need to distinguish between jurisdiction of our expertise and the expertise of our clients. Let's get this straight—we are the experts on communication, cognition, voice, and swallowing. Depending on our work setting, we have specific knowledge and skills commensurate with the people we serve. Our clients and their families are the experts on our clients! They are the experts on living with a child with autism, supporting them, helping them, and knowing what they value. They are the experts on living with aphasia, what they want to do and who they want to do it with, and how they feel about it. Delineating who does what is a process that begins with collaborative goal setting. This is the process of learning what our client's value and ultimately what they want to do. Their part of the goal—what they want to do (I wanna hang out with my friends—which by the way includes interacting with/communicating with them). Our part of the goal—how they do it (what strategies or supports they use) or how they get better at it (intervention approaches to improve skills/reduce impairment). Keeping these basic parameters straight can help you avoid the expert trap.

Step 1: See your clients as experts, which involves acknowledging their inherent competence. It doesn't matter if they are 2 years old or 96 years old, whether they have a simple voice disorder or a severe dementia. Along with acknowledging their competence, learning about who they are and what they value reveals their humanity. They are someone's child, partner, sibling, aunt, uncle, grandparent, and friend. That automatically means they have a personal stake in what they do. **Step 2:** Use a collaborative goal setting framework and supports (see Chapter 4 for use of tangible interview tools like Talking Mats, and see Box 5-5 for the collaborative goal setting framework). The purpose of this approach is to learn what our clients want and need to do within everyday life. **Step 3:** Write goals that include our client's end goals (what they want and need to do—activity and participation goals) and our measures of goal achievement. This may include goal attainment scaling (GAS), which can empower our clients to determine their own progress toward goals and may improve their understanding of/intentionality toward goals. **Step 4:** Apply our expertise (evidence-based practice) to fit their goals. Throughout, we need to employ a collaborator, not fixer, mindset. That means checking in regularly to ensure we remain on the same page.

Keep in mind that there are different kinds of goals. Katarina Haley (2021) identifies four key considerations: (1) real choices (e.g., what you want to work on?), (2) action choices (e.g., how much do you want to work on?), (3) performance goals (e.g., I want to run a marathon in a certain amount of time), and (4) actionable goals (e.g., I'm going to run three times a week, I'm going to run whether it rains or not). Consider these factors as you collaboratively identify goals.

Box 5-5
Collaborative Goal Setting

I sometimes joke around with my students about my lack of dancing skills. In fact, I share a fictitious story about an assessment I developed to examine dancing skills. I call it the Standardized Assessment of Dancing Skills or SADS because my dancing skills are truly sad. Anyway, if you administer the SADS to me, you will see that I score in the 10th percentile, which may lead you to believe I need a dancing intervention. But do I? That depends on whether dancing is a priority for me. Going on a cruise with my wife where there is dancing every evening . . . the need for a dancing intervention goal may increase. One of my daughters is getting married . . . perhaps even greater need for a dancing goal. But, in my current situation, I don't want a dancing goal. Unfortunately, this is exactly how speech-language pathologists often set goals—based on an impairment, rather than an interest, value, or need. Collaborative goal setting is intended to give voice to those interests, values, and needs.

A figure from Hersh et al. (Figure 5-6) eloquently captures the pairing of SMARTER client-centered, collaborative goals with the widely used SMART goals framework. While the SMARTER framework was initially structured around the process for setting goals, the acronym seems to exemplify the goals themselves (D. Hersh, personal communication). A goal could technically be framed as a SMART goal but improved through the SMARTER process by making it truly collaborative. Unfortunately, SMART goals (when they omit the SMARTER process) tend to be clinician led. While this work was framed around individuals with aphasia, it has broader applications. The seven keys to the SMARTER, collaborative goals are:

1. **Shared:** This includes a shared decision-making process where clinicians know the client's values and perspectives, provide real choices and opportunities for negotiating/collaborating on goals, and a collaborative consensus on goals. People want to be involved in decisions about therapy and what is possible within the services being provided. Hersh et al. (2012) argued that it is not enough to just ask what clients want to work on or to invite them to a meeting. They need enough information about the context and process to be partners, along with communication-friendly materials and supports.

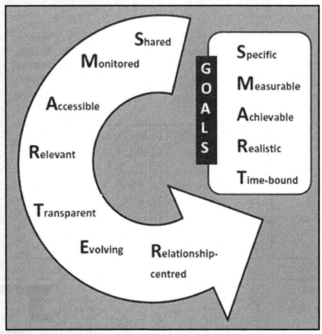

Figure 5-6. SMARTER goal framework.

(continued)

Box 5-5 (continued)
Collaborative Goal Setting

2. **Monitored:** This monitoring should be ongoing, iterative and recognize incremental change, and measurable by the client/family as well as the clinician. This is also intended to facilitate conversations about any need to re-examine the direction of therapy. Progress toward goals should also be collaborative; this means sharing the means of evaluating progress. Goal outcomes do not have to be numerically based and/or should include qualitative descriptors of performance.

3. **Accessible:** Creating communication accessibility is our expertise as speech-language pathologists. So, we've got some work to do here. The concept of goals is foreign to many of our clients. We need to make it clear what we mean by goals (and conversely, what our clients mean by goals) and apply all of our best techniques (supported conversation, rating scales, AAC, etc.) to make it clear what goals are. Tools such as Talking Mats, supported conversation, and the like are necessary to ensure accessibility.

4. **Relevant:** This is one of the primary reasons we need to learn about the values, interests, and goals of our clients. We need to learn what they want to do and what they need to do and how that changed given their communication impairment. In fact, what is relevant or salient to that individual matters from the perspective of neuroplasticity (Kleim & Jones, 2008). Hersh et al. (2012) acknowledge that therapy goals tend to be based upon the results of communication assessment rather than relevance. Clients should have a "supported in-depth interview where possible" (p. 228). They should be able to set goals as challenging and ambitiously as they desire. "The job of the SLP then is to work out with our clients what smaller steps are needed to reach that goal. Being *transparent* is about making that journey to the goal really clear so it can be jointly owned" (D. Hersh, personal communication).

5. **Transparent:** Clients do not always see the relationship between impairment-focused therapy sessions and their goals, which are predominantly activity and participation-based goals (Gustafsson & McLaughlin, 2009). Transparent goals connect the dots between treatment targets and outcomes (i.e., address x at x accuracy level in order to do <u>insert client end goal which is likely to be an activity and participation-based goal</u>).

6. **Evolving:** Effective goals must change over time, as priorities change, as goals are met, as self-awareness improves and as what is feasible is further recognized.

7. **Relationship-centered:** Relationship-centered care acknowledges the client's competence and personhood, giving them a stake in making decisions about themselves whenever possible (Hughes et al., 2008). Hersh et al. (2012) contended that strong, therapeutic relationships should be prioritized over formal assessment whenever possible. That is not to say that formal assessment is not important, as clearly it is critical to communication and swallowing management. Rather, results of formal assessments alone should not drive goal selection. Strong therapeutic relationships support the collaboration necessary to jointly make decisions about goals and selection of personally relevant activities (Hersh et al., 2013).

GOAL COMPONENT:	WHO: Name, Ms., Mrs., Mr., Dr., etc.	SKILL/TARGET: production of /phoneme/, attention to task, orientation to …, recall of …, self-assessment, etc.	PERFORMANCE LEVEL: for X min., for X times, in X context, with X level of accuracy	CONDITION: w/ X type of cues or support, in the presence of X demands, environment	PURPOSE: In order to achieve activity/ participation outcomes
A client might see it more like this (personal communication with Deborah Hersh):					
I want to be able to do x	To do that, I need to practice these sounds/words/ sentences/exercises.	For that, I need x support, with x cues, and practice it x number of times.	I will look at x results on x measure to see if it is getting any better.		

(continued)

> ## Box 5-5 (CONTINUED)
> ### Collaborative Goal Setting
>
> Collaborative goals are a precursor to effective therapeutic alliance and cooperation. Therefore, they are interwoven with all aspects of our disciplinary assessment and intervention, including counseling. For an excellent podcast conversation with Dr. Deborah Hersh regarding SMARTER goals, see Box 5-6.
>
> Later is a rough framework for writing collaborative, person-centered goals. This order works, but you can also change order and maintain necessary goal elements.

> ## Box 5-6
> ### SMARTER Goals
>
> Check out this great podcast conversation on Aphasia Access Conversations Podcast Episode #35 with Dr. Deborah Hersh, as she discusses collaborative goal setting and the SMARTER goals framework.
>
> https://aphasiaaccess.libsyn.com/35-therapy -in-transit-using-lpaa-in-acute-and-sub-acute -settings-a-conversation-with-deborah-hersh -phd

Collaborative goal setting is not only about conjointly developing goals but also in conjointly evaluating outcomes. Using GAS appears to have a positive effect on the development of self-awareness, which allows clients to identify realistic, achievable goals (Doig et al., 2010; Hoepner et al., 2021; Malec, 1999). Medley and Powell (2010) conducted a conceptual review of the literature on self-awareness, which suggested that motivational interviewing may support clients in identifying their ability level and setting goals that balance their abilities and aspirations. Combining GAS with motivational interviewing may help strengthen goal-oriented action as well (Lewis et al., 2017).

What might "counseling" goals in speech-language pathology look like?

- Client will identify their own (re)habilitation goals.
- Client will measure their own goal outcomes.
- Client will reflect/report on their socioemotional status weekly given the support of rating scales and communication supports.
- Partners/caregivers will reflect/report on their socioemotional status weekly.
- Client (and family) will receive education regarding their communication disorder.

Okay, so collaboration and eliciting our client's goals and solutions is important but is there ever a moment to offer advice? Miller and Rollnick (2013) emphasize some clear constraints:

- Engage first and be sure you have a strong foundation of trust and alliance.
- Get permission first.
- Advice should be presented in a clear and specific manner.
- Use in small doses and use sparingly.
- Be aware of and responsive to the client's reactions.
- Use "autonomy-supportive" language that emphasizes personal choice. "Ultimately, it's your decision not mine."
- Offer a menu of options. If you present one suggestion at a time, it invites sustain or resistance talk, whereas multiple options offers choice. Remember to use communication supports in offering those options (e.g., written choice).

Don't Show Your Hand (or at Least Be Careful When You Do)

We all have a little bit of egocentrism within us. A common pitfall of this tendency is showing your hand by letting your opinions and biases emerge (particularly before you know enough about your client's perspectives). Incidentally, this can have a big effect on how others perceive and thus respond to our cultural (in)sensitivity. It is not that we need to remain totally neutral but rather that we pause and delay our responses in favor of listening. Once you say "I think x," you have revealed your perspective. That perspective may conflict with the client's perspective or the client may believe that you are the expert, therefore your perspective is correct. If you begin by finding out about the person's values and perspectives, you can avoid this pitfall. Just pausing and inhibiting the sharing of your perspective can reap benefits, too. A prolonged pause has often saved me from putting my foot in my mouth. It also helps me to be less *blabby* in the future. After all, it is not about us, it is about our clients' values, needs, and perspectives. Following this principle is also central to being culturally responsive. We cannot possibly know the cultural norms and expectations for every culture or individual but we can learn what matters to the individuals we work with. If, however, we say what we think, believe, or expect before learning what they believe and value, we make it difficult (at best) for them to respond honestly, or we unintentionally create a rift in our developing relationship.

So, what about sharing about ourselves? Is it ever appropriate? Let's start with this important distinction: sharing stories from your past is different than sharing personal stories from your own life that relate to your client's current situation. Whenever we contextualize our experience with their current experience, we infer a direction on their part (e.g., "I was in this situation and I did x and it worked really well."). We need to be sensitive to our internal reaction to any such sharing (i.e., do our emotions, affect, and nonverbals suggest that we believe this is the right path or a good example of how to handle a situation?). And we need to be sensitive to our client's reaction. Further, when the focus moves from our client toward us, it loses its value. Miller and Rollnick (2013) frame three additional, important considerations:

1. Is it true? It should be genuine/true but not necessarily the whole truth.

2. Does it have the potential to be harmful? If it is critical to what the client has already done or will do, it could be harmful.

3. Is there a clear reason it will be helpful? Miller and Rollnick (2013) follow with some great potential examples of how self-disclosure could be helpful:

   a. "To promote trust and engagement (Cozby, 1973).

   b. To model openness and encourage reciprocity of disclosure (Sullivan, 1970).

   c. To answer a client question ("Do you have children?; "Have you ever felt like this?").

   d. To affirm; affirmations are a form of self-disclosure, a genuine in-the-moment appreciation of the client's nature or actions" (pp. 150-151).

Addressing Counseling Moments

Unlike a professional counselor-counselee relationship where the client comes to the counselor's office with the express purpose and intent of addressing some sort of counseling issue, speech-language pathologists and their clients come together for a different purpose. While that purpose may revolve around addressing articulation accuracy, voice quality, expressive language, memory, executive dysfunction, dysphagia, or the like, counseling moments arise on a regular basis within those sessions. Across types of clients and across the lifespan, the nature of those moments can differ widely. For instance, some speech-language pathologist-client interactions follow a routine that is similar to the more traditional counselor-counselee relationship. This might occur, for example, when serving a transgender client who is seeking a clear change in not only their verbal communication but a host of non-linguistic changes concurrently. Conversely, counseling moments may happen in the hallways with a parent of a child you are serving, on your way to and from

sessions, or in the notes you exchange with parents in an assignment notebook (paired with hard to come by exchanges at parent-teacher conferences).

How do you know when you're in the midst of a counseling moment? Often, our gut is a pretty good indicator. Johnson, Jilla, and Danhauer (2018) note that in some counseling moments, clinicians fail to respond, while in others they may respond with information, rather than a response that addresses the affective need. They provide excellent examples of counseling moments, paired with "*matched*" (counselor addresses the moment) and "*mismatched*" (counselor either fails to respond or responds with information when the situation calls for an affective response). For example, if the client says, "I feel old when wearing hearing aids," a *mismatched* response could include, "Many working adults use them" (p. 16). A matched response could be, "Tell me more about that . . ." (p. 16). Some situations clearly call for an information response. For instance, if a client asks, "How long do hearing aid batteries last?", a response of, "about 5 to 7 days" (p. 16) would be an effective response. Now, it's your turn. If your client's partner asks, "What is aphasia?", what kind of a response is needed (i.e., affective or informational)? What if they ask, "How do people live with aphasia?"? Suppose they ask, "Is my child ever going to talk?" or "What does it take to diagnose autism?"?

What Does Counseling Look Like for Different Clients?

Some version of this inquiry is common for individuals just beginning to learn about counseling in speech-language pathology. "What do counseling moments look like with a 3-year-old?" "What does counseling look like for a person with early dementia?" "Maybe we only really counsel the parents of children?" "Maybe we only counsel the partners of people with dementia?" These types of questions are often followed by "I have a voice client right now and can clearly see where counseling fits into their sessions but not so much with my 4-year-old articulate client." "We spend a big portion of sessions on counseling with my transgender client, but it's harder to see the application to kids." These are all great questions and comments. Certainly, not all types of clients warrant the same counseling tools or approaches. And even if you could use the same broad approach, you would have to modify how it is implemented. First off, counseling and motivational interviewing are clearly not equivalent. Motivational interviewing shares many of the core skills and assumptions that a counseling approach has more broadly. Other approaches have been used and examined in our disciplinary literature and deserve consideration, particularly for certain "types" of clients. Secondly, motivational interviewing is not mutually exclusive to those other approaches. No one says you cannot mix motivational interviewing with a narrative approach to counseling, positive

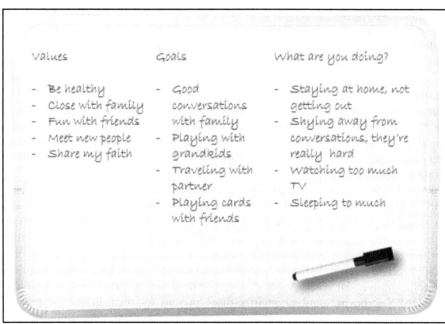

Figure 5-7. Cross mapping values with behaviors/actions.

psychology, or any other techniques applied within our discipline. Understanding and having skill in multiple "types" of counseling would allow you to be more flexible and tailor an approach to individual clients. Those other approaches will be addressed in Chapter 6, whereas the methods for motivational interviewing will be discussed in this chapter.

Value Mapping and Exploring Value-Behavior Discrepancies

Value mapping is a process of identifying core values (see Chapter 4). Exploring value-behavior discrepancies is the process of identifying actions that are congruent and incongruent to a client's desires and goals (and ultimately their core values). When we elicit clients' perspectives about broader life goals and values, we create a reference point for comparison (Figure 5-7). For instance, if one of my life goals/values is to live a long, healthy life, then eating too much, exercising too little, smoking, or drinking would be incompatible/incongruent with the broader life goal/value. If a client wants to engage in social interactions with their family and truly values those moments, it would be incongruent to throw in the towel when it comes to practicing communication strategies. An important thing to remember is that exploring value-behavior discrepancies is not about throwing the incongruent behaviors in their face, it is about fostering their ability to recognize that certain behaviors are incongruent with their life goals and values. Miller and Rollnick (2013) emphasize the use of *self-confrontation* through *self-reflection*, rather than a righting response that throws it back in their face. Self-confrontation can be prompted through open-ended questions and our responses should affirm their feelings, rather than our interpretations. It also requires a safe, supportive context without fear of judgment.

For individuals with communication disorders, it may be helpful to lay out a physical map of their values and behaviors. This includes identifying their goals, core values, and behaviors/actions (including those that are congruent with their agenda and those that are incongruent). This is best achieved through drawing out (eliciting) those elements collaboratively. If you already know some of their values or goals, it is okay to say, "I know you value x, is it okay if I jot that down on the whiteboard?" Remember, a core value of motivational interviewing is to have a conversation, not a transaction—so the end goal isn't to make a list but to process through the relationship between values and behaviors/actions. Restating those relationships is one way to approach this, "You want to meet new people and have good conversations but you find yourself staying at home instead." Or, you can turn it around as a question for them. "How do you think staying at home and shying away from conversations affects your goals and values?"

DARN-CAT

A common misconception about motivational interviewing is that it is only focused on change. When you define change more broadly, you can make more everyday applications of motivational interviewing. Change can come in the form of a specific goal—"I want to read to my grandchildren." Likewise, change can come in the form of identifying one's own solutions to a particular challenge. Change can be increasing the amount of time spent on a given goal or altering the way you approach it. It can be the recognition that some of one's own behaviors are incongruent with their broader life values and goals.

A second misconception is that people need to be convinced of why they should change. Considering the roots of motivational interviewing for treating people with substance abuse, smoking, alcohol, and other addictions, it is important to note that most people recognize particular unhealthy behaviors are not okay. For instance, they realize that smoking causes health problems and do not need us to convince them of that. Any attempt to convince them comes across as patronizing and prescriptive. The same applies to many of our clients who understand why but need to think through the how. Remember, when we make the arguments for change, it puts our clients in the position of arguing against that change.

Every time a client encounters a challenge, we should consider if they wish to address it. When appropriately supported from a communication standpoint, collaborative goal setting addresses the first component of the DARN acronym (Miller & Rollnick, 2013), *desire*. Do they desire to improve the intelligibility of their speech or their ability to communicate through writing, for instance? If they do not, it is not our role to tell them that they have to value improving a specific communication skill. That does not mean that we just give up, but rather, help them to more critically evaluate it through agenda mapping and exploration of value-behavior discrepancies. For instance, if a person says they don't care if their speech isn't clear but say other things that contradict this statement (e.g., "I want to return to my work as a receptionist"), their agendas are not congruent with one another. In this case, getting them to identify that clear speech is necessary to carry out their job is a reason for change, a reason (desire) to work on improving their speech. We prompt this through reflections and self-confrontation (self-evaluation). This is also a great place to use the strategy *double-sided reflection*, "On one hand, you don't care about the clarity of your speech in most situations. On the other hand, you want to return to your job as a receptionist, where speech clarity is important." In this way, you use their words to develop and highlight discrepancy.

Simply desiring something does not mean it can or will happen. I might desire to run a marathon but that does not mean I have the ability or the resources necessary to do so. Thus, examining *ability* is an important step in making change. In the marathon example, I say that I want to run it but that is not congruent with my abilities. This creates another opportunity to have a conversation about that goal area. For instance, "You want to run a marathon but you have not trained for it. You don't want to put the energy into training for the marathon. Do you think you will be able to accomplish it without the training?" In cases, like this, where ability can change but it takes effort (much like working on your speech quality), fostering self-evaluation creates an opportunity to elicit potential change talk. "I really want to run a marathon with my daughter and I know that means I will have to train." Self-evaluation is crucial to autonomy

in decision making, a central component of motivational interviewing. The counselor/speech-language pathologist can more confidently inhibit their righting reflex when they know a prompt for self-evaluation will follow. So, when our client says, "I want to return to work fulltime, next week", we can begin the process of fostering self-evaluation (i.e., "Okay, what will you need to do in order to return to work?" "Are there any potential barriers?"), rather than saying what we may be thinking internally ("Are you serious? There is no way, you have right-sided paralysis, you have severe memory problems, . . .").

Regardless of desire or ability, it is helpful when the client can identify their own *reasons* for change. Sticking with the marathon example, running the race with my daughter is one reason but it is pretty broad. If I can identify specific reasons why I want to run with my daughter, it increases my likelihood of following through. When the person identifies reasons for change, you have elicited change talk. You reflect and summarize those reasons for them in your response, "You want to run a marathon with your daughter because . . . and you know it will mean some hard work on your part."

Once you have established a desire, ability, and reasons for taking on a given goal, it is helpful when it fulfills a purpose or *need*. If it is just a nice thing but is not really needed, it will rightfully be in competition with things that you need to do. For instance, you need to work, eat, sleep, and pay the bills. If that does not leave time for preparing for a marathon, it is not likely to happen. Need could be a perceived need to spend time with the daughter or a need to become healthier. Establishing what that need is becomes crucial to follow-through.

After you have established DARN, you can begin to collaborate on eliciting the client's own words of *commitment, activation, and taking steps* (mobilizing change talk). Methods for eliciting and evoking change talk are discussed further later. Part of that "talk" is language of commitment. Rating scales can be a very important tool for addressing commitment. The Readiness Ruler (Rollnick et al., 1999) is a simple rating scale used for examining readiness for change and can be a powerful tool in monitoring ongoing progress (Figure 5-8). A core element of evoking in motivational interviewing is the idea of fostering incremental (achievable) change. Rating scales can help us to elicit client's change talk at an achievable increment. Using the same rating scale format, you can ask clients to rate confidence and commitment to goals. Open-ended questions like, "Why did you choose 7?" followed by, "Why not a 6 or less?" and, "What would it take to move to an 8?" Asking why they didn't select a lower number typically prompts change talk, as they describe why they rated it higher (e.g., "I didn't rate my readiness as a 2 because I do want to change, I just know it will take a lot of work"). You respond by reflecting, "On one hand, you want to change but on the other hand, you recognize this will take some work." Likewise, when you ask them what it would take to increase readiness or confidence rating, they typically use change language (e.g., "To move from a 7 to an 8, all I would

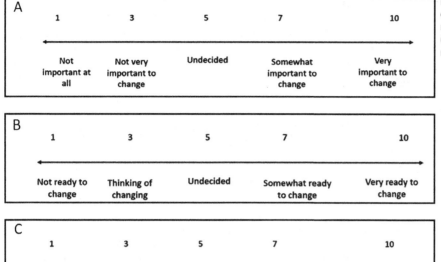

Figure 5-8. (A) Commitment ruler. "Rate your commitment to make a change." (B) Readiness ruler. "Rate your readiness to make a change." (C) Confidence ruler. "Rate your confidence in making a change."

have to do is . . ."). In this manner, you evoke tangible, concrete steps toward change. Again, you affirm them by saying "It sounds like you recognize what you need to do to change. Doing x will help you move to an 8." Along with the rating scale, use other communication supports (e.g., written choice) to ensure a means of response. In their responses to these questions, listen for language of *activation* (moving toward action). This includes statements like "I'm ready to . . .", "Having x will help me get started . . .", and the like. Finally, *taking initial steps* toward action further attests to commitment to change. Please complete the exercise in Box 5-7 regarding the readiness, commitment, and confidence rulers.

The Method of Motivational Interviewing

Implementing motivational interviewing in the context of typical speech-language pathology clinical sessions requires a strong understanding of the underlying principles. While we sometimes discuss the approach in a linear fashion, beginning with engaging, then focusing, followed by evoking and planning, more often we weave in and out of these stages. Nonetheless, understanding the stages, basic techniques, and terminology can help you navigate less traditional counseling moments. Understand the techniques and terminology helps you to be more intentional about your approach, which is even more crucial when you are not following a linear sequence.

Box 5-7
Thought Exercise

What is something that you know you should do but you're not very good at following through? How committed, ready, confident on a scale of 1 to 10 are you in completing it? Use the Readiness Ruler for this. Once you answer, consider why you didn't rate it lower (if possible) or what it would take to increase confidence by one point.

Next, think of something that you are very good at following through with consistently. How committed, ready, confident are you with doing that? Once you answer, consider why you didn't rate it lower (if possible) or what it would take to increase confidence by one point.

OARS

Open-Ended Questions

These are an effective way to turn the power over to our clients (Miller & Rollnick, 2013). Some may find it intuitive to ask a close ended question, particularly for persons with communication impairments, seeking a response that is a bit easier for most to respond to in the moment. As tempting as that is, closed-ended questions put the power on the person asking the question and tend to constrain or even end topics. Open ended questions, while broader and more challenging to respond to in the moment can be scaffolded with communication supports (e.g., pause/wait time, written choices) in order to allow the client to control the direction of the

Box 5-8
Open-Ended Versus Closed-Ended Questions

OPEN-ENDED QUESTIONS	CLOSED-ENDED VERSIONS
• What recreation activities do you enjoy?	• Do you like canoeing? Fishing? Cross country skiing?
• Where do you like to go out for dinner?	• Do you like the Olive Garden?
• What are your goals for therapy?	• Do you want to work on naming?

conversation. Aside from framing your questions as open ended, there are some other common pitfalls when asking open-ended questions. Add-ons and revisions are common missteps. This simply means, you ask a well-formed open-ended question but you feel compelled to repair it. Often, if we have the perception that the question is too broad, we may narrow it with a closed-ended add-on. Similarly, if we ask an open-ended question we perceive as imperfect, we may revise it with several follow-up revisions or versions of the same question. Responding to multiple versions of the same question is challenging for everyone but particularly challenging for people with cognitive or communication impairments. Another common pitfall is double-barreled questions. Even if both components are open ended, it is more difficult to answer two at the same time (e.g., What do you think about therapy and working on going back to school?). Simply put, less syntactically complex and shorter questions make responding easier. Box 5-8 compares open-ended and closed-ended questions.

Beyond recognizing how to frame open-ended questions, there are a handful of questions that are good to have at the ready. You may wish to rephrase them to fit your counseling voice but they are good generic questions. Here are some go to questions: "What do you think?", "How would you approach it?", "What has worked in the past?", "Tell me more.", "Are there strategies you could use to address this?" (phrased as a closed-ended question but typically draws an open-ended response), and "What help would (do) you need?". Of course, in novel interactions you will need other questions as well.

Active listening can become almost cliché in the realm of counseling practices. I have heard several people say, counseling is all about being a good listener. That is not to say listening is not important, as it is of the utmost importance for successful therapeutic relationships. Simply saying, I'm an active or good listener, however, is not enough. Evidence of active listening includes non-linguistic elements such as

forward leaning, open stance/sitting, attentiveness, and nodding. Perhaps even more important and powerful are the final three elements of OARS. Each of the elements (affirmation, reflection, and summary) demonstrate active listening in a specific manner.

Affirmations

Affirmations are the act of acknowledging someone's feelings, perspectives, and responses to a situation (Miller & Rollnick, 2013). When we genuinely affirm people's feelings, perspectives, ideas, frustrations, and reactions to a situation, we demonstrate active listening. A common pitfall for affirmation moments is to either console or correct the person. The *consoling trap* is a human tendency to want to make people feel better. The response "you'll be okay" or "it will all work out" fails to acknowledge and affirm the person's feelings and perspectives in that moment. Not consoling does not equate to not being empathetic. Rather, your affirmations of a person's feelings demonstrate your empathy. Another common human response is to contend their feelings or perspectives are somehow wrong, "it wasn't a stupid idea" or "you don't really feel that way." If you have a hard time letting things go that you believe are incorrect, this might be challenging. Here's a silly example: I went to a home improvement store to purchase some incandescent light bulbs. Because I was carrying too much stuff, the package of light bulbs fell from my arms and one of the bulbs exploded as I tried to set my stuff on the checkout counter. The clerk said, "That wouldn't happen if you bought LED bulbs." I responded, "I know, right, but those bulbs give me a headache" (actually, I was purchasing them for my wife and they bother her). The response was stunning, "No, they don't." I actually prefer LED bulbs, so I may agree that scientifically, they have not been linked to headaches. However, the principle of the response is what I and probably most human beings would rebel against. The same is true when we correct our clients, whether we are right or not—it doesn't really matter. Of course, there are situations where right or wrong matters but in the case of a client's feelings, our response should be an affirmation. We may have them self-assess (self-confront) at some point but correcting them is likely to result in push back. Box 5-9 provides examples of how to frame affirmations and an affirmations exercise.

As we move into reflections and summaries, this is a crucial time for us to self-assess. How do we recognize change talk when it happens? In order to do that, we need to recognize resistance talk, sustain talk, ambivalence, and change talk, too (Figure 5-9). See Box 5-10 for examples of each type of talk. Refer back to Chapter 4 to address ways to assess readiness to change (e.g., Readiness Ruler, agenda mapping). Finally, recognize that the change you are looking for will not always come in the form of changing a specific behavior. It can come in the form of talking or thinking through the situation. If you are successful in getting the client to think out loud, you have likely been successful in evoking their ideas for change.

Box 5-9

Affirmations

Let's consider some simple examples of affirmation. There are endless permutations, so do not feel like you have to respond the same way as others do or follow the examples here. Find a counseling voice for affirmations that fits you. If you are comfortable, you will be more confident and effective in delivering affirmations.

Here are some different ways of framing affirmations:

- Sounds like . . .
- I'm hearing that . . .
- You're feeling like . . .
- It seems that . . .
- It's really important to you that . . .
- It's really frustrating for you that . . .

Exercise: Try making a consoling and/or correcting response for each statement below. Then, make an affirmation for each statement in your own counseling voice (C = client, Y = you).

C: I'm really upset about the way you handled things.

Y: You feel frustrated by the way I handled the situation.

C: Having a brain injury really sucks. I can't do anything like I used to do it.

Y: It is very hard to have brain injury because it feels like you can't do things like you used to.

C: My mom is just stupid, I cannot stand the way she treats me. It should be my decision whether or not to come to therapy.

Y: You're frustrated with your mom because she made the decision to send you to therapy and you wish you had a say.

C: I'm happy with my choice. It was a good decision.

Y: You're glad you did it and feel good about the decision.

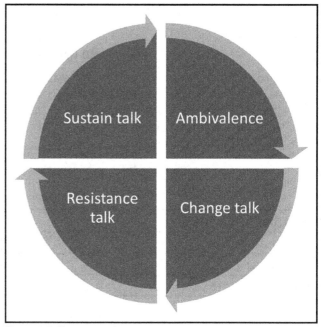

Figure 5-9. Change continuum.

say does not need to be in a verbal modality, they may use high-, low-, or no-tech AAC; gesture; drawing; writing; or other modalities to convey their idea. We reiterate or reflect that statement by verbalizing it (typically) but may also reflect in multiple modalities. Typically, reflections are "you" statements. Box 5-11 provides examples of client statements and clinician reflections.

Summaries

Summaries are used to collect and concisely reflect and restate the client's own potential solutions and reasons for change (Miller & Rollnick, 2013). Miller and Rollnick (2013) describe the process of pulling together those solutions and reasons as creating a "bouquet of change talk." Common pitfalls for delivering effective summaries include struggles with identifying change talk and struggles with recalling what the client said in order to summarize it. Identifying change talk begins with developing an ear for evidence of shifting perspectives from resistance to ambivalence toward readiness for change. Recalling what the client says often relies on effective notetaking. Consider the following strategies: 1) don't attempt to write everything down verbatim, 2) identify key information, and 3) make it collaborative. To make the process of note taking collaborative, often it helps to say/ask, "Is it okay if I take some notes to make sure I capture what your ideas are accurately?" Give them an opportunity to verify and contribute to the notes as well. "Does this look right? Anything we should add?" Effective notes allow you to summarize their ideas, solutions, and reasons for change effectively. Restating their words reiterates their change talk and you should emphasize these are their words. Often, clients thank you for the solutions and the best part

Reflections

Reflections are simply a restatement of a client's own words (Miller & Rollnick, 2013). It may help to follow the mantra, *saying is believing*. Reflections are like saying it again, as we reiterate their ideas, potential solutions, and reasons for change. In the case of reflecting statements by persons with communication disorders, we either expand a bit or make statements more concisely. Note that what they

---

Box 5-10

An Eye and Ear for Change Talk

It's hard to discretely separate types of statements into types of talk, as there is more of a continuum across statements. For instance, *probably* is closer to change talk than *maybe*, and *I think* is closer to ambivalence than *I know* or *obviously*. That being said, these types of statements give you a sense of a person's readiness for change.

Resistance talk — Sustain talk — Ambivalence — Change talk

RESISTANCE TALK	AMBIVALENCE
• I can't	• I guess, but
• I won't	• I might, but
• I don't care	• Maybe
	• Probably, but

SUSTAIN TALK	CHANGE TALK
• It's working fine	• I think
• I'm doing alright	• I know
	• I recognize
	• Clearly
	• Obviously

Box 5-11

Reflections

C: Need to practice more.

Y: You know that you need to spend more time practicing these techniques.

C: I will only get better if I do more work on it. Like when I'm trying to say something it helps to have notes or a plan, like the script you talk about. That's how I get my point across when people don't get what I mean.

Y: You recognize that having a scripted response or taking time to think before responding will make your response clearer.

C: [Points to message on AAC board about family and gestures more.]

Y: You want to spend more time with your family. Is that right?

---

is responding, "These are your ideas, not mine. I'm just reminding you of what you said." Complete the summarizing exercise in Box 5-12.

The "Steps" of Motivational Interviewing

Engaging

Engaging is closely associated with therapeutic alliance and rapport (Miller & Rollnick, 2013). Recall our discussion of interactional money in the bank or interactional capital from Chapter 3 (McMorrow, 2003). Building positive relationships and interactions can help as we inevitably ask clients to do difficult things. It may help to think about engaging in two ways, the long haul and the present moments. Once a relationship has been established, there is carryover of rapport and therapeutic alliance from past successes. Engaging is a key way to establish that alliance, rapport, and trust in the first place. Harkening back to the discussion of eliciting person-centered information about what our client's value, enjoy, and their goals, engaging is a way of directly

Box 5-12
Summary

Exercise: Practice summarizing these statements in your own words (your own counseling voice). Identify the change talk within each client's statements. What key words would you write down to help you summarize each client's statements?

C: I don't know what to do. I find myself forgetting things all of the time. If I don't write things down, I don't remember them. Flat out don't even know that they happened or that I'm supposed to do something. It's just hard because writing everything down makes me look like a total idiot, like a moron. Depending upon who is around, I just refuse to do it.

Y: While you recognize that you need to write things down in order to remember them, it is still hard to do because you feel like it makes you look foolish. You feel more comfortable writing things down around some people more than others.

C: I just get so anxious in class and pray that the teacher doesn't call on me and that I don't have to talk. I mean, I want to talk with my classmates but some of them just don't get it. I guess it is okay if I stutter because it doesn't mean I'm not smart. I mean, I get good grades and my teachers know that. Some teachers can't even make eye contact with me.

Y: You know that it is okay to stutter and it has nothing to do with your intelligence or worth but you still get nervous sometimes in class. Some of your teachers and classmates don't know how to respond or help. Does that sound right?

likely to get into some challenging conversations, it's a good number to keep in mind. Also, if you know you are going to put your client in challenging situations (like pronouncing words accurately when it is hard to do so, such as using semantic feature analysis to identify the right words), the proportion probably still holds true as well.

A key element of engaging is the idea of maintaining a positive, non-directional conversation. The client may make statements that lead toward a particular topic of focus but do your best to remain in engaging for a few minutes before moving on. Having go-to phrases that fit your counseling voice are helpful. This includes statements like, "It sounds like that may be something you want to discuss more. Let's come back to that." A common pitfall is diving into a deep conversation before you've established a recent/current positive interaction to draw upon. Of course, there are times when it is necessary to dive right into that difficult conversation but if given the opportunity, try to pause that conversation for a few moments. See Box 5-13 for some examples of engaging and conversation starters.

Focusing

Focusing is the process of selecting a topic to discuss, a problem to solve, a direction, or a goal to address (Miller & Rollnick, 2013). Once you have clearly established a client's goals, you may return to this focus on a day-to-day basis. As we know from collaborative goal-setting principles, person-centered goals are those we draw out of our clients. Once we have collaboratively established their goals, it is still worthwhile verifying and re-evaluating those goals over time. Finding out is this still their priority is part of the ongoing negotiation of the focus for the session or a conversation. That being said, a part of our role is to stick to their focus, rather than constantly shifting focus without accomplishing anything. A common pitfall in the focusing phase is **assumptions**. We make assumptions about what people would value, what they mean, and how they intend to address challenges. It is especially crucial when interacting with people with communication disorders to verify that what we think they want is actually what they want. There are far fewer missteps when we verify a client's focus. Further, when we ask verification questions, it often helps to solidify and bring clarity to the client's commitment to that focus. Also, make sure that their focus is in line with their overarching values and goals. Finally, make it tangible and reviewable. Using a whiteboard or simply writing it down on a shared document keeps the focus clear.

Agenda mapping is a helpful process for achieving focus (Miller & Rollnick, 2013). Basically, it follows the format of a multiparameter sort. You could use icons/cards from Talking Mats (https://www.talkingmats.com/), Activity Card Sort (Baum & Edwards, 2008), LIV Cards (Haley et al., 2013), or a homegrown sort to achieve this. This involves two philosophical decisions: to sort more traditional speech-language or swallowing targets (e.g., articulation, naming,

identifying what matters to our clients and the process of authentically inquiring about this information builds trust. Not to say that friendships can be fickle but there is a definite recency effect. Even when you have established a history of therapeutic alliance, trust, and rapport, there is a need to revisit engaging on a regular basis. Whenever we ask people to do something that is difficult or uncomfortable, it is useful to have a more recent experience of alliance and rapport to draw upon.

Rollnick suggests engaging for about 10% to 20% of your total time, so if you have a 30-minute session, that means 3 to 6 minutes at the start. Note that speech-language pathology sessions are different than a full-fledged counseling session, so this proportion is not a perfect fit. If you know you're

Box 5-13
Engaging

Engaging is more than chitchat, although it sometimes begins that way. It may sound more like a conversation with a friend than a client (while keeping it professional). This is your opportunity to relate and share a bit about yourself, as long as your story doesn't become the focus. Rogers (1965) emphasized sharing when you know it is congruent with your client and a genuine experience of yours. So, when the client says, "I saw a great movie," you can say, "I heard that was good." Or when they say, "I went fishing with my dad," you can say, "That sounds like fun, I used to love doing that with my dad too." The key is keeping it positive and non-directional for a bit.

Common starters could include:

- What have you been up to? (when you already know the person)
- What do you like to do in your spare time? (if you're getting to know the person)
- How have things been going at home? School? Work? (unless you know that this will trigger an upset)
- How's that home improvement project going?

The direction you go with engaging depends on what you know about a client. If you know that certain topics are sensitive or triggers, they are not a good choice to begin engaging. For instance, I once observed this attempt at engaging as I ended a session with a person with a traumatic brain injury and the chaplain stopped by for a conversation. She said, "So, I hear you like snowmobiling," which could be a fine way to start that conversation. In this case, the gentleman sustained his head injury in a snowmobile accident. I could see the look of terror on her face when the words left her mouth. The good news is, there is always a path to repair, even when we slip up, which we ALL do. She nervously laughed and followed up with "Okay, that was a sensitive place to start, do you have any other hobbies before we start talking about snowmobiling." Perfect save, I thought as I walked out of the room.

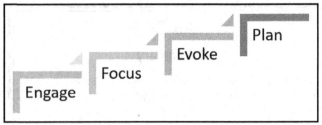

Figure 5-10. Motivational interviewing steps.

diet/consistency) or more activity and participation-focused goals (e.g., visiting with friends, posting on social media, dining out). Recall that motivational interviewing emphasizes a client's goals, values, and abilities, rather than their impairments. Thus, an agenda mapping sort of activities and participations may best align with a motivational interviewing approach. Other potential agenda (focus) items may include those related to psychosocial well-being (see Figure 5-11 for a communication-accessible example). Remember, in motivational interviewing, the process of focusing is meant to be a conversation, not a transaction. A potential pitfall of a topic sort like the one shown in Figure 5-10, is becoming procedural or transactional. This can be addressed by having a conversation about the sort. This process may lead to identification of one topic or you may sort and prioritize topics if the person indicates a desire to address more than one. A simple rating scale sort would work for this (Figure 5-12). Note that beyond the hierarchy of priority achieved through the topic sort, you will want to negotiate and put words to why. For example, the client's relationship with their spouse might be of utmost importance to them but may not be a priority of discussion on a given day. Likewise, financial security may not be a relevant topic, as the person may have already achieved financial security—not identifying it as a topic of discussion doesn't reduce its overall value to that individual. Identifying family relationships and emotional health as priority topics may indicate importance or potentially an area of concern/struggle. Thus, follow-up conversations about those selections are important to ensure a mutual understanding of why they were identified. Box 5-14 provides examples of focusing questions.

Evoking

Evoking is emblematic of the underlying philosophy of motivational interviewing. The function of evoking is to elicit a person's own potential solutions for a problem and/or their own reasons to change (Miller & Rollnick, 2013). A major pitfall in the evoking stage is *asking and then telling*. Asking an initial evoking question is the relatively easy part. Again, human nature is to expect a response (especially when we can already see potential solutions) before the person has time to think about or develop a response. This is true for everyone but especially true for people with communication disorders. "What are some potential solutions?" followed by, "hearing none, here are my solutions for you." or, "What are

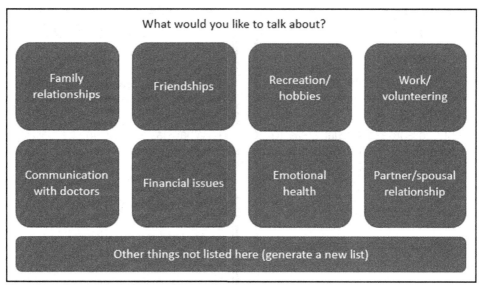

Figure 5-11. Communicatively accessible agenda mapping.

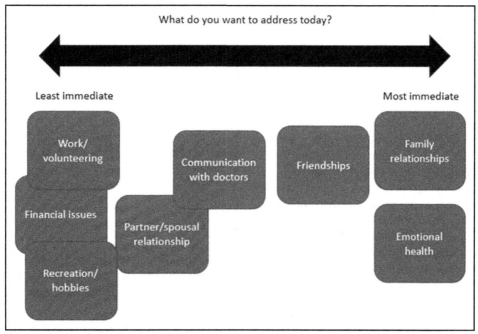

Figure 5-12. Agenda sort rated for priorities.

some reasons to change?" followed by, "hearing none, here are the reasons you should change." Waiting for and scaffolding a person with a communication disorder to respond should be what we as speech-language pathologists should do best. This is our use of supported conversation, choices, augmentative communication strategies, and tangible sorting techniques. It also requires becoming comfortable with some dead airtime. Pausing can feel uncomfortable, like far more time is passing than in reality. As such, we need to be mindful of our wait time (probably not by watching the second hand on your wristwatch, but have a strategy). Often, when we wait, it pays off. Having an anchor to ensure waiting would be helpful. I know this is lame but in my office, I slowly unscrew the cover to my water bottle, take a sip, screw

the cover on, and set it back down (you'll need a strategy that works for you). Let's return to Aura Kagan's (1998) principle of revealing competence. By definition, part of revealing competence is ensuring a means of response. So, if we get a prolonged blank stare or a verbal indication like, "I don't know," it may be because we haven't ensured a means of response. That either means we need to provide an alternative means of communication (e.g., written choice, Talking Mats, a picture sort, AAC device) or we may need to reframe our question (i.e., from one that is too vague or too syntactically complex toward one that is more specific or contextualized and/or is less syntactically complex). As a reminder, we may just need to wait for the client to formulate their response (Leaman & Archer, 2022).

Box 5-14
Focusing

Focusing is intended to identify the client's agenda and achievable goals. These goals should be congruent with their values.

- You have identified some potential areas to focus on. Is x the one you want to address?
- Which goal would you like to address first? Which one is your biggest priority?
- It sounds like you want to focus on x, is that right?

Evoking is intended to address ambivalence and establish a positive change in direction and motivation. As such, it is crucial that we elicit the client's reasons for change and avoid (inhibit) providing our reasons that they should change. Box 5-15 provides several examples of evoking questions and strategies.

Planning

The broad purpose of motivational interviewing is to help our clients develop an actionable plan (Miller & Rollnick, 2013). Once we evoke their own solutions for addressing the problem, it can feel like we are finished. A common pitfall is just stopping there (ideas ≠ plan). Effective planning takes that idea a step or two further—**take some tangible steps**. In fact, the more steps you can take toward the goal/plan, the better. For instance, if the solution we evoked was for the client to join a fitness club, having them take the first few steps will increase the likelihood that they follow through. So instead of accepting "I'll join a fitness club," have them call to make an appointment or sign up for the fitness club. The more incremental and actionable the plan, the better. This allows us to collaboratively address barriers, which would delay or derail follow-through. For example, they call and find out that the monthly cost is $200 and they cannot afford that rate.

Identify potential barriers to implementing the plan (e.g., time, money, support). Consider what your client needs in order to carry out the plan. Identify and utilize facilitators to goal completion (e.g., having a friend collaborate for accountability, having time set aside each day to complete tasks, using a to do list). Here's an example I've seen play out in the past—the client says, "I'll get a calendar/planning app to help remind me what to do and when to do them." When asked about the app in the next session, the client says, "I don't know how to get the app," or, "I wasn't sure which app to get," or, "I didn't get around to choosing an app," or, "I couldn't figure out how to use the app I purchased." All of these barriers were avoidable, if the speech-language

---

Box 5-15
Evoking

With evoking, we elicit our client's goals and change talk. Here are some examples of evoking questions.

- What has worked in the past? (*looking back strategy*)
- Was there a time, in the past, when you were successful in overcoming this challenge? (*looking back strategy*)
- What might work in the future? (*looking forward strategy*)
- What are some potential barriers to achieving this goal (addressing this challenge)? What are some potential facilitators for achieving this goal? (*exploring sustain talk and eliciting change talk strategies*)
- Let's brainstorm, what are some potential solutions? ideas? (*evocative questions strategy*)
- What are some reasons you would like to change? What are some reasons for continuing in your same path? (*eliciting change talk and exploring sustain talk*)
- What do you hope our work together will accomplish? (*exploring goals and values*)
- What do you think you might be able to change? (*using evocative questions*)
- What might be good things about making this change? (*using evocative questions*)
- How important is it for you to make this change? (*exploring goals and values, Readiness Ruler*)

---

pathologist simply encourages the client to take these steps within the session. Perhaps even more commonly, you verbally discuss a plan with the client and ask them to try it out/get started and report back to you in your next session. Then you get to the next session and ask, "So how did it go?" and they admit, "I couldn't remember," or, "I wasn't sure what I was supposed to do." That leads us to our next planning tool, making it tangible and reviewable.

Put it on paper, either physically or metaphorically. As you elicit a client's plan, it is crucial to write down that plan. Given the principle of point-of-service documentation, this can be a very collaborative process. In fact, I have witnessed some physicians who are very good at it and who are probably not aware what a powerful counseling technique this is. Because the person being "counseled" is using their energy to think of solutions and to communicate them, I typically

---

Box 5-16
Planning

Planning tools include blank paper, black markers/Sharpies, Word documents, phones, photos, and your best supported conversation/communication supports.

Questions you might ask in planning include:

- What are some things that might get in the way of completing this plan? Or, simply stated, What might mess up the plan?

- What are some things that might help or increase the likelihood of completing this plan? Or, simply stated, What might help with the plan?

- What do you need (what kinds of supports, people, materials, technologies, etc.) to complete this plan effectively?

- What are the steps involved in completing this plan?

- Does the plan we've written down make sense? seem accurate? need any changes?

Box 5-17
Summary of Communication (Cognition) Strategies and Modifications

- **Always acknowledge competence.** This is true beyond individuals with communication disorders but definitely crucial for those individuals who may not be recognized by others as deserving a seat at the decision-making table. Our clients and their families are the experts on living with communication disorders.

- **Offer multiple modalities of communication.** This may include but is not limited to: written choice, rating scales, drawing, self-generated photos, AAC systems, Talking Mats/LIV Cards/Activity Card Sort/homegrown multiparameter visual sorts, speaking valves, writing, scanning, object selection, etc.

- **Put it on paper.** Provide visible, tangible, and reviewable information to enhance comprehension and support memory/processing. Dry erase boards, tablets, and computer screens can work in the same way.

- **Just wait.** Increase pause and wait time to account for processing and language impairments.

- **Take the first few steps together.** Like many of the adaptations suggested here, this one is particularly important for persons with communication disorders, as it helps clients to make it beyond the first few hurdles and barriers.

- **Avoid assumptions.** For people without communication disorders, assumptions are often made due to poor communication. It is better to ask than assume. In this case we need to ask using communication supports that fit the individual.

---

suggest the speech-language pathologist takes on the role of the scribe, but that can differ across clients. This accomplishes a few things: (1) Documents the plan for them, so that they can refer to it outside of the session; (2) documents the plan for you (this may require scanning, copying and pasting, photographing, or printing a copy) to put in the client's chart; (3) reviews the plan with them that day, which allows you to reiterate it, clarify/verify it, and refine it, and it also makes it clear that it is their plan, not yours (and at best, you had a collaborative role); and (4) returns to the plan in subsequent sessions to check-in on progress (or completion), updates or changes, challenges they may have encountered, and whether it remains relevant. Again, give a copy to them and retain a copy for yourself. Box 5-16 provides several examples of planning questions and tools.

Chapter Summary

Motivational interviewing is one of many counseling techniques. It is built on the principles of collaboration and empowering our clients to determine their own plan based upon their own interest, goals, and values (Miller & Rollnick, 2013). Central to motivational interviewing is creating a space where clients can talk through and think through their current situation. For persons with communication disorders, this talking through and thinking through remains possible when we support communication. Modifications to the approach primarily involve the provision of other modalities or means of communication, visible-tangible-reviewable artifacts and scaffolds to make accessing and reviewing those thoughts more possible, and a strong adherence to the belief that individuals with communication disorders have a stake in making decisions about their own lives (personhood and acknowledging competence). Box 5-17 highlights keys to making communication accessible to individuals cognitive and communication impairments.

Pulling It All Together

Motivational interviewing can seem like a lot of skills to pull together initially. Miller and Rollnick's acronyms can be a helpful reminder, as you begin to apply these methods to practice. While there is no substitute for experiential learning in real counseling moments, considering common counseling moments and applying motivational interviewing approaches can be useful (see Box 5-18).

Key Takeaways

- The **righting reflex** is the human tendency to want to provide solutions or correct others. It is often met with pushback, another human tendency to resist being told what to do and how to do it.
- Most clinicians need to actively **resist or inhibit** their righting reflex, in order to gain and maintain therapeutic alliance with our clients.
- The **expert trap** is one way that speech-language pathologists get drawn back into the righting reflex. Given our professional training, we are misled to think that we are the experts and thus know what our clients should do or even what they should prioritize in terms of goals. In reality, our clients are the experts when it comes to what they want and need to do.
- **Collaborative goal setting** is a method for shared decision making and planning regarding treatment goals. It is a crucial step in achieving therapeutic alliance and collaboration in treatment.
- Counseling, including motivational interviewing, is the process of helping our clients to identify their **own solutions and reasons to change**. As such, our approach should be tailored to each individual we serve.
- We can explore **readiness to change** and **confidence to change** through tools like the **Readiness Ruler.**

- **Value sorts** and **agenda mapping** can help us identify what the client wants and needs to do, along with their core values.

- As we elicit what our clients want and need to do, we can begin to map our client's beliefs, interests, and values onto the therapy targets and goals we address (i.e., **value mapping**). When we effectively learn what our client's value, we can hold them to their own standards and help them to identify incongruencies between their goals/values and their actions/behaviors (**exploring discrepancy**).
- When we observe a discrepancy between core values and behaviors, we should prompt self-evaluation (**self-confrontation**) rather than pointing out the discrepancy. **Double-sided reflections** can also help highlight discrepancy (e.g., "on one hand . . . , on the other hand . . .").
- Before we identify goals, it is important for us to understand our clients' desires, ability, needs, and reasons for change (**DARN**).
- Once goals are identified, we collaboratively establish commitment, activation, and take steps (**CAT**).
- **OARS** allow us to elicit and respond to client communication. This set of techniques is a fairly common core across counseling approaches.
- **Stages of change** or readiness to change loosely align with the continuum of change talk. Further, recognizing the nature of talk on this continuum (resistance talk to sustain talk to ambivalence and finally change talk), allows us to reiterate change talk when we hear it being produced.
- When we make the arguments for change, we put our clients in the position of **arguing against that change**.
- **Engaging** allows us to establish positive, non-directional conversation before diving into a specific goal or challenge.
- **Focusing** is the process of collaboratively establishing a direction for therapy.
- **Evoking** is the process of eliciting a client's own potential solutions and reasons for change.
- **Planning** is the process of solidifying and initiating an actionable process for addressing barriers to goals and ultimately carrying out incremental steps toward goals.
- A number of tools exist, within our discipline and more broadly, that can make motivational interviewing **accessible** to individuals with communication disorders.

Box 5-18

Practical Examples

Scenario #1. An autistic student hates algebra, says he's dumb and horrible at math. Communication breakdown between the student and math teacher are common, which may provide an opportunity to work on self-advocacy skills. *Note: autistic people prefer identity-first language.

DARN—Do a little investigating. Does the student have the desire to improve his algebra performance? Does he have the ability? (Have you seen him be successful in the past? What helped him in that situation?) Can he identify reasons for improving? (Can he make connections between his agenda—what he wants to do, what type of profession he sees himself working in, etc. and algebra?). Is there a need? (Can he connect the dots, with or without your scaffolding, between algebra and other things he wants to do?)

CAT—If he has DARN, you can collaborate with him to identify a commitment, evoke a plan of action, and take steps toward making that improvement. You can do this through implementation of OARS techniques and the steps of motivational interviewing.

OARS—To begin the conversation, ask open-ended questions, affirm his feelings (acknowledges competence and shows you are really listening), reflect and summarize his potential solutions and change talk.

O: p1. Why do you say/think you're dumb? p2. Why do you believe you are horrible at math? p3. How effective is your communication with your teacher?

A: p1. S: "Because I suck in class, I get bad grades, I don't get it." Y: "You feel dumb because you struggle in class and don't get good grades." p2. S: "Math is the worst. I know how to do it but not when the teacher makes these dumb stories. I don't understand why we can't just do the math problems." Y: "You're frustrated because you know how to do the calculations but really struggle with word problems." p3. S: "She doesn't listen." Y: "You feel like she doesn't listen.", follow up with another open-ended question, Y: "What do you say to her?" S: "I tell her it is stupid, no one is ever going to do these stupid stories." Y: "How effective is that?" (closed ended but foster self-assessment, self-confrontation). S: "Not." Y: "Can you think of a time when you were successful? What worked?" (now, I'm evoking) S: "One time, we mapped out the math problem to the story. That worked." Y: "Wow, that sounds interesting, tell me more." (now, I'm evoking more change talk) S: "I told her, I know how to do the math problem, I don't see how that connects with the story. She helped me find the parts in the story that gave me clues about the problem. It was like the only time I've ever gotten it." Y: "Again, wow, that sounds like a terrific approach. It sounds like the two of you worked together really well that time." Y: "How might you approach that in the future?" (now, I'm evoking again) S: "I could ask her to help me find the parts of the story that give me clues to the type of calculations I need to make."

R/S: Y: "You recognize that it helps when the teacher helps you find part of the story that help you know which calculations to make. Also, you recognize that asking her to help you with that could really help with your math work." (restating and reinforcing the student's change talk)

Steps of motivational interviewing—Engaging helps you to develop and maintain therapeutic alliance and have recent, positive interactions to draw upon when asking the student to do something that is difficult. In this case, you know that the student is struggling with algebra, so you can begin by verifying that this is an area of frustration. Next, you move into evoking the student's perspectives on the experience and potential solutions. Change talk comes as he identifies his own potential solutions. This is the point we left off in the reflections and summaries previously. Now that you have evoked a reasonable and actionable solution from the student, it's time to begin collaborative planning. This includes making a plan for how he is going to ask the teacher (perhaps a script), when he will ask (next class, meeting, etc.), and perhaps even take the first steps (e.g., sending an email to the teacher to initiate a meeting to discuss his request for help).

(continued)

Scenario #2. Counseling is necessary for all clients speech-language pathologists work with. For individuals beginning to use AAC and developing language, it's still possible to use motivational interviewing techniques—it just looks a little different. A client you are working with who is nonverbal and learning to use AAC is showing signs of distress. She has a tense facial expression, fists clenched, and vocalizations suggesting being upset.

In this case, start by roughly running through principles of **DARN** in your head. Does the student want to control their frustration/behave in an appropriate manner? The assumption is, yes. Does the student have the ability to control their frustration/behave positively? Consider past scenarios when you know they were successful and what that took or looked like. Does the student have reasons to behave appropriately? Hopefully, this is internally driven—they want to do well, rather than externally driven (i.e., they'll get punished if they don't control their frustration or they get a reward when they do). Need—do they recognize the potential impact of dealing with this moment to their success in other contexts? This is where our scaffolding comes in handy.

Here's how you might use **OARS** to help problem-solve the situation.

O: Asking open-ended questions and giving an opportunity to respond, scaffolding with choices when needed for language development/reducing linguistic demands.

A: Making sure to affirm feelings in the moment.

R/S: Reflecting and summarizing as a counseling approach, but also helps model more complex language for the student.

Bolded words suggest words you might highlight/model using the individual's AAC system as you go.

"I'm seeing that your **face** is tense, your **fists** are clenched, and it **sounds** like something is upsetting you. **How are you feeling**? Are you feeling **sad, mad, frustrated,** or something else?"

Student selects **frustrated** on AAC system.

"You're feeling **frustrated. It's okay** to feel that way. What made you **frustrated**?"

Student selects **loud.**

"Yeah—that assembly we were just at was really **loud**. I can see how the **loud noises** would make you feel **frustrated** or **overwhelmed**. When we feel **frustrated,** we can **do** some things to help us **calm down**. What would you like to do (preferred activities)—**take a break, do a puzzle,** or **other?**"

Student selects **take a break.**

"I think that's a great idea. You're feeling **frustrated** from the **loud** noises so you can **take a quiet break** to **calm down**."

Steps of motivational interviewing—Engaging allows you to have a therapeutic alliance with the client and also allows you to help predict what they might be trying to express when language is limited. Building on past experiences and what worked well for the client allows you to offer helpful choices—while also giving the option for "other." Evoking how the student felt and what made them feel that way allows you to collaboratively come up with a solution. In this situation, change talk is when the student suggests a coping strategy that would be beneficial for them. Moving forward, you can model for the student how they can express "I'm frustrated from loud noise, I need to take a break." This plan allows for a more independent and effective moment of emotional regulation in the future.

CAT—When loud, busy, and overwhelming situations take place, we can predict moments where a communication strategy and action (i.e., take a break) are eminent. Having a written plan or scripted response can help. Put action steps in place in anticipation of similar circumstances in the future.

*Case by Aspen Townsend

References

Baum, C., & Edwards D. F. (2008). *Activity card sort* (2nd ed.). American Occupational Therapy Association (AOTA Press).

Cook, D. A., & Artino Jr, A. R. (2016). Motivation to learn: An overview of contemporary theories. *Medical Education, 50*(10), 997-1014.

Cozby, P. C. (1973). Self-disclosure: A literature review. *Psychological Bulletin, 79*(2), 73.

Deci, E. L., & Ryan, R. M. (2012). *Self-determination theory.* In P. A. M. Van Lange, A. W. Kruglanski, & E. T. Higgins (Eds.), *Handbook of theories of social psychology* (pp. 416-436). Sage Publications Ltd. https://doi.org/10.4135/9781446249215.n21

Doig, E., Fleming, J., Kuipers, P., & Cornwell, P. L. (2010). Clinical utility of the combined use of the Canadian Occupational Performance Measure and Goal Attainment Scaling. *American Journal of Occupational Therapy, 64*(6), 904-914.

Ginsberg, J. I. D., Mann, R. E., Rotgers, F., & Weekes, J. R. (2002). Motivational interviewing: Preparing people for change. *Motivational interviewing with criminal justice populations, New York.*

Gustafsson, L., & McLaughlin, K. (2009). An exploration of clients' goals during inpatient and outpatient stroke rehabilitation. *International Journal of Therapy and Rehabilitation, 16*(6), 324-330. https://doi.org/10.12968/ijtr.2009.16.6.42435

Haley, K. L. (2021). Aphasia access distinguished speaker's series. https://www.aphasiaaccess.org/speakerseries/

Haley, K. L., Womack, J., Helm-Estabrooks, N., Lovette, B., & Goff, R. (2013). Supporting autonomy for people with aphasia: Use of the Life Interests and Values (LIV) cards. *Topics in Stroke Rehabilitation, 20*(1), 22-35. https://doi.org/10.1310/tsr2001-22

Hersh, D., Newitt, R., & Barnett, F. (2018). Change talk when talk has changed: Theoretical and practical insights into motivational interviewing in aphasia. *Aphasiology, 32*(Suppl. 1), 85-87.

Hersh, D., Worrall, L., Howe, T., Sherratt, S., & Davidson, B. (2012). SMARTER goal setting in aphasia rehabilitation. *Aphasiology, 26*(2), 220-233.

Hersh, D., Worrall, L., O'Halloran, R., Brown, K., Grohn, B. & Rodriguez, A. (2013). Assess for success: Evidence for therapeutic assessment. In N. Simmons-Mackie, J. King, & D. Beukelman (Eds.), *Supporting ommunication for adults with acute and chronic aphasia* (pp. 145-164). Brookes Publishing.

Hoepner, J. K., Sievert, A., & Guenther, K. (2021). Joint video self-modeling for persons with traumatic brain injury and their partners: A case series. *American Journal of Speech-Language Pathology, 30*(2S), 863-882.

Hughes, J. C., Bamford, C., & May, C. (2008). Types of centredness in health care: Themes and concepts. *Medicine, Health Care and Philosophy, 11*(4), 455-463. https://doi.org/10.1007/s11019-008-9131-5

Johnson, C. E., Jilla, A. M., & Danhauer, J. L. (2018). Developing foundational counseling skills for addressing adherence issues in auditory rehabilitation. *Seminars in Hearing, 39*(1), 13-31.

Kagan, A. (1998). Supported conversation for adults with aphasia: Methods and resources for training conversation partners. *Aphasiology, 12*(9), 816-830.

Kleim, J. A., & Jones, T. A. (2008). Principles of experience-dependent neural plasticity: Implications for rehabilitation after brain damage. *Journal of Speech, Language, and Hearing Research, 51*(1), S225-S239.

Lewis, T. F., Larson, M. F., & Korcuska, J. S. (2017). Strengthening the planning process of motivational interviewing using goal attainment scaling. *Journal of Mental Health Counseling, 39*(3), 195-210.

Malec, J. F. (1999). Goal attainment scaling in rehabilitation. *Neuropsychological Rehabilitation, 9*(3-4), 253-275.

Markland, D., Ryan, R. M., Tobin, V. J., & Rollnick, S. (2005). Motivational interviewing and self-determination theory. *Journal of Social and Clinical Psychology, 24*(6), 811-831.

McMorrow, M. J. (2003). *Getting ready to help: A primer on interacting in human service.* Paul H. Brookes Publishing.

Medley, A. R., & Powell, T. (2010). Motivational interviewing to promote self-awareness and engagement in rehabilitation following acquired brain injury: A conceptual review. *Neuropsychological Rehabilitation, 20*(4), 481-508.

Miller, W. R., & Rollnick, S. (2013). *Motivational interviewing: Helping people change.* Guilford Press.

Prochaska, J. O., & DiClemente, C. C. (2005). The transtheoretical approach. In J. C. Norcross & M. R. Goldfried (Eds.), *Handbook of psychotherapy integration* (pp. 147-171). Oxford University Press.

Rogers, C. R. (1965). *Client-centered therapy.* Houghton Mifflin.

Rollnick, S., Mason, P., & Butler, C. (1999). *Health behavior change: A guide for practitioners.* Churchill Livingstone.

Ryan, R. M., & Deci, E. L. (2000). Self-determination theory and the facilitation of intrinsic motivation, social development, and well-being. *American Psychologist, 55*(1), 68.

Sullivan, H. S. (1970). *The psychiatric interview.* Springer.

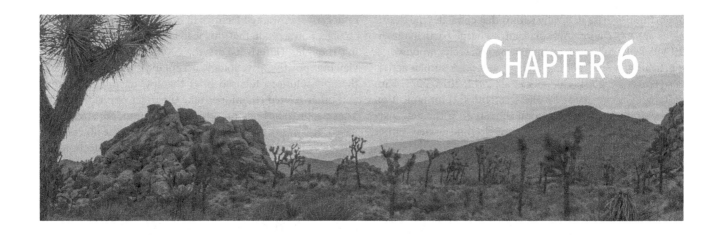

CHAPTER 6

Other Counseling Approaches in Speech-Language Pathology

Jerry K. Hoepner, PhD, CCC-SLP

Small steps can change a vicious cycle of problem maintenance to a virtuous cycle of problem resolution ~ John Wheeler

In the absence of meaningful engagement in chosen life activities, all interventions will ultimately fail. ~ Mark Ylvisaker

While motivational interviewing is a focus of this text, there is evidence for several other useful counseling approaches in speech-language pathology. For the most part, these approaches are not mutually exclusive or fundamentally dif erent from motivational interviewing. Many share the same core values and techniques. Having a sound knowledge and skills in multiple techniques will allow you to be flexible in meeting the needs of individual clients. Some approaches are likely a better fit for certain client types and age groups.

Behavioral Activation

While you may not think of behavioral activation as a counseling approach, it fits within Kneebone's (2016) Level 2 of the stepped care model of collaborative psychosocial care. Behavioral activation includes (1) activity scheduling, (2) mood monitoring, (3) graded task assignments (i.e., breaking complex tasks into manageable steps), (4) problem solving (i.e., identification of barriers to activity and reinforcement), and (5) promoting attention to the experience within the moment (e.g., mindfulness, meditation, and yoga practices). It can be delivered to individuals or groups. Many participation-based interventions and service delivery frameworks use behavioral activation (e.g., Life Participation Approach to Aphasia [Chapey et al., 2000], biopsychosocial models such as the World Health Organization's International Classification of Functioning, Disability and Health framework [2001]). Behavioral activation has relevance to any individuals and their partners/families who are at risk for social isolation due to their communication impairments and dif erences. This includes but is not limited to aphasia, dementias, stuttering, transgender communication, dysphagia, and any self-isolating individuals. In this approach, intervention is focused on increasing participation in personally relevant, personally selected, and personally meaningful activities. Once engaged in the activities, communication

Hoepner, J. K. (Ed.). *Counseling and Motivational Interviewing in Speech–Language Pathology* (pp. 95-114). © 2024 Taylor& Francis Group.

opportunities arise naturally within that context. One example is aphasia camps. Aphasia camps engage participants in activities like hiking, canoeing, kayaking, crafts, woodworking, fishing, sailing, golfing, archery, and other similar activities (Fox et al., 2004; Hoepner et al., 2012, 2016, 2021; Kim & Renzo Garcia, 2019). In these activities, communication is a byproduct of the behavioral activation. Ultimately, participation is believed to reduce depression and anxiety. Other examples include project-based interventions, intensive programs (e.g., intensive comprehensive aphasia programs, intensive comprehensive stuttering programs), and peer support groups.

Cognitive Behavioral Therapy

We will start with cognitive behavioral therapy (CBT) and put a small asterisk beside this topic. I believe it is fundamentally different from motivational interviewing and the remainder of the common approaches used in speech-language pathology. Secondly, while I feel pretty comfortable with scope of practice and the ability of well-trained speech-language pathologists to deliver motivational interviewing and each of the remaining techniques in this chapter, I caution speech-language pathologists that CBT lands solidly in the stepped care model Levels 3 and 4, although it is included as well in Level 2 (recall that most trained speech-language pathologists should feel comfortable in Levels 1 and 2; Kneebone, 2016). In my interpretation, CBT lands more firmly in the psychotherapy domain, which is not delivered by nonprofessional counselors unless they have specialized training and perhaps certification. That being said, Menzies et al. (2009) make a compelling argument that speech-language pathologists have been using many CBT techniques for years as a part of stuttering interventions. Likewise, Ylvisaker and Feeney (2000) advocated for a holistic approach to cognitive rehabilitation that draws upon psychotherapy principles and CBT, along with addressing cognition, communication, and behaviors in context. Given their bent toward positive psychology and positive routines, I think Ylvisaker and Feeney would approach CBT with some caution as well. One way that they addressed this was a shift toward separating irrational behaviors (in the case of brain injuries, caused by impaired self-awareness and self-regulation) from the individual's identity/sense of self. This is an important shift in theoretical and philosophical mindset, as it shifts the focus from ridding oneself of negative behaviors toward fostering positive behaviors. This includes the use of a positive model of self through metaphor (Ylvisaker & Feeney, 2000; Ylvisaker et al., 2008).

CBT is fundamentally different from most other counseling techniques used by speech-language pathologists and found in prior disciplinary research. The crux of that difference is the premise that CBT trains clients to rid themselves of negative, unwanted feelings in order to facilitate behavior change. Some argue that this leads to avoiding and repressing thoughts (Eifert & Forsyth, 2005). Motivational interviewing, positive psychology, acceptance and commitment therapy, solutions-focused brief therapy, narrative therapy, and other related techniques take the exact opposite stance. Those approaches rely on self-determination, are strengths-based, and even embrace acknowledgment of the illness narrative. That is not to say that CBT is not a valid technique, it just does not align as clearly with a person-centered, relationship-based, strengths-based approach, which are all central to the underlying approaches discussed in this text. CBT is an approach designed to address different kinds of mental health challenges, including those that are deeply entrained and perhaps less responsive to other approaches discussed here. Further, I do believe your philosophical mindset matters when approaching CBT.

CBT was initially developed for the treatment of depression (Beck, 1967). CBT is a psychological intervention that attempts to change thinking patterns. It is built on the premise that psychological problems are based on automatic, negative, faulty, or unhelpful ways of thinking. This results in learned patterns of negative or unhelpful behaviors. CBT is intended to teach better ways of coping with those behaviors and reducing their symptoms. In the case of acquired communication impairments, such as traumatic brain injuries, awareness of one's deficits and self-regulation are often impaired. For instance, irrational thoughts might include believing one can return to work when cognitive and/or physical status is not currently compatible with that goal. Ylvisaker and Feeney (2000, 2001, 2005) posited that CBT, along with a holistic, contextualized approach, can be used as a way to address those "irrational" thoughts in context.

CBT consists of three core techniques: cognitive restructuring, coping skills training, and problem solving (Frojan-Parga et al., 2009). **Cognitive restructuring** is the process of identifying and evaluating automatic thoughts and distortions, contrasting them with objective observations. **Automatic thoughts** are immediate, reflexive internal thoughts that are dysfunctional or negative. These thoughts can apply to oneself, the world, or the future (Gladding, 2009). For example, "I'll never be able to walk again," or "I'm worthless, it would have been better if I hadn't survived the accident." Many of these automatic thoughts contain cognitive distortions. **Cognitive distortions** are irrational or maladaptive thoughts. These include all-or-nothing thinking (e.g., "If I can't work, I might as well not live"), overgeneralizations (e.g., "None of the other kids stutter"), magnifications/catastrophizing (e.g., "If I can't talk fluently, I'll never get a job"), magical thinking (e.g., "If I can just get back home, I'll be fine"), dismissing positives (e.g., "That was just luck, it won't happen again"), and emotional reasoning (e.g., "I know I did worse than last time, because it felt really hard").

Cognitive restructuring involves four steps: (1) identify automatic thoughts, (2) address cognitive distortions, (3) identify and dispute irrational or maladaptive thoughts,

---

Box 6-1

Cognitive Restructuring Sequences

Overgeneralizations are <u>underlined</u>. Dismissing positives are *italicized*.

Minicase #1: It's a little more straight forward when their fears are irrational. For instance, a person who stutters who believes that "all" others will laugh at their stutter.

Identifying automatic thoughts—You ask, "What are you worried about?" Client replies, "<u>Everyone</u> will think I'm stupid and laugh at me."

Addressing cognitive distortions—You ask, "How likely is your worst fear to come true?" You could have them rate the likelihood, or you could have them rate how often they experience this response.

Identify and dispute irrational or maladaptive thoughts—You ask, "If your worst fear does come true, what is likely to happen?" Client replies, "I'll feel embarrassed."

Accept rational conclusions—Few people are likely to think I'm stupid and laugh at me.

Minicase #2: It gets a little muddier when their fears are at least somewhat rational or likely to happen. For instance, a person with aphasia fears falling out of the conversation because "nobody" will wait for them to talk.

Identifying automatic thoughts—You ask, "What are you worried about?" Client responds, "<u>Nobody</u> will wait for me to talk."

Addressing cognitive distortions—How likely is your worst fear to come true? "Some people don't wait." You could also have them rate likelihood on a rating scale. Follow-up question: Do some people wait? "*Yes, those that understand my aphasia.*"

Identify and dispute irrational or maladaptive thoughts—You ask, "If your worst fear does come true, what is likely to happen?" Client responds, "I just won't have a conversation with those people." You ask, "Is it possible to let them know about your aphasia, so they understand?" Client responds, "I suppose."

Accept rational conclusions—You ask, "What do you think about this statement? 'When people understand my aphasia, they are better at waiting for me to get my thoughts out.'" You could have them rate likelihood on a rating scale.

Of course, there is a little bit of truth in both "all" and "nobody" kinds of statements. It is an overgeneralization, but in both cases, they have likely experienced those responses.

---

and (4) accept rational conclusions (Hope et al., 2010). See Box 6-1 for two brief examples of cognitive restructuring sequences. This process is typically carried out through dialogue, role plays, and homework. Role plays are structured by the clinician, so they can be tailored to an appropriate level of challenge and to relate specifically to client goals. Homework is intended to foster exposure and practice in more real-life contexts. Menzies et al. (2009) used worksheets to challenge negative thoughts associated with stuttering. Two excellent worksheets are available in Appendices A and B of Menzies et al. (2009), which include prompts for predictions and actual outcomes. This parallels Ylvisaker and Feeney's (1998, 2009) obstacle-goal-plan-do-review framework for planning and self-evaluating performance in context, which is discussed further in Chapter 8.

Some automatic thoughts are more surface-level and make better choices for early targets. Others are deep seated and have become a part of a client's core cognitive schema, so they should not be addressed in early treatment (Heimberg & Becker, 2002). The Unhelpful Thoughts and Beliefs About

Stuttering checklist is a helpful tool for identifying negative and intrusive thoughts about stuttering (St. Clare et al., 2009).

Exposure therapy is another common CBT approach. This involves incrementally increasing exposure to triggers. In speech-language pathology, this includes pseudostuttering or voluntary stuttering (Menzies et al., 2008, 2009; Scheurich et al., 2019). Menzies et al. (2009) suggested moving from low-level fear situations toward more difficult tasks. Suggestions include use of the telephone, talking to respected people/people in authority, meeting people for the first time, meeting friends they haven't seen for a long time, and group presentations. Perhaps the client's irrational fear is that everyone will laugh at them. Following the exposure exercise, the client and clinician can reflect directly on this concrete experience (e.g., did everyone laugh at you?). Another application of exposure therapy could include engaging in a social conversation at a cofee shop, knowing you will experience word finding difficulties and other problems expressing yourself clearly—instead of avoiding the context

Box 6-2
Focusing on Strengths Does Not Mean Avoiding Weaknesses

This is a common scenario that student volunteers encounter/experience at our aphasia camp—a rustic, residential camp experience for adults with aphasia and their partners. Students start up a casual conversation with a camper with aphasia and you can just see the avoidance. Internally, they are thinking "Don't ask about their job, they can't do that anymore," or "don't ask about their hobbies, it might make them feel bad if they can't do them anymore." Those internal thoughts that prevent them from starting a conversation on those topics are at least partially the product of an impairment-focused mindset. In reality, those types of things (jobs, hobbies, etc.) are inseparable from their identity. For instance, I am a dad, husband, speech-language pathologist, and professor who likes fishing, woodworking, and traveling. If something alters my ability to participate in those roles, they remain a part of my identity. So, lean into those conversations in a compassionate, empathetic way but know that these are things that matter to them. This may help you uncover things that they can return to doing as well.

because it is a difficult context for interacting. This approach can begin with imagining/guided imagery and structured role plays before moving into real-life contexts. Ylvisaker and Feeney (1998, 2005, 2009) use the obstacle-goal-plan-do-review framework as a type of behavioral experiment to evaluate actual outcomes in context. This allows clients to self-confront irrational behavior. For instance, at the outset, in the client's prediction, they may say, "I can complete this [work related] task in 10 minutes with no errors," but upon completion, they may see that it took longer to complete and that they made several errors. If set up well, the client makes these assessments and realization about their "faulty" thinking, rather than receiving negative input from the clinician. Beyond therapy sessions, these type of behavioral experiments must be carried out in everyday environments as well (Ylvisaker & Feeney, 2005).

Self-paced computerized CBT treatment has been used to address social anxiety in stuttering (Helgadottir et al., 2014; Menzies et al., 2016). The approach uses information gathered in pretreatment assessment to develop personalized behavioral experiments and exposure tasks. **Behavioral experiments** help clients to calibrate actual probability estimates because the client conducts the experiment. For example, if a client voluntarily stutters with friends, they can measure how often the response corresponds with their fear (e.g., how often voluntarily stuttering results in a friend laughing at them).

CBT has been used extensively to treat tinnitus, often being paired with masking therapy and sound treatment. It has been shown to be efficacious (Li et al., 2019) and several meta-analyses exist (Hesser et al., 2011; Landry et al., 2020).

Positive Psychology and Coaching

Traditional psychology theories have a focus or emphasis on pathology. Positive psychology is a relatively new theoretical stance, built upon the basic principles of positive emotions and personal strengths. A number of individuals and theories have contributed to the development of positive psychology, including Rogers's principles of the fully functioning person (1965), Maslow's self-actualization (1954-1971), Deci and Ryan's self-determination theory (1985), Csikszentmihalyi and Csikszentmihalyi's concept of flow (1990), and Ryf and Singer's psychological well-being (1996). Martin Seligman, however, is often credited as being the founder of positive psychology, given his work on learned helplessness, optimism, and authentic happiness (1991 to 2006).

Seligman suggests that rather than focusing on positives (e.g., relatively good mental health, quality of life, contentment, and satisfaction), we often overfocus on problems (e.g., addressing mental health problems). This myopic view overlooks a focus on well-being. In speech-language pathology, there is a clear parallel to theoretical perspectives on the individuals we serve. An impairment-based approach in speech-language pathology focuses on the articulation errors, word finding problems, memory problems, dysphagia, and other impairments, rather than identifying what the person can do through a strengths-based approach. See Box 6-2 for an example of how this has become engrained in our way of thinking. Participation-based approaches, such as the Life Participation Approach (Chapey et al., 2000), emphasize engaging in personally selected activities as the starting point. This type of approach flips the table, focusing on re-engaging with a whatever-it-takes (strengths-based) mindset. Engaging in personally selected and meaningful activity provides opportunities for practicing communication in context, rather than within contrived tasks. Such approaches align well with a positive psychology approach.

Seligman (2011) identified five elements that compose well-being in the **PERMA** model (Positive emotion, Engagement, Relationships, Meaning, and Accomplishment). These elements are measurable and correlate strongly with subjective well-being—achieving them enables people to flourish, find happiness, and thrive. Further, these elements moderately correlate with one another (Goodman et al., 2017). Let's explore the model and consider how it may be applied within speech-language pathology. ***Positive emotion*** is a mindset of positive affect. Achieving and maintaining positive affect relies on recalling the good things from one's past, engaging in pleasurable moments within the present moment, and having a positive outlook or expectations for the future. Of course, problems such as communication disorders can disrupt those positive emotions and divert attention toward negative emotions. Positive psychology interventions designed to foster a positive mindset, optimism, gratitude, and well-being are discussed following this PERMA section.

Engagement is the process of participating in personally selected activities. This is more about doing something you want to do than doing something well. Becoming absorbed in an activity, losing sense of time, and perhaps forgetting about those challenges and negative emotions for a while is often described as a state of ***flow*** (Csikszentmihalyi & Csikszentmihalyi, 1990). Fostering engagement and providing necessary scaffolding to achieve a relative match between level of challenge and ability (with supports) can help people to achieve ***flow***. Fostering ***flow*** requires attention to environmental factors that support engagement and considering the balance of skill and challenge in meaningful life activities (Sather et al., 2017). This includes modifying the environment and providing scaffolding for successful participation, such as supported conversation techniques or physical access supports. Following a similar framework, the environmental press model (Lawton & Nahemow, 1973), Hoepner et al. (2018) suggested it is necessary to balance the level of challenge and support to optimize participation. Simply stated, too much challenge without enough support results in less-than-optimal participation. Likewise, insufficient challenge can result in less-than-optimal participation, as clients may feel patronized, bored, or unstimulated by the task. Our role in this type of situation is to collaboratively identify meaningful activity, fostering appropriate choices about level of challenge and scaffolding success with whatever supports are needed.

Relationships are crucial to well-being. Maintaining and nurturing authentic connections with others requires some form of communication. Janice Light (1997), in a seminal paper on communication and augmentative and alternative communication (AAC), emphasized the importance of developing social closeness for individuals with communication impairments. This is achieved not only through supported communication but through mutual engagement in meaningful activity. It's not the quantity but the quality that people desire; feeling alone in a crowd is still feeling alone (Dalemans et al., 2010).

Finding ***meaning*** includes a sense of belonging and/or contributing to something meaningful. Levasseur et al. (2010) developed a taxonomy of social experiences, which emphasized the overlap between relationships and sense of purpose or meaning (Figure 6-1). Simply being with others is on the lower end of the hierarchy of social experiences, while helping others or more broadly contributing to society

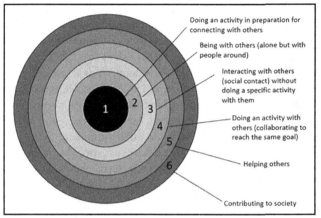

Figure 6-1. Taxonomy of Social Experiences (Reproduced with permission from Levasseur, M., Desrosiers, J., & Whiteneck, G. (2010). Accomplishment level and satisfaction with social participation of older adults: Association with quality of life and best correlates. *Quality of Life Research, 19*(5), 665-675.).

are more fulfilling. Behn (2016) suggested that project-based interventions can help achieve this desire for purpose and meaning, as they are situated between levels 4 and 5. Behn et al. (2016) argued the importance of this approach in developing self-worth and improving quality of life. Among the tenets of project-based interventions is the production of a concrete product that is meaningful to the client, who takes on the expert role, collaborating with others to produce something designed to help others (Feeney & Capo, 2010; Ylvisaker et al., 2007). In fact, Feeney and Capo (2010) identified the central purpose of project-based interventions as ***meaning making***.

This all connects to the final element of PERMA, ***accomplishment***. The pursuit and achievement of goals for their own sake is central to intrinsic motivation. Setting and meeting goals begins with the process of collaborative goal setting and in many cases, fostering self-assessment and improved self-awareness in order to jointly identify actionable and achievable goals. This includes not only self-identification of goals but self-evaluation of goals. The use of self-assessed goal attainment scales may improve self-awareness (Doig et al., 2010; Hoepner et al., 2021; Malec, 1999). Conjointly examining outcomes gives clients a direct role in measuring outcomes. Making those accomplishments meaningful is at the heart of person-centered care, collaborative goal setting (discussed previously in Chapters 4 and 5), and project-based interventions (Behn, 2016; Behn et al., 2016, Feeney & Capo, 2010; Ylvisaker et al., 2007).

Positive Psychology Exercises and Interventions

There are a number of established and evidence-based positive psychology interventions. Bolier et al. (2013) provided an exceptional review of positive psychology interventions in their meta-analysis of 39 investigations. In particular, readers are directed toward Table 2 (Bolier et al., 2013, pp. 7-10) for an overview of interventions and outcomes. What follows is not an exhaustive list but an intentionally selected list for consideration as a part of your interactional toolbox. Note that Holland and Nelson (2020) dedicated a great deal more discussion to positive psychology and included a number of useful exercises and ideas, some that are included here and others unique to their text. It may help to think of these exercises as prophylactic, in that they preempt negative thought by fostering positive thought and establishing a positive mindset. The intent is to cultivate a client's sense of gratitude, optimism, and well-being. This makes these interventions relatively easy to combine with other communication and counseling interventions.

- **Count your blessings** involves keeping a gratitude journal, given the following prompt, "There are many things in our lives to be grateful about. Think back over the past week and write down on the lines below up to five things in your life that you are grateful or thankful for" (Emmons & McCullough, 2003). This approach has been used with people without specific impairments and those with impairments such as neuromuscular disease. In all conditions, individuals in the counting blessings condition demonstrated greater positive af ect, more optimism, and a better connection to others than the control condition or the alternate condition—listing hassles. Positive ef ects have been noted with adolescents as well (Froh et al., 2008; Huebner et al., 2000).

- **Three good things** asks people to identify three good things that happened over the course of a week and identify the contributors to these positive events (e.g., I lost 3 pounds because I went on daily walks). Positive ef ects of this intervention were not immediate but appeared 3 to 6 months later (Seligman et al., 2005).

- **Grateful self-reflection** asks people to meditate on these questions weekly: "What did I receive? What did I give? What more could I do?" (Chan, 2010).

- **Practicing optimism** asks people to journal about "their best possible life in the future" (Boehm et al., 2011).

- **Gratitude letters** asks people to write letters of appreciation to people to whom they are grateful. It has more value when sent than when simply written and not sent (Boehm et al., 2011).

- **Gratitude visits** asks people to deliver their letters of appreciation in person. Ef ects were stronger and more enduring when they deliver the letter in person than when they simply write the letter (Seligman et al., 2005). See Pickering's examples in Chapter 8.

In summary, PERMA (Seligman, 2011) can be supported by positive psychology strategies and common speech-language pathology interventions:

- Positive emotions can be fostered by helping clients to recognize and savor positive moments. This can be approached through gratitude and optimism exercises.

- Increasing engagement can help clients to identify and use their strengths. Goal setting and monitoring approaches can help them recognize their abilities.

- Encouraging development and maintenance of relationships can be facilitated through communication partner training.

- Life participation approaches and project-based interventions can help clients find meaning and a sense of accomplishment.

Acceptance and Commitment Therapy

Acceptance and commitment therapy (ACT) is a counseling intervention that blends mindfulness and acceptance processes with commitment and behavior change processes (Hayes et al., 1999; Hayes, 2004). The goal is to work toward psychological flexibility. Our external behaviors (what we do in the world) can be a reflection of our internal behaviors (what we think in our minds). While some of our external behaviors can be adaptive (e.g., avoiding challenging situations), these behaviors can be harmful when they become part of our internal thought processes. This relates to the concept of *experiential avoidance*, whereby avoiding thoughts or behaviors leads to less resolution and exacerbation of the problem (Hayes et al., 1996). If we avoid everything that feels frustrating, makes us angry, makes us feel down or depressed, or makes us feel anxious, our range of remaining activities becomes highly restricted, and we become increasingly isolated. *Cognitive fusion* occurs when we connect a thought to an experience (Hayes, 1989). For example, we associate an amusement park with fear or school with anxiety. A key element of ACT is becoming mindful of our thoughts and values. This helps us to make a choice about when to act on our thoughts—when our thoughts align with our values. This helps us to move toward psychological flexibility, a state where we are comfortable with both good and bad feelings, which allows us to control our behaviors and live a meaningful life. These ideas are eloquently captured in the ACT Hexaflex: being present, acceptance, defusion, self-as-context, committed action, and values, which result in psychological flexibility (Figure 6-2).

ACT values continuous, nonjudgmental connections between psychological (our thoughts) and environment (our physical context) in the moment. This allows us to *be present* in the moment, rather than ruminating on the past or worrying about the future. There is increasing attention to the principles of mindfulness in speech-language pathology. We are better positioned to engage in the interactions of the moment and respond to them when we are mindful. Meditation and deep breathing have been used to help persons who stutter remain present in the moment and decrease avoidance of speaking situations (Beilby & Byrnes, 2012; Beilby & Yarus, 2018; Plexico & Sandage, 2011).

Acceptance is a willingness to embrace all that the moment brings, the good and the bad, the joyful and the painful. This is fundamentally different from resignation, the idea that this is their lot in life and that they should just give up. Instead, clients are encouraged to feel their struggles and then let them go. They are also encouraged to feel their successes and joys, rather than overlooking them by avoiding the moment. This recognizes that we won't/can't be happy all of the time.

Let's return for a moment to the concept of feeling and letting go of struggles. Whereas cognitive behavioral therapy compels clients to rid themselves of negative thoughts, ACT asks clients to feel them and let them go (Hayes, 2008). As humans, we tend to attach significance to our thoughts (cognitive fusion). *Defusion* is the process of creating separation between the client and their thoughts (Hayes & Wilson, 1994). A classic defusion technique is the *Milk, Milk, Milk* exercise, whereby you have the client explore properties of the word milk. The word is then repeated in chorus by the client and clinician for about a minute. The word begins to lose meaning, just becoming a sound. The point is to separate thoughts from their meanings. This is the idea that even in the face of sad, frustrating, or challenging thoughts/feelings, the client can continue to interact with the world in a manner consistent with their values. You might think of this process as evaluating or vetting your thoughts. One strategy is to identify "silly thoughts." For instance, you might say to yourself, "I had a silly thought. I keep thinking that I'm not good enough to do this before I've really even tried." or conversely, "I think I can do this; I might as well try." We may need to prompt, "What's the flip side?" Another approach is having clients identify their thoughts, "I'm having the thought that there is just too much to overcome; it's just not possible." and conversely, "I'm having the thought that this is a lot to take on; I've got to break this down into achievable steps." Again, we may need to prompt, "What would it take to overcome it?" Learning to appreciate but move forward from difficult moments can help defuse negative thoughts. When we recognize a client is overwhelmed by their thoughts, we may scaffold this defusion by prompting, "Tell me what you're thinking right now." The client might respond "For a moment, I felt like the world was really crashing down on me. I had to step back and recognize that the moment would pass to be able to think about moving forward." The idea is becoming aware that one's thoughts can derail their actions, so taking a moment to take stock can allow us to avoid being led by our emotional responses to a moment. For instance, Beilby and Byrnes (2012) encouraged people who stutter to notice their thoughts, specifically their negative thoughts associated with stuttering. By recognizing those negative reactions as thoughts, persons who stutter can manage their emotional responses, in part by recognizing that they are an unavoidable response to stuttering (Beilby & Byrnes, 2012; Beilby & Yaruss, 2018). In this way, the person accepts the stutter and emotions associated with it, rather than avoiding the interaction and withdrawing.

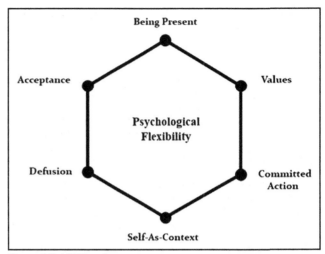

Figure 6-2. ACT Hexaflex.

We all have a tendency to conceptualize ourselves, having a strong sense of who we are. This can certainly be constructive but it can also inadvertently create limitations or fixations on who we are or are not. For instance, I recently heard my nephew say, "I'm not a school person. School does not agree with me." This assumes that "school" is a uniform experience and that he cannot adapt. Hayes (2004) calls this a *I-here-now frame*, whereby *I* experienced this thought *here* and *now*, so it becomes a pattern of thinking—the here and now are cognitively fused to the thought. ACT attempts to move clients toward *self-as-context* (perspective taking), where they let go of their attachment to who they are in situations where that conceptualization is limiting or harmful (Hayes et al., 2004). Again, ACT encourages us think about ourselves as independent evaluators. If we step back to the observational role, what do we see? ACT has been used to explore emotions that persons associate with being "a person who stutters" (Beilby & Byrnes, 2012; Beilby & Yaruss, 2018). The intent is to separate the emotions associated with the experience of stuttering from their view of being a person who stutters (Beilby & Byrnes, 2012; Beilby & Yaruss, 2018). In this way, they can view themselves with more objectivity, reducing or eliminating the emotional biases associated with being a person who stutters.

Committed action is demonstrated through development of larger patterns of behavior, which are tied to the client's values. This is inherently tied to the collaborative goal setting process, helping us to collaboratively set achievable goals and address barriers to goal achievement. We can explore those values through structured interviews, as described in depth in Chapter 4.

Hayes et al. (2004) provide an excellent framework for thinking through individual client cases. Five distinct steps are identified as crucial to developing a treatment plan:

1. Analyze the scope and nature of the presenting problem.
2. Assess factors affecting the client's level of motivation for change.

3. Analyze the factors that detract from the client's psychological flexibility.

4. Assess factors that are promoting psychological flexibility.

5. Develop a treatment goal and associated set of interventions.

This can be summed up as identifying *the problem* (e.g., feelings about stuttering, word finding difficulties, and memory problems that would lead to avoidance or withdrawal), *motivation factors* (e.g., self-efficacy to improve—I can/can't, tangible intrinsic reasons to participate like enjoyment, extrinsic ideas like fear of consequences like dismissal from rehab, history of rule following—"I should" mindset, or belief in the rationale for treatment), *barriers to flexibility* (e.g., avoidance, poor persistence or self-regulation, negative self-assessments, maladaptive coping behaviors—substance use/self-mutilation/over- or under-eating/suicide attempts, or thought fusion), and *goal setting*. A number of assessment and intervention tools are available through ACT and relational frame theory websites (www.acceptanceandcommitmenttherapy.com and www.relationalframetheory.com). This includes the Automatic Thoughts Questionnaire, Child and Adolescent Specific ACT Measures, Comprehensive Assessment of Acceptance and Commitment Therapy Processes, Emotion Efficacy Scale, Fusion Measures, Hexaflex Measure, Mindfulness Measures, Self-Care Monitoring Forms, State Self Compassion Scale, Values Measure, and more.

Solutions Focused Brief Therapy

Solutions focused brief therapy (SFBT) helps clients to envision their preferred future; recognize positive signs of change; and explore resources, skills, and resilience (de Shazer, 1988; Ratner et al., 2012). As the name implies, SFBT is designed to be delivered in three to eight sessions. SFBT is intended to be a conversation. It begins by asking clients questions about how they define the way they would like their lives to be and how they will know if they have achieved that preferred life. This begins by developing a focus and direction for the conversation that addresses what the client wants. Once we've established a direction, we need to elicit from them a detailed description of their preferred future or best hopes.

Wheeler (2001) eloquently describes the basic assumptions of SFBT:

SFBT ASSUMPTIONS	HOEPNER'S IMPLICATIONS
Presenting problems are seldom static—they usually vary in frequency and intensity.	If something is not a big deal today, it doesn't mean it won't be tomorrow and vice versa.
Clients often have resources to deal with their difficulties.	Assume they have resources and expertise to deal with problems.
Small steps can change a vicious cycle of problem maintenance to a virtuous cycle of problem resolution.	Accept incremental changes and encourage clients to do the same. Small changes can foster a ripple effect.
The clinician's responsibility is not to offer the client solutions but to help them find their own.	Elicit the client's solutions, rather than prescribing ours.
Problems fluctuate in their severity and exceptions are waiting to be found.	Have an eye for exceptions and scaffold client's ability to self-identify them by freeze framing in context, playing back videos or audio, debriefing about successes.

Two additional assumptions are central to SFBT. Clients are considered to be *experts* of their own lives, being competent and coequal to the clinician (Hanton, 2011; Jones-Smith, 2012; Lipchik et al., 2012). Because the client is the expert, the clinician follows a *not-knowing* approach (De Jong & Berg, 2013). In a *not-knowing* stance, the clinician demonstrates genuine curiosity in their client and takes an interpretive approach to client descriptions of their experiences. Further, the clinician asks not-knowing questions to dig deep into client experiences (e.g., "Tell me more" or "What do you mean by this?" or "Help me to understand this better"). These questions can be helpful in withholding judgment and our tendency to provide expert advice or solutions (Iveson & McKergow, 2015).

SFBT is composed of several techniques. *Problem-free talk* is an approach to eliciting talk about aspects of the client's life outside of their problems (Wheeler, 2001). This includes talking about coping, work, and aspects of life where they enjoy success. For instance, "Let's set x challenges aside for a moment, tell me about some things that are working or going well." *Goal clarification* is the process of guiding a client toward envisioning a future without their current problem. Key questions about this preferred future include "What would be different from your current life?", "How would you know if you had achieved your preferred life?", "How will others know?", "How would your partner respond differently to you?", and "How will your interactions be different?" Our follow-up questions dig deeper into each of these questions, seeking as much detail as possible. This begins to construct an alternative narrative of the future and what it would look like. The entire conversation is built around three key ideas: (1) how you will know, (2) how others will know, and (3) embedding the preferred future into their everyday patterns of interaction. Sometimes, parents or clients themselves become so focused on problems that they forget successes (Wheeler, 2001). White (1995) calls this **problem saturated thinking**. A process of **illuminating the exception** is used to identify a time or times when the problem was overcome or didn't happen and what actions or factors made this possible. Essentially the focus becomes solutions, rather than the problem (Jones-Smith, 2012). SFBT encourages clients to do more of what works, and if it is not working, to do something different (Jones-Smith, 2012). SFBT places one foot in possibility while maintaining the other foot in acknowledgment of the problem (O'Hanlon & Beadle, 1997). This includes acknowledging the emotional impact of the problem.

Much of the power of SFBT comes from the questions asked, so considering how you make those questions communicatively accessible is important. Northcott et al. (2015) suggested modifications such as simple syntactic structures, sign-posted topic changes, and chunking information into short phrases. Further, repeating back parts of the client's messages as you understood them and using closed ended questions to confirm meaning provide a means of verification. As a rule, it is easier for people to respond to clarifications in the moment. Therefore, respectful, periodic interruptions are often necessary, rather than letting the person go on extensively, which makes it harder for them to recall and reflect on the context. Additionally, SFBT values preserving as many of the client's exact words as possible when repeating back statements for confirmation and verification. This assures reiteration of the client's solutions for best hopes/preferred future.

Some common language and techniques used for goal oriented and future-oriented thinking include:

- **A great night's sleep/Miracle question:** A hallmark question used with SFBT is de Shazer's (1988) **miracle question,** "Now, I want to ask you a strange question. Suppose that while you are sleeping tonight and the entire house is quiet, a miracle happens. The miracle is that the problem which brought you here is solved. However, because you are sleeping, you don't know that the miracle has happened. So, when you wake up tomorrow morning, what will be different that will tell you that a miracle has happened and the problem which brought you here is solved?" (p. 5). This can also be addressed as one's best hopes or preferred future. Northcott et al.

(2015) modified the miracle question to make it more communicatively accessible to persons with aphasia, "Suppose when you go to sleep tonight, a miracle happens and the problems that brought you here today are solved. But since you are asleep, you don't know the miracle has happened until you wake up tomorrow; what will be different tomorrow that will tell you that the miracle has happened?" (p. 13). In length alone, the prompt was cut from 79 to 51 words, not to mention decreasing linguistic complexity. However, it was still too complex and was thought that being cured was an unrealistic hope. Therefore, it was replaced by the **tomorrow question**, "Let's imagine tomorrow everything goes really well [pause]. What is the first thing you'll notice?" (p. 14). We have retained all three versions here, as you may wish to create your own version to suit clients. It is more about the concept than the wording, so choose something that makes sense for your clients.

  ∘ Write, gesture, draw, find photos, or take photos of what your life looks like with a miracle or preferred future. Northcott et al. (2015) also used objects in the environment, clients' phones, and Talking Mats.
  ∘ Who is there to support you and how?
  ∘ What have you done to make it happen?

- **Experiment invitation/Exception questions:** Invite clients to build upon what is already working. Using experiments to find out what is working also provides learning about what is not working, so those approaches can be eliminated.

  ∘ When were things better?
  ∘ What were you doing differently?
  ∘ What else was different?
  ∘ What would you have to do to have more times like this?

- **Coping questions:** This gets at resiliency and puts them in the expert role.

  ∘ What helped you through these struggles?
  ∘ What have you done to make it through?
  ∘ What helps?

- **Scaling questions/Rating scales:** Use a simple rating scale, from 1 to 10 (1 = worst, 10 = best) to respond to questions about your life. Northcott et al. (2015) replaced the anchor *best hopes realized* for 10 with *living with aphasia the best way you can*. The intent was to make a more concrete association with the client's personal challenges and goals. The key is to personalize and ensure comprehension of the anchors.

  ∘ Rate your ability/opposite of the problem (e.g., ability to talk clearly, ability to remember, organization, etc.) today.

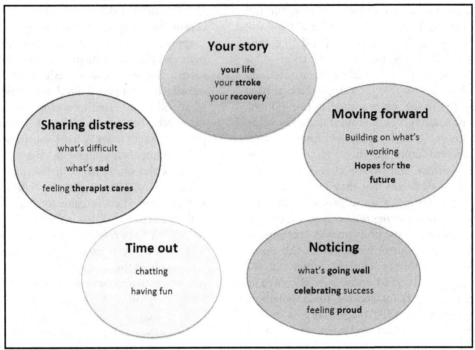

Figure 6-3. Proposed components of an adapted SFBT program for aphasia. (Northcott et al. / desaturated from original / CC BY 4.0).

Box 6-3

Solutions Focused Brief Therapy

Check out this great podcast conversation on Aphasia Access Conversations Podcast Episode #64 with Dr. Sarah Northcott as she discusses SFBT and the SOFIA trial.

https://aphasiaaccess.libsyn.com/solution -focused-brief-therapy-a-counseling-approach -for-slps-in-conversation-with-sarah-northcott

---

° Rate your ability 1 or 2 days ago, 1 or 2 months ago, 1 or 2 years ago. What was happening/what was different when it was higher?

° When your ability decreases, what strategies do you use to improve things?

° What is a reasonable goal for your ability in 1 month (or whatever time frame you choose)?

° What would it take to move you up one point on the scale? How would you know when you were one point better?

° What strategies, skills, and abilities do you have that would help you move up on the scale?

° What have you learned about yourself from previous experiences?

Northcott et al. (2021) examined the perceptions of individuals with aphasia regarding the SOFIA trial using SFBT. In this work they share the framework for the proposed elements of their adapted SFBT program (Figure 6-3). The five-component framework includes Your Story, Moving Forward, Noticing, Time Out, and Sharing Distress. The framework appears to be a simple but eloquent tool for implementing SFBT with individuals with aphasia, and likely other communication disorders. The study found that individuals with aphasia all believed that an adapted SFBT approach could be used with individuals with aphasia. Two overarching themes were identified, including valued therapy components (exploring hopes, noticing achievements, companionship, sharing feelings, and relationship with the therapist) and perceptions of progress (in terms of mood, identity, communication, relationships, and independence). Specifically, they valued opportunities to discuss their hopes, achievements, and experiences, given communication supports. After SFBT, individuals with aphasia felt better about themselves, with increased confidence to begin or return to personal activities such as conversations with friends and family, taking the garbage out, use public transportation, or starting a volunteer position. There were four categories of participants, the "changed" group (therapy had a meaningful impact on their life), the "connected" group (therapy was valued primarily for companionship), the "complemental" group (where SFBT was a complement to other things they were doing to improve), and the "discordant" group (who wanted to engage in impairment-based communication work rather than SFBT). The relationship with the therapist was key to their experience and outcomes. This adapted framework appears to have good potential to help individuals with aphasia, and may also be a good fit for other communication disorders. For a great podcast conversation with Dr. Sarah Northcott on SFBT, see the link in Box 6-3.

Action plans are a helpful tool for making multistep goals tangible and trackable. A variety of tools exist that prompt information about end goals, pie-in-the-sky goals (best hopes), actionable steps, resources needed to meet the goals, and indicators of success. Some include prompts to identify strengths and challenges. Rating scales can be included to track confidence.

Can Solutions Focused Brief Therapy Be Modified for Use With Children?

Several articles address specific implementation issues (Lloyd & Dallos, 2006; Wheeler, 2001). Research evidence includes a recent meta-analysis of SFBT in children and adolescents (Hsu et al., 2021) and several systematic reviews (Bond et al., 2013; Woods et al. 2011). The National Society for Prevention of Cruelty to Children has created a very accessible and easy to follow toolkit for working with children ages 5 to 19 years old (Bazalgette et al., 2015). The toolkit is available at https://learning.nspcc.org.uk/research-resources/2015/solution-focused-practice-toolkit. All of the techniques are cross referenced to evidence-based applications of SFBT with children (Berg & Steiner, 2003; Milner & Bateman, 2011; Ratner et al., 2012; Shennan & Wells, 2014). It includes tools for explaining and implementing SFBT, including "My Journey," "Ladders and Tool Bags," and cartoon stories. All are accompanied by child-friendly graphics and text. *My Journey* includes questions and prompts, such as "What am I already doing well?", "What can I do differently to help me get to my goal?", and "What are my hopes?" (Bazalgette et al., 2015, p. 8). *Ladders and Tool Bags* is a Chutes and Ladders–like game that prompts questions about skills and strengths. *Jamie's Cartoon Story* explores strengths and interests, along with child-friendly versions of common SFBT prompts. For example, "Imagine a time machine that you can take into the future . . ." (like a TARDIS) and the *Crystal Ball* can be used to explore best hopes (pp. 12-13, 30-31). Scaling techniques are also used, very much like they are for standard SFBT. The *My Likes and Strengths* tool explores interests through drawing and questions. Strengths can also be explored through sorting strengths cards. There are a number of drawing and writing exercises that explore strengths and interests, including a special camera that catches clients doing things they're good at and a mind map/spider diagram of the things they like about themselves. Several of the exercises use metaphors to explore growth. Exploring goals and growth can be augmented using the *Traffic Lights* activity (red = worst, yellow = now, green = where you want to go). Likewise, the *Change the Channel* drawing exercise explores what life might be like if things were better for you. For younger children, the *Talking Through Puppets* exercise allows them to talk about themselves in the third person, particularly if they're shy or reticent to share directly. Preferred future is explored through *Waving a Magic Wand*, the *Miracle Day*, *Time Machine*, and other similar tools. Achievements that show how the child will know they have met their goals include metaphors such as ***climbing a mountain***, ***climbing a ladder***, or ***taking off*** with a rocket ship. Physical objects such as a staircase or hopscotch can be used if a more concrete visual is needed. Achievement walls and scrapbooks can be used to track goals and achievements. A ***salt jar*** can be used to represent strategies, with different colored salt or sand is added in layers within the jar to represent strategies. Altogether, this toolkit is a great resource for structuring SFBT with children, particularly because it includes activities to fit a range of ages and interests.

Narrative Approach

The fundamental, underlying impetus for the narrative approach relates to the tendency of traditional psychology and society for that matter, to focus on impairments, shortcomings, or differences (particularly undesirable differences). A basic premise of the narrative approach is that we are all story tellers. We construct our own stories but our stories are typically coconstructed by the people who surround us. The stories that we tell about ourselves and the stories others tell about us shape our behaviors and sense of self (Neimeyer, 1995). In this manner, personal narratives synthesize meaning from experiences, both past and future (Dimaggio et al., 2003). Our story becomes our identity, so the way we plan and respond to our future relates to the identity we've created, making it somewhat predictable. Sometimes, however, outside people or events influence our story lines in ways that are undesirable or limiting (Neimeyer, 1995). This includes cultural stereotypes and expectations, which can begin to dominate a client's personal narrative and thus the way they interpret their world (Wolter et al., 2006). People often seek or are referred to therapy when their impairments become their identity (Neimeyer, 1995). These defeatist, hopeless, and limiting thoughts are sometimes imposed by others as the result of assessment results that emphasize impairments rather than abilities (Stacey, 1997). When such thoughts become a person's dominant narrative, they have the potential to profoundly affect motivation and the way people look at the future. White and Epston (1990) described the language such individuals use in describing their life as ***problem-saturated*** and ***thin descriptions*** because events, details, and things not related to their disorder are left out. For instance, DiLollo et al. (2005) found that individuals who stutter attribute little or no meaning to periods of fluent speech and successful therapy, which contributed to stuttering persistence. So, this all begs the question, how do we turn the tables on defeatist attitudes and identities?

Neimeyer (2001) suggested that narratives can be a mechanism for adaptation and renegotiating identity when people experience loss. Our role is to help redirect clients in moving their narratives from passive to active and thus be in control of how their future story unfolds (Randall, 1995), for example, "this happened to me" vs. "I did this." Tools for scaffolding sharing of personal narratives include *Your Life: Looking Back, Moving Forward*, which includes pictographic supports (Sinden, 2015). Strong and Shadden (2020) emphasize reconstructing identity through personal narrative and life stories. Consistent with Wolter et al. (2006), principles of externalizing the problem, identifying the influence of the problem, and then reconstructing/reshaping the storylines, Strong and Shadden (2020) suggested directly tackling how the problem (stroke and aphasia) impacts a person's life story. This includes fostering the sharing and validation of illness narratives, then using small stories and anecdotes in shaping reconstruction. "The power of story lies in the fact that stories are dynamic and subject to change. Stories are told and retold, and during the retelling, the storyteller may view the content of the story differently and ultimately view how the situation has impacted his or her life" (Strong & Shadden, 2020, p. 373). We all do this, right? "I didn't get into X university," becomes "not getting into X university made me realize what great opportunities Y university offered," becomes "Even though I had hoped to get accepted at X university, I've decided Y university was actually a better fit for me." The intent is for identity to shift toward one that includes the problem but rewrites the future in a positive, aspirational manner. This can be accomplished through small stories/everyday narratives, illness narratives, and big stories/life story narratives (Bamberg, 2010; Strong & Shadden, 2020). An important point is that this is more than a "silver lining" kind of thing, which could be perceived as patronizing. This is a reshaping and reimagining of one's present and future identity. See Box 6-4 for a real-life application of this approach.

Wolter et al. (2006) identified three basic elements of the narrative approach to counseling:

1. **Externalize the problem:** The intent here is to separate the problem from personal identity, to the extent possible. This includes modeling externalizing language. An interesting example of this comes in an advertisement campaign by coaches against cancer. Coaches in the commercials make statements like "I hate you, cancer," "You're going down, cancer," and even "expletive you, cancer" that exemplify the attempt to model the mindset of overcoming the problem. What if we did this, perhaps without the expletives, for our clients? This encourages our clients to give the problem a name and talk about it in the third person.

2. **Map the influence of the problem on the life of the person:** Our role is to encourage "thick" description and listen for clues to alternative storylines. Remember, "thin" descriptions are problem-saturated and leave out things not related to the problem. Thick descriptions encourage clients to provide detailed information about the impact of the problem on all aspects of their lives. Of course, providing more information can provide clues for inconsistencies, positive experiences, and alternative storylines.

3. **Map the influence of the person on the problem:** This is where we begin to redirect narratives from passive to active, putting them in control of their lives.

   ○ **Unique outcome questions:** Can you think of times when . . . the problem was absent? You forgot about the problem? You overcame the problem? This helps the person begin to recognize when they dealt with the problem successfully. For example, the client says, "I had a really good day yesterday, I didn't have any trouble finding words." You respond by eliciting details about why, "What was different about yesterday?" or "What do you think led to such a great day?" That may elicit things like, "I haven't been sleeping well. Finally, (2 nights ago) I got some good rest," or "I took more breaks," or "I was mindful of my strategies," and the like. Those responses are tangible examples of why they were successful and how they took control, preempted problems, and overcame.

   ○ **Unique account questions:** Were there other times when . . . the problem was absent? Forgotten? Overcome? Explore what factors led to that difference (that success). Begin to systematically map and make sense of the times when they were successful, took control, preempted problems, and overcame. This may be a strategies kind of conversation, a conversation about environmental modifications, and/or a conversation about preparation. Put this on paper, make the mapping of success (absent problem, ignored problem, overcome problem) to the client's actions/behaviors (the things they did leading up to or in the moment of being successful).

   ○ **Unique redescription questions:** Drawing upon those unique accounts, help move your client toward developing meaning about who they now are, "I do well when I prepare for upcoming interactions," or "If I have a script, I feel as though my (aphasia, anomia, stuttering, memory challenges, etc.) aren't noticeable." In this way, successes/formulas for success become a part of their identity, "I'm good at preparing so my (aphasia, anomia, stuttering, memory, etc.) is not a problem."

   ○ **Unique possibility questions:** Encourage clients to aspire to a life that was successful like they were in their unique accounts and redescriptions. Differentiate the "problem's" plans for the future and their own aspirational plans (emerging alternative story), "The problem (my aphasia, anomia, stuttering, memory challenge, etc.) has these plans for my future *but* my plans for the future are different" or "I see myself accomplishing . . ."

   ○ **Unique circulation questions:** Identify key people with whom to share their emerging alternative story. This creates accountability and support in following through with their aspirations. Find out, who

---

Box 6-4
Ted's Excellent Routine

Ted is a 60-year-old man who has survived two brain injuries and cancer. He has good days and bad days, depending on his energy level and fluctuations in cognition from day to day. To gauge how much to do on a given day, he does a daily self-assessment to determine his physical and mental status. This includes a thinking task, like a crossword puzzle, and a simple physical task, like throwing darts to get a sense of how the day may go. If he does really well, he knows he can put more on his schedule, and if he struggles, he knows not to set high expectations. In either case, he stops doing his chores and other tasks around the house by 4 p.m. each day. That way, he can review his "to do list" for the day, transfer unfinished tasks to the next day, and journal about the day. He also reserves the right to bump that 4 o'clock time to any point earlier in the day if necessary. He often remarks, "My 4 o'clock might happen at 4 p.m. or it might happen at 10 a.m. Either way, I know when I've reached my 4 o'clock that it's time to call it quits for the day." He also uses the strategy of taking it easy during the day, resting prophylactically if he knows he has a big event in the evening. That way he can be sure he is at his best when he attends an evening event, thus delaying his 4 o'clock to sometime later in the evening.

Each evening, prior to bed, Ted reads through his journal from previous days. This allows him to see what he did on previous successful days and what was different on days when his 4 o'clock arrived early. Implicitly and explicitly, he has learned the ingredients of successful days when he overcame his challenges and how to avoid things that bring on his 4 o'clock earlier. Ted is so good at the self-assessment piece and routine that he rarely experiences unexpected troubles. It pays to plan ahead, Ted!

The best part of Ted's dedication to routine and reflection is this—it has become his legacy and alternate story. He is an overcomer who conquered two brain injuries, conquered cancer, and became a peer mentor and advocate. He helped found a church service for people with disabilities, and he has spoken about brain injury nationally and internationally. When a new attendee comes to our brain injury group, it is inevitable that Ted or another member will say, "It's past my 4 o'clock," which leads to the resharing of Ted's success story.

---

are those key people—partners, parents, children, family, coworkers, and/or friends?

° **Questions that historicize unique outcomes:** Ask questions to link aspects of past stories to their alternative story, "What inner, tenacious characteristics from before your problem helped you overcome the problem?", "Can you think of examples of when you overcame the problem?" This helps to create a memorable, positive history of the alternative story.

° **Tools of the trade to make all of this communication-friendly:** Rating scales, visuals, daily journals/reflections/check-ins. (See Box 6-4 for Ted's Excellent Routine.)

Thinking about how you'll pull together all of the Wolter et al. (2006) steps? The structure above is certainly a great starting point. You may also wish to refer to the "My Story" Project (Strong, 2015). The framework asks the questions *"Who was I before my stroke and aphasia?", "My stroke and aphasia", "Who I am today",* and *"My future goals."* Note that stroke and aphasia could easily be swapped out for other acquired neurogenic disorders like traumatic brain injury. Four individual sessions are devoted to story construction, one to rehearsing the story, and one group session to tell the story.

Development of the story was supported by incorporating client artifacts such as photos and other memorabilia. A slide show is used to organize and record personal narratives. The coconstruction process creates a context for reflecting upon changes to identity and life following stroke and aphasia (Strong et al., 2018). This reframing helped to facilitate a positive outlook on life. The process changes how people view their life. Part of this shift in how one views oneself was facilitated by an opportunity to discuss things that had been weighing heavily upon their minds. This highlights the importance of creating a safe space for sharing their feelings and concerns. Other important outcomes include a sense of meaning in providing hope to others, along with gains in communication confidence. For a fantastic podcast conversation with Dr. Katie Strong about the "My Story" Project, see Box 6-5.

Another potential model for implementing Wolter et al.'s (2006) narrative counseling approach is metaphoric identity mapping. Ylvisaker et al. (2000, 2008) introduced the idea of metaphoric identity mapping, where clients are encouraged to consider "possible selves" through a process of reauthoring alternative narratives. Markus and Nurius (1986) defined "positive selves" as complex representations of what people would like to become ("hoped-for selves") and what they fear

Box 6-5
The Power of a Story

Check out this great podcast conversation on Aphasia Access Conversations Podcast Episode #55 with Dr. Katie Strong as she discusses the "My Story" project.

https://aphasiaaccess.libsyn.com/the-power-of-a-story-a-conversation-with-katie-strong

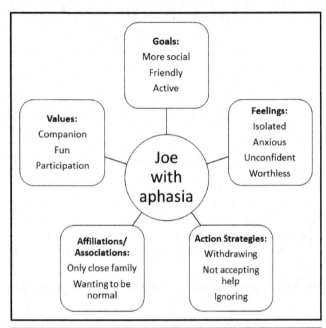

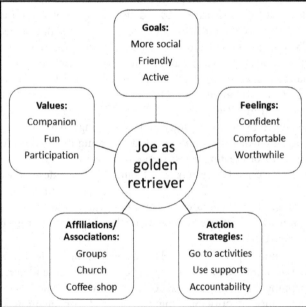

Figures 6-4a and 6-4b. Current and aspirational-positive metaphoric identity maps. (Note: Golden retriever was identified as a positive metaphor, given their social and gregarious companionship.)

becoming ("feared selves"). In this way, the concept of "positive selves" can be used to evaluate a person's current identity or sense of self. Ylvisaker et al. (2008) provide a framework for implementing metaphoric identity mapping that begins with initially establishing a therapeutic relationship, collaborative goal setting, overcoming chronic resistance and obstacles, and potential referral to formal psychotherapy (see pp. 722-724 for the full procedures). In this process, clients collaborate to develop their current identity map and a positive map that incorporates a metaphoric "hoped-for-self" (Figure 6-4). Refer to Chapter 4 to revisit the parallels with Fish et al. (2021) formulations frameworks.

Group Therapy

There is a rich history of group therapy evidence within psychotherapy and mental health counseling literature. It is beyond the scope or purpose of this text to address that literature. Instead, we will discuss the use of groups within the speech-language pathology discipline as a context where counseling moments arise, either by design or spontaneously.

Groups are a powerful context for counseling, including what we deliver incidentally but particularly for peer-to-peer counseling, often scaffolded by us. Peers are able to deliver something that we cannot. Inherently, there is a power differential between therapist and client. We hold the power in that we can ask about all of their personal information, but they do not have equal access to ours. Peers have equal power and sharing is more completely bidirectional. Secondly, peers share an experience that we do not share with our clients. Not all experiences are the same but they have enough in common, certainly more in common than we do with our clients, to empathetically relate on a level that we cannot. So, do we have a role in this context? Absolutely, we often play a key role in helping to shape, reflect, and summarize peer-to-peer feedback. Motivational interviewing or any of the previously discussed counseling approaches are very useful in this context. Imagine a peer who delivers on target but linguistically incohesive feedback to a peer. We can take that feedback and repackage it as cohesive and concise phrases that validate the peer who is delivering it and makes it accessible to the peer who is being supported. Now imagine a context where a peer delivers on target but not fully expanded or formulated feedback to a peer. We can take that feedback, expand upon a broken and incomplete message with the specificity and details needed, "I think what Shelby is saying is . . . , is that right, Shelby?" Again, this validates Shelby and makes the feedback meaningful to the peer who is being supported. Another bonus, peers can say things to peers that we cannot. Tough love and direct advice have some serious limitations, as we have discussed throughout this text. That being said, a little direct feedback and reality checking from the right person can be effective, particularly when trust and mutual respect has already been established. Box 6-6 illustrates the importance and accessibility of peer-to-peer support.

Box 6-6
Only Peers Will Do

Bentley was an 18-year-old male who was attending his first session of our community brain injury support group, which took place via Zoom. His parents had attended the previous session but wanted to give Bentley some space for his first session. To his left sat his girlfriend. When Bentley joined the group, all of the group members reached out to warmly greet and graciously welcome him. We began with introductions from other group members. I noted that, "Bentley may just listen in for his first meeting," and my group regulars know that means to give him some space and follow our lead. Meanwhile, I chatted privately with Bentley (a real silver lining of the telegroup context) to get a sense of his level of comfort. I let him know that we would follow his lead asking, "Would you prefer to just listen in or jump into the discussion?" He shared that he preferred to just listen in for this first session. He left his webcam off and mic muted. By the time all members had introduced themselves, he turned his webcam on and said, "I guess I can introduce myself as well." This included sharing about his accident, revealing that his best friend was a passenger and that he had died in the accident. After the introduction, he turned his webcam off again and muted his mic. The group began its project-based intervention work. Midway through the session, Bentley turned his webcam back on, unmuted his mic, and shared, "As a first timer, what drew me to the group was that people kept telling me, you should go to the group, you'll see that you're not the only one and that there's hope, that's what made me come." Clearly, Bentley was warming up to the group. He left his webcam on and continued to listen in. As we approached the end of the session, Bentley unmuted and interrupted to ask a question, "I'm wondering if I can get some advice from all of you. It's about prom. I wanted to ask tonight because we don't have our next group until after prom. How should I respond to people when they say, 'I'm sorry about your buddy'? I don't want to talk about it, especially with people who aren't my friends. I mean, not my close friends. I feel really uncomfortable when they say that kind of stuff. What should I do?" On cue, group members responded with kindness, empathy, and grace. No "you should do x" responses but a lot of follow-up questions, affirmations, and reflections. Basically, they helped guide him to *do whatever is comfortable to you and feels right. It's not about your making your friends and classmates feel good, it's about doing what feels right for you.* And kaboom, therein lies the power of groups.

Self-Anchored Rating Scales

Rating scales are a common tool in many counseling approaches and should be a standard element of an adapted approach for individuals with communication disorders. Berg and de Shazer (1993) developed the self-anchored rating scales (SARS) technique as a part of SFBT. SARS can be used in several different ways (Franklin et al., 1997). See Table 6-1 for purposes and potential dialogues.

Self-Anchored Rating Scales for Couples and Families

SARS can be a helpful tool for working with partners and parents as well (Fox, 2012; Fox et al., 2012; Franklin et al., 1997; Nelson, 2004). Central to use with partners or parents is the principle of accepting multiple truths, realities, and potential solutions (Fox, 2012; Fox et al., 2012; Franklin et al., 1997; Nelson, 2004). Fox et al.'s work was with adults with aphasia and their partners, whereas Franklin et al's. and Nelson's work was with parents and children. There is value in having both clients and partners/parents respond to questions, such as those identified in Table 6-1, using SARS. The intent is not to corroborate ratings of the client against their partner/parent, but rather to explore their individual realities, thus eliciting self-anchored responses. As Fox (2012) eloquently describes, "the clinician listens without judgment and accepts that each partner's 'truth' makes sense from the perspective of his or her own lived experience" (p. 137). The clinician then clarifies to reach a better understanding of the different opinions of the person with aphasia and their spouse/partner. This allows the clinician to summarize each person's perspective, without judgment, so that the person with aphasia and spouse/partner can understand each other's perspectives. In this manner, each individual (person with aphasia and partner) "gains a better understanding of the other's reality, and the stakeholders establish a norm that difference of opinion will be openly discussed and accepted" (p. 137). Since collaboration is crucial to successful dyadic/ couple interactions, understanding those perspectives is critical. This establishes a space where all parties can more honestly examine all potential solutions.

TABLE 6-1
Self-Anchored Rating Scales Purposes

PURPOSE	DIALOGUE	FOLLOW-UP QUESTIONS
Outcome measure	"Rate your performance level today."	"What is your goal level?" or "What level would you like to reach?"
Using the scale to discuss and identify best hopes realized	"What rating would you make if your best hopes were realized?"	"How would others know?" or "What would be different?"
Having the client identify where they are now in relation to resolution or best outcome	"If your best hopes are a 10 on this scale, what would you rate yourself today?"	"What do you need to do to get closer to a 10?"
Using the scale to identify exceptions to the problem	"You rated yourself a 3, why not a 2 or less?"	"Tell me more about those times when you had success."
Using the scale to discuss and identify solutions	"You moved from a 4 last week to a 5 this week. What was different that made the change?" or "Has there ever been a time when it was higher than 5? What was the difference?"	"Tell me more about that time when you were so successful. Who was there … what was different … what did you do …"

Adapted from Franklin, C., Corcoran, J., Nowicki, J., & Streeter, C. (1997). Using client self-anchored scales to measure outcomes in solution-focused therapy. *Journal of Systemic Therapies, 16*(3), 246-265.

Establishing the phrasing for implementation of SARS is crucial. Fox et al. (2012) and Nelson (2004) have a number of useful dialogues that may help you to develop phrasing options that fit with your counseling voice. While we cannot include the full dialogues here, some key phrases are referenced:

- Introducing SARS, "I'm going to create a scale that will help us track how your communication changes over the next few weeks. I'll place the number 10 at the top and the number 0 at the bottom of this line. Tell me what communication was like for the two of you immediately after . . . his stroke?" (Fox et al., 2021, p. 20).

- "On a 0 to 10 scale, with 0 being no speech and 10 being good enough communication that [person with aphasia] no longer needs therapy, how would you rate communication immediately after his stroke?" (Fox et al., 2021, p. 20).

- Other assessment questions, "What would be good enough?", "What does communication look like now?" (Fox et al., 2021, pp. 20-21).

- Intervention questions, "What would a small change in communication look like?" or, "OK. Let's say your communication is currently at about a 5 or 5.5 on your scale. What would it take to bump it up by half a point or so? What would it look like if things got just a little better?" (Fox et al., 2021, p. 22).

- Introducing SARS, "Let's say that '10' stands for what you hope you get out of therapy, and '0' stands for how things were when you called for an appointment. How

do you think your child will be able to communicate when he is at a '10'?" (Nelson, 2004, p. 16).

- Assessment questions, "So when he's a 10, he'll be able to use some words to ask for things, right?" or, "So when he's at a 10, he'll be asking for things by saying their names and playing with kids using action words." or, "Now, let's talk about how he was communicating when you called for an appointment." (Nelson, 2004, p. 16).

- Intervention questions, "Yes, he's already made some nice changes in noticing language and using a word. Let's put him at a '2.' Let's suppose that at our next session, you tell me that he's moved from a '2' to a '3.' What would you tell me he is doing differently?" or, "Are there times when this is happening [he is using 2 new words], even a little bit, now?" [eliciting exceptions] "What did you do to make that happen?" (Nelson, 2004, p. 16).

Notice how both Fox et al. (2012) and Nelson (2004) work with the client and partners/parents to calibrate the scale. Specifically, they calibrate small increments of change on the scale, so that stakeholders can recognize change (progress). This helps stakeholders to see that problems are solved one small step at a time (De Shazer & Molnar, 1987). Further, the assessment questions help to collaboratively develop goals that are important to the couples/families. This moves partners and parents from being bystanders in therapy to change agents (Andrews & Andrews, 2000; Nelson, 2004). Boles and Lewis (2003) use the SFBT framework to deliver SARS to individuals with aphasia and their partners. Because the intervention is focused on everyday interactions, questions relate to ease and satisfaction of dialogue within the couple.

Sample SARS questions include, "How easy is it to talk about 'deeper' issues?", "How much do you enjoy sitting and chatting?", "How satisfied are you with your relationship?", and "How easy is expressing emotion to each other?" (Boles & Lewis, 2003). The *Aphasia Couples Therapy Workbook* (Boles, 2010), is a nice resource for structuring these interactions and includes several additional SARS questions.

Self-Management and Self-Coaching

In this age of technology, a number of tools have emerged that have the potential to augment counseling and coaching interventions. While it is not the intent or purpose of this brief summary to identify best options for self-help, web-based, or app-based self-management and self-coaching tools, it is good for speech-language pathologists to be aware that these are possibilities. It is with this in mind that I share a few examples here, with the caveat that these are simply examples, not recommendations. Some app-based tools include Noom (CBT), CBT-I Coach, CBT Companion, What's Up (CBT and ACT), Mood Kit (CBT), Self-Help for Anxiety Management, CBT Thought Record Diary, Headspace (mindfulness and meditation), Mindfulness Coach, Calm (mindfulness), Breathe2Relax, and much more. They vary in cost from free to more expensive monthly subscriptions. As technology is constantly changing, you will need to stay on top of latest changes if you recommend app- or web-based supports for your clients.

Chapter Summary

A variety of methods exist for counseling individuals with communication disorders that are supported by research evidence within and outside of the discipline. Most of these approaches share common core features, which align well with person-centered care. Additionally, the approaches are not mutually exclusive and can be used across the lifespan and disorders. Some approaches may be a better fit for certain types of clients or ages.

Key Takeaways

- Several evidence-based counseling approaches can be used within speech-language pathology.
- These approaches are not mutually exclusive and can be combined to meet the needs of clients.
- Some approaches may be a better fit for certain clientele.
- Knowing about different approaches may allow you to be more flexible in implementing counseling.

References

Andrews, J. R., & Andrews, M. A. (2000). *Family-based treatment in communicative disorders: A systemic approach.* Janelle Publications, Incorporated.

Bamberg, M. (2010). Who am I ? Narration and its contribution to self and identity. *Theory & Psychology, 21*(1), 1-22.

Bazalgette, L., Emilsson, M., Breslin, S., Modder, A., Clunas, M., Brown, A., & Anderson, N. (2015). *Solution-focused practice: A toolkit for working with children and young people.* The National Society for Prevention of Cruelty to Children (NSPCC). https://learning.nspcc.org.uk/research-resources/2015/solution-focused-practice-toolkit

Beck, A. T. (1967). *Depression: Clinical, experimental, and theoretical aspects.* Hoeber Medical Division, Harper & Row.

Behn, N. (2016). *Communication and quality of life outcomes in people with acquired brain injury following project-based treatment* [Unpublished Doctoral thesis]. City University London.

Behn, N., Cruice, M., Marshall, J., & Togher, L. (2016). A feasibility study investigating the use of project-based treatment to improve communication skills and quality-of-life (QoL) in people with ABI. *Brain Injury, 30*(5-6), 500.

Beilby, J. M., & Byrnes, M. L. (2012). Acceptance and commitment therapy for people who stutter. *Perspectives on Fluency and Fluency Disorders, 22*(1), 34-46. https://doi.org/10.1044/ffd22.1.34

Beilby, J. M., Byrnes, M. L., & Yaruss, J. S. (2012). Acceptance and commitment therapy for adults who stutter: Psychosocial adjustment and speech fluency. *Journal of Fluency Disorders, 37*(4), 289-299. https://doi.org/10.1016/j.jfludis.2012.05.003

Beilby, J. M., & Yaruss, J. S. (2018). Acceptance and commitment therapy for stuttering disorders. In B. A. Amster & E. R. Klein (Eds.), *More than fluency: The social, emotional, and cognitive dimensions of stuttering.* Plural Publishing.

Berg, I. K., & de Shazer, S. (1993). Making numbers talk: Language in therapy. In S. Friedman (Ed.), *The new language of change: Constructive collaboration in psychotherapy*, (pp. 5-24). Guilford Press.

Berg, I. K., & Steiner, T. (2003). *Children's solution work.* Norton.

Boehm, J. K., Lyubomirsky, S., & Sheldon, K. M. (2011). A longitudinal experimental study comparing the effectiveness of happiness-enhancing strategies in Anglo Americans and Asian Americans. *Cognition & Emotion, 25*(7), 1263-1272.

Bolier, L., Haverman, M., Westerhof, G., Riper, H., Smit, F., & Bohlmeijer, E. (2013). Positive psychology interventions: A meta-analysis of randomized controlled studies. *BMC Public Health, 13*, 119.

Boles, L. (2010). *Aphasia couples therapy workbook.* Plural Publishing.

Boles, L., & Lewis, M. (2003). Working with couples: Solution focused aphasia therapy. *Asia Pacific Journal of Speech, Language and Hearing, 8*(3), 153-159. https://doi.org/10.1179/136132803805576110

Bond, C., Woods, K., Humphrey, N., Symes, W., & Green, L. (2013). Practitioner review: The effectiveness of solution focused brief therapy with children and families: A systematic and critical evaluation of the literature from 1990-2010. *Journal of Child Psychology and Psychiatry, 54*(7), 707-723.

Chan, D. W. (2010). Gratitude, gratitude intervention and subjective well-being among Chinese school teachers in Hong Kong. *Educational Psychology, 30*(2), 139-153.

Chapey, R., Duchan, J. F., Elman, R. J., Garcia, L. J., Kagan, A., Lyon, J. G., & Simmons Mackie, N. (2000). Life participation approach to aphasia: A statement of values for the future. *The ASHA Leader, 5*(3), 4-6.

Csikszentmihalyi, M., & Csikszentmihalyi, M. (1990). *Flow: The psychology of optimal experience.* Harper & Row.

Dalemans, R. J., De Witte, L., Wade, D., & van den Heuvel, W. (2010). Social participation through the eyes of people with aphasia. *International Journal of Language & Communication Disorders, 45*(5), 537-550.

Deci, E. L., & Ryan, R. M. (1985). Conceptualizations of intrinsic motivation and self-determination. In *Intrinsic motivation and self-determination in human behavior* (pp. 11-40). Springer.

De Jong, P., & Berg, I. K. (2013). *Interviewing for solutions* (4th ed.). Brooks/Cole, Cengage Learning.

De Shazer, S. (1988). *Clues: Investigating solutions in brief therapy.* WW Norton & Co.

Dilollo, A., Manning, W. H., & Neimeyer, R. A. (2005). Cognitive complexity as a function of speaker role for adult persons who stutter. *Journal of Constructivist Psychology, 18*(3), 215-236.

Dimaggio, G., Salvatore, G., Azzara, C., & Catania, D. (2003). Rewriting self-narratives: The therapeutic process. *Journal of Constructivist Psychology, 16*(2), 155-181.

Doig, E., Fleming, J., Kuipers, P., & Cornwell, P. L. (2010). Clinical utility of the combined use of the Canadian Occupational Performance Measure and Goal Attainment Scaling. *American Journal of Occupational Therapy, 64*(6), 904-914.

Eifert, G. H., & Forsyth, J. P. (2005). *Acceptance and commitment therapy for anxiety disorders: A practitioner's treatment guide to using mindfulness, acceptance, and values-based behavior change strategies.* New Harbinger.

Emmons, R. A., & McCullough, M. E. (2003). Counting blessings versus burdens. *Journal of Personality and Social Psychology, 84*(2), 377-389.

Feeney, T. J. & Capo, M. (2010). Making meaning: the use of project-based supports for individuals with brain injury. *Journal of Behavioral and Neuroscience Research, 8,* 70-80.

Fish, J., McIntosh, J., Lack, V., & Betteridge, S. (2021). *Seeing the wood and the trees: Social cognition, social communication, and cognitive communication after brain injury.* Cognitive Communication Symposium. Manchester, UK.

Fox, L. E. (2012). AAC collaboration using the Self-anchored rating scales (SARS): An aphasia case study. *Perspectives on Augmentative and Alternative Communication, 21*(4), 136-143.

Fox, L. E., Andrews, M. A., & Andrews, J. (2012). Self-anchored rating scales: Creating partnerships for post-aphasia change. *Perspectives on Neurophysiology and Neurogenic Speech and Language Disorders, 22*(1), 18-27.

Franklin, C., Corcoran, J., Nowicki, J., & Streeter, C. (1997). Using client self-anchored scales to measure outcomes in solution-focused therapy. *Journal of Systemic Therapies, 16*(3), 246-265.

Froh, J. J., Sefick, W. J., & Emmons, R. A. (2008). Counting blessings in early adolescents: An experimental study of gratitude and subjective well-being. *Journal of School Psychology, 46*(2), 213-233.

Frojan-Parga M.X., Calero-Elvira A. & Montano-Fidalgo M. (2009). Analysis of the therapist's verbal behavior during cognitive restructuring debates: A case study. *Psychotherapy Research, 19*(1), 30-41. https://doi.org/10.1080/10503300802326046

Gladding, S. (2009). *Counseling: A comprehensive review* (6th ed.). Pearson Education Inc.

Goodman, F., Disabato, D., Kashdan, T., & Kauffman, S. (2017). Measuring well-being: A comparison of subjective wellbeing and PERMA. *The Journal of Positive Psychology, 13*(4), 1-12. https://doi.org/10.1080/17439760.2017.1388434

Hanton, P. (2011). *Skills in solution focused brief counselling and psychotherapy.* Sage.

Hayes, S. C. (Ed.). (1989). *Rule-governed behavior: Cognition, contingencies, and instructional control.* Plenum.

Hayes, S. C. (2004). Acceptance and commitment therapy, relational frame theory, and the third wave of behavioral and cognitive therapies. *Behavior Therapy, 35*(4), 639-665.

Hayes, S. C. (2008). Climbing our hills: A beginning conversation on the comparison of acceptance and commitment therapy and traditional cognitive behavioral therapy. *Clinical Psychology: Science and Practice, 15*(4), 286-295.

Hayes, S. C., Strosahl, K. D., Luoma, J., Smith, A. A., & Wilson, K. G. (2004). ACT case formulation. In *A practical guide to acceptance and commitment therapy* (pp. 59-73). Springer.

Hayes, S. C., Strosahl, K. D., & Wilson, K. G. (1999). *Acceptance and commitment therapy: An experiential approach to behavior change.* Guilford Press.

Hayes, S. C., & Wilson, K. G. (1994). Acceptance and commitment therapy: Altering the verbal support for experiential avoidance. *The Behavior Analyst, 17*(2), 289-303.

Hayes, S. C., Wilson, K. G., Gifford, E. V., Follette, V. M., & Strosahl, K. (1996). Experiential avoidance and behavioral disorders: A functional dimensional approach to diagnosis and treatment. *Journal of Consulting and Clinical Psychology, 64*(6), 1152.

Heimberg R. G., Dodge C. S., Hope D. A., Kennedy C. R., Zollo L., & Becker, R. E. (1990). Cognitive-behavioral group treatment for social phobia: Comparison to a credible placebo control. *Cognitive Therapy and Research. 14,* 1-23. https://doi.org/10.1007/BF01173521

Helgadottir, F., Menzies, R., Onslow, M., Packman, A., & O'Brian, S. (2014). A standalone Internet cognitive behavior therapy treatment for social anxiety in adults who stutter: CBTpsych. *Journal of Fluency Disorders, 41,* 47-54. https://doi.org/10.1016/j.jfludis.2014.04.001

Hesser, H., Weise, C., Westin, V. Z., & Andersson, G. (2011). A systematic review and meta-analysis of randomized controlled trials of cognitive-behavioral therapy for tinnitus distress. *Clinical Psychology Review, 31*(4), 545-553.

Hoepner, J. K., Buhr, H., Johnson, M., Sather, T., & Clark, M. B. (2018). Interactions between the environment, physical demands, and social engagement at an Aphasia Camp. *Journal of Interactional Research in Communication Disorders, 9*(1), 44-75.

Hoepner, J. K., Sievert, A., & Guenther, K. (2021). Joint video self-modeling for persons with traumatic brain injury and their partners: A case series. *American Journal of Speech-Language Pathology, 30*(2S), 863-882.

Holland, A. L., & Nelson, R. L. (2018). *Counseling in communication disorders: A wellness perspective.* Plural Publishing.

Hope, D. A., Burns, J. A., Hyes, S. A., Herbert, J. D., & Warner, M. D. (2010). Automatic thoughts and cognitive restructuring in cognitive behavioral group therapy for social anxiety disorder. *Cognitive Therapy Research, 34,* 1-12. https://doi.org/10.1007/s10608-007-9147-9

Huebner, E. S., Drane, W., & Valois, R. F. (2000). Levels and demographic correlates of adolescent life satisfaction reports. *School Psychology International, 21*(3), 281-292.

Hsu, K. S., Eads, R., Lee, M. Y., & Wen, Z. (2021). Solution-focused brief therapy for behavior problems in children and adolescents: A meta-analysis of treatment effectiveness and family involvement. *Children and Youth Services Review, 120,* 105620. https://doi.org/10.1016/j.childyouth.2020.105620

Iveson, C., & McKergow, M. (2015). Brief therapy: Focused description development. *Journal of Solution-Focused Brief Therapy, 2*(1), 1-17.

Jones-Smith, E. (2012). *Theories of counseling and psychotherapy: An integrative approach.* SAGE Publications.

Kneebone, I. I. (2016). Stepped psychological care after stroke. *Disability and Rehabilitation, 38*(18), 1836-1843.

Landry, E. C., Sandoval, X. C. R., Simeone, C. N., Tidball, G., Lea, J., & Westerberg, B. D. (2020). Systematic review and network meta-analysis of cognitive and/or behavioral therapies (CBT) for tinnitus. *Otology & Neurotology, 41*(2), 153-166.

Lawton, M. P., & Nahemow, L. (1973). Ecology and the aging process. In C. Eisdorfer & M. P. Lawton (Eds.), *The psychology of adult development and aging* (pp. 619-674). American Psychological Association. https://doi.org/10.1037/10044-020

Levasseur, M., Desrosiers, J., & Whiteneck, G. (2010). Accomplishment level and satisfaction with social participation of older adults: Association with quality of life and best correlates. *Quality of Life Research, 19*(5), 665-675.

Li, J., Jin, J., Xi, S., Zhu, Q., Chen, Y., Huang, M., & He, C. (2019). Clinical efficacy of cognitive behavioral therapy for chronic subjective tinnitus. *American Journal of Otolaryngology, 40*(2), 253-256.

Light, J. (1997). "Communication is the essence of human life": Reflections on communicative competence. *Augmentative and Alternative Communication, 13*(2), 61-70.

Lloyd, H., & Dallos, R. (2006). Solution-focused brief therapy with families who have a child with intellectual disabilities: A description of the content of initial sessions and the processes. *Clinical Child Psychology and Psychiatry, 11*(3), 367-386.

Malec, J. F. (1999). Goal attainment scaling in rehabilitation. *Neuropsychological Rehabilitation, 9*(3-4), 253-275.

Maslow, A. H. (1954). *Motivation and personality.* Harper.

Menzies, R., O'Brian, S., Lowe, R., Packman, A., & Onslow, M. (2016). International Phase II clinical trial of CBTPsych: A standalone internet social anxiety treatment for adults who stutter. *Journal of Fluency Disorders, 48*, 35-43. https://doi.org/10.1016/j.jfludis.2016.06.002

Menzies, R. G., O'Brian, S., Onslow, M., Packman, A., St. Clare, T., & Block, S. (2008). An experimental clinical trial of a cognitive-behavior therapy package for chronic stuttering. *Journal of Speech, Language, and Hearing Research, 51*(6), 1451-1464. https://doi.org/10.1044/1092-4388(2008/07-0070)

Menzies, R. G., Onslow, M., Packman, A., & O'Brian, S. (2009). Cognitive behavior therapy for adults who stutter: A tutorial for speech-language pathologists. *Journal of Fluency Disorders, 34*(3), 187-200. https://doi.org/10.1016/j.jfludis.2009.09.002

Milner, J., & Bateman, J. (2011). *Working with children and teenagers using solution focused approaches: Enabling children to overcome challenges and achieve their potential.* Jessica Kingsley Publishers.

Molnar, A., & de Shazer, S. (1987). Solution-focused therapy: Toward the identification of therapeutic tasks. *Journal of Marital and Family Therapy, 13*(4), 349-358.

Neimeyer, R. A. (1995). Client-generated narratives in psychotherapy. In R. A. Neimeyer & M. J. Mahoney (Eds.), *Constructivism in psychotherapy* (pp. 231-246). American Psychological Association. https://doi.org/10.1037/10170-010

Neimeyer, R. A. (2001). Reauthoring life narratives: Grief therapy as meaning reconstruction. *The Israel Journal of Psychiatry and Related Sciences, 38*(3/4), 171.

Nelson, L. J. (2004). Clinical issues: Using self-anchored rating scales in family-centered treatment. *Perspectives on Language Learning and Education, 11*(1), 14-17.

Northcott, S., Burns, K., Simpson, A., & Hilari, K. (2015). 'Living with aphasia the best way I can': A feasibility study exploring solution-focused brief therapy for people with aphasia. *Folia Phoniatrica et Logopaedica, 67*(3), 156-167.

Northcott S., Simpson A., Thomas S., Barnard, R., Burns, K., Hirani, S. P., & Hilari, K. (2021). "Now I am myself": Exploring how people with poststroke aphasia experienced solution-focused brief therapy within the SOFIA trial. *Qualitative Health Research, 31*(11), 2041-2055. https://doi.org/10.1177/10497323211020290

O'Hanlon, W. H., & Beadle, S. (1997). *A field guide to possibilityland: Possibility therapy methods.* BT Press.

Plexico, L. W., & Sandage, M. J. (2011). A mindful approach to stuttering intervention. *Perspectives on Fluency and Fluency Disorders, 21*(2), 43-49.

Randall, W. (1995). *The stories we are: An essay on self-creation.* University of Toronto Press.

Ratner, H., George, E., & Iveson, C. (2012). *Solution focused brief therapy: 100 key points and techniques.* Routledge.

Rogers, C. R. (1965). The concept of the fully functioning person. *Pastoral Psychology, 16*(3), 21-33.

Ryff, C. D., & Singer, B. (1996). Psychological well-being: Meaning, measurement, and implications for psychotherapy research. *Psychotherapy and Psychosomatics, 65*(1), 14-23.

Sather, T. W., Howe, T., Nelson, N. W., & Lagerwey, M. (2017). Optimizing the experience of flow for adults with aphasia. *Topics in Language Disorders, 37*(1), 25-37.

Scheurich, J. A., Beidel, D. C., & Vanryckeghem, M. (2019). Exposure therapy for social anxiety disorder in people who stutter: An exploratory multiple baseline design. *Journal of Fluency Disorders, 59*, 21-32. https://doi.org/10.1016/j.jfludis.2018.12.001

Seligman, M. E. P. (2006). *Learned optimism: How to change your mind and your life.* Vintage.

Seligman, M. E. P. (2011). *Flourish.* Free Press.

Seligman, M. E. P., Steen, T. A., Park, N., & Peterson, C. (2005). Positive psychology progress: Empirical validation of interventions. *American Psychologist, 60*(5), 410.

Shennan, G., & Wells, J. (2014). Solution-focused practice and song—An overture: The best part of us. *International Journal of Solution-Focused Practices, 2*(1), 24-31.

Sinden, E. (2015). *Your life: Looking back, moving forward.* The Aphasia Institute.

Stacey, K. (1997). From imposition to collaboration: Generating stories of competence. In C. Smith & D. Nylund (Eds.), *Narrative therapies with children and adolescents* (pp. 221-254). Guilford Press.

St. Clare, T., Menzies, R. G., Onslow, M., Packman, A., Thompson, R., & Block, S. (2009). Unhelpful thoughts and beliefs linked to social anxiety in stuttering: Development of a measure. *International Journal of Language & Communication Disorders, 44*(3), 338-351.

Strong, K. A. (2015). *Co-construction of personal narratives in supporting identity and communication in adults with aphasia.* The 'My Story' Project.

Strong, K. A., Lagerwey, M. D., & Shadden, B. B. (2018). More than a story: My life came back to life. *American Journal of Speech-Language Pathology, 27*(1S), 464-476.

Strong, K. A., & Shadden, B. B. (2020). The power of story in identity renegotiation: Clinical approaches to supporting persons living with aphasia. *Perspectives of the ASHA Special Interest Groups, 5*(2), 371-383.

Wheeler, J. (2001). A helping hand: Solution-focused brief therapy and child and adolescent mental health. *Clinical Child Psychology and Psychiatry, 6*(2), 293-306.

White, M. K. (1995). *Re-authoring lives: Interviews & essays* (pp. 3-21). Dulwich Centre Publications.

White, M., & Epston, D. (1990). *Narrative means to therapeutic ends.* Norton.

Wolter, J. A., DiLollo, A., & Apel, K. (2006). A narrative therapy approach to counseling: A model for working with adolescents and adults with language-literacy deficits. *Language, Speech, and Hearing Services in the Schools, 37*(3),168-177.

Woods, K., Bond, C., Humphrey, N., Symes, W., & Green, L. (2011). *Systematic review of Solution Focused Brief Therapy (SFBT) with children and families.* Department for Education.

Ylvisaker, M., & Feeney, T. J. (1998). *Collaborative brain injury intervention: Positive everyday routines.* Singular Publishing Group.

Ylvisaker, M., & Feeney, T. (2000). Reflections on Dobermanns, poodles, and social rehabilitation for difficult-to-serve individuals with traumatic brain injury. *Aphasiology, 14*(4), 407-431.

Ylvisaker, M., & Feeney, T. (2001). Supported behavior and supported cognition: An integrated, positive approach to serving students with disabilities. *Educational Psychology in Scotland, 6*(1), 17-30.

Ylvisaker, M., & Feeney, T. (2005). School success after brain injury: Behavioral, social, and academic issues. In L. W. Braga, L. W. & A. C. da Paz (Eds.), *The child with cerebral palsy, acquired brain injury and developmental delay: A family-based approach to neurodevelopment.* Taylor and Francis.

Ylvisaker, M., & Feeney, T. (2009). Apprenticeship in self-regulation: Supports and interventions for individuals with self-regulatory impairments. *Developmental Neurorehabilitation, 12*(5), 370-379.

Ylvisaker, M., Feeney, T., & Capo, M. (2007). Long-term community supports for individuals with co-occurring disabilities after traumatic brain injury: Cost effectiveness and project-based intervention. *Brain Impairment, 8*(3), 276.

Ylvisaker, M., McPherson, K., Kayes, N., & Pellett, E. (2008). Metaphoric identity mapping: Facilitating goal setting and engagement in rehabilitation after traumatic brain injury. *Neuropsychological Rehabilitation, 18*(5-6), 713-741.

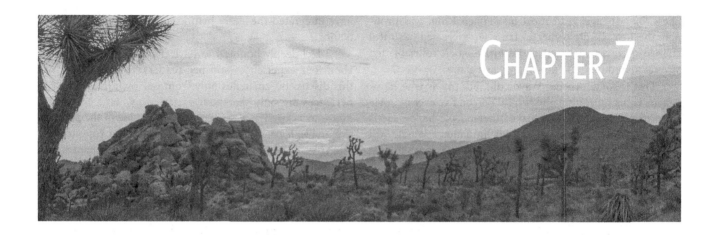

CHAPTER 7

The Lived Experience
Lessons From the Experts

CeCelia and Wayne Zorn; Wendy and Nicholas Allen; and Derek Daniels, PhD, CCC-SLP

I am not what happened to me, I am what I chose to become. ~ Carl Jung

Prologue

This chapter shares the first-hand stories of five experts (CeCelia and Wayne, Wendy and Nick, and Derek). These are direct reflections about the lived experience of individuals living with a communication disorder, from the perspective of a partner, parent, and individual themselves. In recent years, there has been increasing emphasis on amplifying these voices. To effectively amplify those voices, it is important that we do not curate or modify their words. So as much as possible, what follows is their words, their truths.

Wayne and CeCelia's Story

A Little Background About Wayne and CeCelia Zorn

Coming from very different sides of the railroad track, CeCelia and Wayne met in high school in rural northeastern Wisconsin. They got married in the mid-1970s, lived in Southern California for 5 years, and have been in western Wisconsin since 1980. Wayne was diagnosed with primary progressive aphasia (PPA) about 8 years ago.

Wayne has always enjoyed a variety of work and lots of play. He owned his own woodworking business, drove a tour bus across the United States, and worked as a first-rate bartender. He was an envied ballroom dancer and an awesome athlete, and he loved his motorcycle, as well as national and international travel. Wayne never refused any table game,

Hoepner, J. K. (Ed.). *Counseling and Motivational Interviewing in Speech-Language Pathology* (pp. 115-132).
© 2024 Taylor& Francis Group.

chess, or cribbage, read most of Stephen King, was probably the first Kindle owner in the region, created beautiful stained-glass artwork, skied the Birkebeiner, roller-bladed several marathons, and golfed a wicked game.

That is some of what Wayne did, but this is who he is: Wayne is the most kind and helpful person I've ever met. He loves to please others and make other people happy. He is courageous—even now, with all his limitations, Wayne will try to do most anything. He loves to learn new songs to sing and he sees the silly all around him. Still . . . and still . . . Wayne brings people close to him—kids, teens, and adults of all ages.

CeCelia brings a three-fold background to this experience. She is a registered nurse, a lifelong writer, and has been an award-winning university professor for 32 years. CeCelia shares many of Wayne's interests, such as travel, biking, tent camping, and the arts (but not golf, fishing, or assembling jigsaw puzzles). She reads voraciously and is relearning how to play the flute—taking individual lessons, playing in two community bands, and auditing a university music history class. She volunteers at a local free clinic and is an active member of the board of directors for Wayne's memory choir. On a daily basis, CeCelia strives toward a life enriched by kindness, joy, perseverance, curiosity, patience, and collaboration. But she will be the first to tell you: "Some days are easy, but some days I just crash." Yet, every day counts because every day she reminds herself, "Life isn't about waiting for the storm to pass. It's about learning to dance in the rain."

A Shore Behind and a Shore Before

CeCelia and Wayne Zorn

As in the life and work of seamen and their shantysongs: *There is forward motion, there is a purpose learned, a shore behind and a shore before.*

My husband, Wayne, and I have been living with his PPA for about 8 years. There has always been a shore behind and a shore before—both have shadow sides and both have provided us with reinforcements. It may seem a bit peculiar, even fabricated, to think the shore before sustains us, but I'm convinced it does.

In this essay, I initially planned to describe two major components of our experience as they may relate to speech-language pathology—what helped, and what were the gaps and how might they be addressed. Cut and dried—just like that, I thought. With careful reflection and greater honesty, however, our experiences have not been either/or. Therefore, I would like to discuss our experiences in various shades, more real, more human. I will focus on the following aspects: (1) feelings of grief and loss, (2) response to others, (3) need to learn, (4) role reversal, and (5) the influence of speech-language pathologists. In differing degrees, these experiences

have integrated the shore behind and envisioned the shore before.

I feel deeply honored to have the opportunity to write about our experiences and beg readers to understand that this discussion emanates only from our own lives. Our experiences are only that—our experiences—and, of course, everyone's experiences are equally valid. One of the primary things I've learned, mostly from online support groups but also from our community aphasia groups, is the mantra that "everyone is different." That mantra invites us but it also shelters us.

The relationships we have established and maintained with members of our community aphasia groups sustain us. Acceptance, support, and role modeling approaches to communication, as well as learning from and about others, have transformed these relationships into timeworn yet robust friendships. These are friendships where others add energy, conversation never really ends, and silence is navigated as easily as words. We are received with openness and there is little need to be on guard or be "right." Our thanks to all these friends!

Finally, I commend your expertise as speech-language pathology clinicians; abilities as scholars, teachers, and leaders; and ambitions as students. Beyond any words possible, I am grateful to you and your profession. There is no doubt that the quality of life Wayne and I currently enjoy would be negligible without the speech-language pathologists in our lives. Your commitment to us as individuals and your leadership in our aphasia groups, as well as in educational and other local and national settings, are gifts we shall cherish always.

Look, Rather Than Look Away

We need you to persist in your looking, rather than look away. We need you to jump in the trenches with us (albeit cautiously) even though it's cold and muddy down here, painful and sad. I've always believed, in my own practice as a registered nurse, that one must approach a sacred place on foot—reverently, perhaps with awe, even with trepidation. Admittedly, it wasn't always easy for me, and I know that many times I failed miserably. Nonetheless, one must approach.

Over the past years, I really had no one with whom I could fully share my feelings of loss and grief, a grief that can hardly be spoken. I didn't want to disclose my sorrow with family or friends. I'm not sure why—maybe I thought others have their own life challenges and didn't need to hear mine. Maybe it's the cloak of stoicism I inherited from family and absorbed from common Midwest culture. I did share a painful incident around our PPA experience with a close family member a time or two; each time she asked briskly, "Could it be worse?" Did I mention family stoicism?

For me, her comment abruptly ended that conversation. Yes, it could be worse and, therefore, the message I heard was to stop complaining! Barriers to full and honest sharing rear their heads in bewildering ways.

Truthfully, though, comments from a few others held me over some rough patches. The night of our 45th wedding anniversary, Wayne and I were tent camping in an isolated wooded area in southern Wisconsin. He was sleeping next to me and had no idea it was our anniversary. I desperately needed to reach out to someone so I texted a special nephew, late at night, from deep inside our sleeping bag. I felt his love and compassion, stirred from his sound sleep 200 miles away and revealed in his drowsy text shorthand. "yul b ok, AC (his abbreviation for Aunt CeCelia) . . . . yer the only married cuple I no who luv ech othr so much . . . wsh I coud do more for u."

That night I realized the avalanche of loss. I would never again receive holiday or special celebratory wishes from Wayne. I would never again hear his "oooooh" and see his grimace when I held my head deep in a migraine or accidently banged against the cupboard door. I would never again hear his prideful comment about something I accomplished in my professional or personal life. Wayne was always a romantic—a man who gave me fresh flowers at least a half dozen times a year for nearly 50 years. He booked a surprise flight for us to Washington, DC, so I could be there in person to receive a teaching award. This avalanche of loss grows daily, stripping more as it descends the slope.

So, yes please, look rather than look away. Ask us about our loss—*I know things are changing, you are losing a lot, how is this for you? Who are you able to share the hardest things with? When are especially painful times for you?* It may help to simply open the door, to ask us about the shore behind: *Other families living with PPA have told me it's particularly hard to think about things they no longer enjoy—how is this for you? What do you miss most of all?*

Just because someone carries it all so well doesn't mean it isn't heavy. Sometimes when I've said, "I'm okay," I wanted someone to look me in the eyes, hug me tight, and say, "I know you're not." Over the years, I've had one, maybe two people come close to that. Our long-term, dear neighbor held me close one day and said, "I really miss the old Wayne . . . but I bet nowhere near how much you miss him!"

Our music-coach friend recently offered to teach Wayne "Three Times a Lady" written by Lionel Richie:

> *Thanks for the times that you've given me*
> *The memories are all in my mind*
> *And now that we've come to the end of our rainbow*
> *There's something I must say out loud.*
> *You're once*
> *Twice*
> *Three times a lady*
> *And I love you.*

Wayne essentially has no speech now except for minimal counting and a repetitive phrase ("yeah, but like that"). Yet, with time, repetition, and extensive, focused music coaching, he is still able to sing in a basic, uncomplicated way. He has always been a happy, confident, amateur singer—singing in choral groups and solos at family gatherings. The first time

our friend sang Richie's ballad for us while she played the piano felt like my life's fabric was ripping to shreds.

Might a speech-language pathologist begin by approaching that sacred place? Thank you for not looking away.

What Do I Say?

I'm never sure how to respond to others' reaction to our situation. I suspect there is no answer, but I'm frequently left feeling unsettled, troubled. Maybe if I had a response or at least an opportunity to unlayer some interactions with others, that feeling wouldn't linger—festering like an embedded sliver for months, sometimes years.

I'm reminded of a comment made by neuroanatomist and stroke survivor Dr. Jill Bolte Taylor, "Although many of us think of ourselves as thinking creatures that feel, biologically we are feeling creatures that think." Perhaps there is some value in recognizing the dominance of feelings over thoughts, a dominance that takes precedence on some days.

I'll share a couple examples of those embedded slivers. Countless people have told me, "He's so lucky to have you" and then often add a comment about the benefit of my nursing skills. I never know what to say; I simply shrug, smile, and say something empty like, "I guess so" or "I don't know." What, exactly, is the intent of their comment? Is it that Wayne should be expressing some "luckiness?" Is it a wispy, shallow compliment to me (when the speaker really has no idea about the dailyness in our lives)? Is it merely others' hazy effort to be kind and supportive? Most often, others quickly follow their comment with an experience from their own lives (e.g., their mother or a friend whose husband has Alzheimer's disease). This switch to their lives is nearly as predictable as night follows day. I find myself listening to their story, supporting them with my understanding. I always have a mixed silent reaction to this very common interaction, believe others' intention is not to hurt or insult, and, frankly, change the subject ASAP.

Sometimes people would start side conversations when Wayne took time to communicate using the whiteboard on his iPad or when he was showing three or four photos from his iPad photo collection. One friend left our restaurant table, presumably to use the bathroom, when Wayne was taking extra time to place our food order. I admit, it can be horribly uncomfortable to witness Wayne's losses, and I certainly may only be speculating that going to the bathroom was related to his communication, but still . . .

Then there was the time a family member gave Wayne a wrapped gift. He opened it quickly (as he usually does), tearing away the paper and ribbon and tossing them to the floor with lots of joy and energy. The person said, right there in front of both of us, "Just like a child!" I clutched my chair so I wouldn't run away and weep.

After seeing a picture of Wayne golfing, another friend told me, "Be glad he's able to golf yet. And a breather for you." Two things about this still gnaw at me, 2 years later. First, was this an instance when others were telling me how to feel: "Be glad!" I began to second-guess myself—maybe I wasn't feeling "glad" enough? Did I need to show more "glad?"

Second, when Wayne golfs, it is *not* at all a "breather" for me. I worry about everything every minute of his 9 or 18 holes or his time on the driving range. First, I worry about the suitability of the clothes I've selected for him to wear, whether he has the golf balls and tees he needs, and if his golf cleats and towel are appropriately clean. Whaaat? . . . you say . . . that sounds like overkill! You may be right, but those are precisely the things that were always critical for Wayne. He methodically attended to all of them—his detailed preparation was part of the event, and now I want to do all I can to honor his joy. This is a man who still takes several minutes to perfectly line up our grocery cart when he returns it to the parking lot cart corral, despite a nasty blizzard or pouring rain. And, throughout his woodworking business, there never was a more perfectly mitered corner, a more velvety-sanded and stained cabinet. If at all possible, I don't want to dismiss even a moment of what was central for him.

Then, too, I worry (1) about his toileting, (2) if his social skills will be sufficient to not to embarrass himself or others, (3) whether his partner feels it's his duty to golf with Wayne, perhaps a "burden," (4) if he's had too much or too little to drink, and (5) if his shorter-distance golf swings indicate a loss of strength and muscle mass. The answer to the strength and muscle loss question is probably "yes"—and then I worry about how I might help with that.

So, no, when Wayne golfs, it is not at all a "breather" for me! In truth, when Wayne is involved in any activity that may appear to be independent from me, it is never, ever a "breather." I fully realize this perspective may change over time.

Finally, and this experience may be one of the most awkward and unique. Because Wayne and I are not affiliated with any religion, I feel especially uneasy when someone tells us, "You are in my prayers," "I'll pray for you," or "God will help you," or sends us religiously affiliated greeting cards, or signs their communication with religious wishes. Of course, this issue existed for years before Wayne's PPA diagnosis, but it now seems more front and center. It's as though our health situation has flung the doors wide open for others to use their own religious beliefs to console or "give us strength." Dare I ask if this carries a hint of others' self-absorption?

Again, I believe there is no ill intent, and I certainly respect the rights of others to hold dear their religious values and convictions. But, in my view, when any personal communication meant to support Wayne and me is marked with a religious reference, it reflects an unconcerned, presumptuous conclusion. I do not feel comforted or reassured. I feel rebuffed and hurt, and I want to look away in any way possible.

Might it be helpful for a speech-language pathologist to help unearth the layers of these and other interactions? Maybe this uncovering would offer a different lens, a constructive angle, through which to frame a common occurrence. Maybe it would help expose the delicate balance between thinking and feeling. Or, realizing I did not share most of these interactions when they occurred, maybe a key approach is simply asking wisely and then listening thoughtfully.

Need to Know

At the appointment when Wayne's diagnosis was confirmed, the neurologist hurriedly handed me one academic-heavy article about PPA from a neuro journal. In this article, the language was complex, multiple variants of PPA were described, and the focus was clearly aimed at a specialist reader. As he stood to leave, with his hand on the door, the neurologist also mentioned the importance of activity and a healthy diet. If I'm not mistaken, he referred to the Mediterranean diet, identifying blueberries and red wine (both of which I love, so I was in luck!).

It was a speech-language pathologist shortly after the diagnosis who interpreted some key points in that article and shared other basic explanatory handouts that, as I remember, focused on loss of speech and specific brain area involvement. In subsequent sessions over the years, I always noted when our speech-language pathologist would comment, "that is part of this," or "that's to be expected," or nod in understanding after I told her something I was observing (e.g., less smiling, loss in comprehending spoken language). Early on, I remember asking the speech-language pathologist, "Will there be a time when Wayne won't be able to talk at all?" She looked at me with a full heart and said, "Yes."

I clung to her honesty, her "knowing," and the teaching. I found myself trying to read between the lines. I wished for much more.

A friend whose husband was diagnosed with PPA about 1 year before Wayne and already had significant losses told me about a large, active online group (Primary Progressive Aphasia Support Group). It is from her and that group that I first remember learning about the dementia associated with PPA. That wakening helped me begin to piece our own picture together. I read those detailed online posts "on the slant," wanting and needing to know but, at the same time, feeling my future pain and glancing back to the here and now. I feel like a child watching a horror movie through the open fingers of my hands covering my eyes.

I'm now finding myself returning to some family and friends to correct and redescribe what is happening. Initially, I presented PPA as a loss of speech. Obviously, PPA is not only a loss of speech—it results in severe cognitive and physical loss. When others witness this in Wayne, they are confused, and I feel I've been dishonest. This has resulted in quite an awkward situation. I wish I had understood the significance of dementia from the start so that my explanation to others would have been more complete.

I admit, maybe the neurologist and speech-language pathologist addressed the dementia, and I just didn't or couldn't hear it. Please tell us gently but openly and honestly. Please use the term "dementia." Please tell us as many times as needed.

Some specific questions may be effective. Where are you learning about PPA? What are you telling your friends and family? Other patients and families living with PPA have asked about X and I've told them that. . . . In the past, other family members have told me they are not sleeping well—how is this for you? What keeps you awake at night? I know you've been attending Group X—what is that like?

Now I Need to Do What?

Role reversal seems like an antiquated phrase. I suspect the language around this concept has developed a hundred-fold but the issue still exists—big time—at least for me. I'm assuming responsibility for tasks and activities that I've never done before. The most challenging have been the car, bike, and small engine maintenance; lawn care; snow removal; TV and its various functions; tech problems; and assorted home repairs, all of which Wayne did more precisely than you can imagine. Initially, of course, Wayne was able to do most things, then some things, but now he's able to do only a very few basics, and only with detailed, stand-by cueing.

I've plowed through this, as most people do. However, with some early planning, I would have been more prepared had I established a list of names and contact info for major needs (e.g., plumber, electrician, tech support, small engine repair service, and general handyman). In that way, I wouldn't have been scurrying about during every minicrisis. The "breakdowns" themselves (which often seem to "pile up") and then the scurrying about for help are both extremely stressful for me.

A few chuckles happened along the way. Well, at least I chuckle about them now. By mistake, I called the plumber about an electrical problem. I imagined his pipe wrench in hand when I heard his smile over the phone, "I'd help you if I could." This was the same plumber who jumped our dead truck battery when he came to fix the kitchen faucet. Now I will drive the truck every 2 weeks to keep things charged, exactly as the plumber advised!

Then there was the day our garage door wouldn't open. I began to panic just a smidgin, as I couldn't get either vehicle out of the garage in an emergency. I glanced over to our neighbor, but couldn't tell if she was home—my panic cranked up a notch. It turned out to be a broken spring, as diagnosed a couple hours later by the handyman. When the garage door repairman came the next morning, he warned, "Ya know, that second spring could go any day. Better replace 'em both." Two new springs are still on order, going on 2 months, thanks to the COVID-19 supply chain disruptions. In the meantime, there's a clamp (a mighty skimpy one, in my view) holding together the broken spring on a heavy door that I cannot budge. I didn't think to ask the repairman if he ever places a clamp on a spring to **prevent** a break. I'm thinking here about his warning and the value of a clamp on the unbroken spring. Lots of focus on prevention in health care—might it also work with garage door openers?

There was also the broken light bulb incident. In the light fixture hanging over our dinner table, the base of the bulb was broken in the socket, so I couldn't remove the bulb to put in a new one. Like many other things that I'll never know, I have no idea how the bulb got broken but I do know it involved Wayne—another story for another time. Anyway, I texted a friend, thinking he would come to fix it. He promptly texted me this long process about shutting off the appropriate circuit breaker (which I couldn't reliably identify) and then using a raw potato to "turn out" the broken lightbulb base. I kid you not—he wrote "raw potato" and added "you may need to use a couple of potatoes before it works. Let me know if you need help." I thought I just did that???? With all due respect to potatoes, by then the electrician and I were on a first-name basis. A 2-minute house call and $40 later, all was good. I consoled myself, "It's all about supporting local business."

All chuckles aside, I'm not sure exactly what might be the implications for speech-language pathologists related to role reversal. Perhaps it is an intentional focus early on and regularly thereafter to discuss responsibilities for tasks and activities as they change throughout the progression. What are you doing that is new or different for you? How is that going? What do you wish you had help with? How and when are you asking for help? What help might you need in the next few months, or longer? Maybe this is a clear example of "forward motion . . . the shore before."

Naturally, usual practices and skills vary among individuals and households. In our experience, detailed preparation with securing names and contact info ahead of time (based on others' recommendations) would have been helpful. This process in itself takes time, contact with friends, and verification (e.g., "Who have you used? Who would you recommend, or not? Are they still in business—their contact info? Are they taking new requests?"). This, of course, is needed for each service—electrical, plumbing, lawn care, handyman, small engine maintenance, and tech assistance.

I suspect you may be asking: "Yes . . . obviously . . . and why didn't you think about doing this at the start?" Admittedly, I wasn't thinking. To be honest, thinking about a broken garage door opener or buying a new lawn mower or arranging for a microwave replacement that needs electrical and cabinetry renovation didn't come to the top of my list until I faced them head on.

Bolte Taylor's perspective that we are feeling creatures that think seems relevant here. I was feeling more than I was thinking. Maybe I was feeling . . . maybe I was feeling there may possibly, just possibly, come a time when Wayne will be able to once again assume these responsibilities.

Maybe I wasn't thinking.

Speech-Language Pathologists: One Life Influencing Another

Many speech-language pathologists, as well as undergraduate and graduate speech-language pathology students, have shared with us their expertise, compassion, scholarship, leadership, and motivation to learn. They are based primarily in practice, higher education, or the larger community. Although grounded in one of these major systems, they have forged an extraordinary network of constructive professional and personal partnerships that could serve as a national model, bar none.

Wayne and I are incredibly fortunate not only to be served by this network but also to have a fundamental understanding of these systems—their goals, language, activities, and individuals in key positions. We feel privileged to live in a university town, recently progressive in many ways, that is a health care hub in a large rural area. We also have basic financial stability that provides access to health care services and to other elements that enhance the quality of our lives. We fully recognize all of these privileges. Our goal is to do all we can to understand, respect, include, and actively support others in our family and our community who are in different circumstances.

In many striking ways—far too numerous to count—speech-language pathologists and students help Wayne and me live with PPA. I'll highlight a few.

It is invaluable to hear speech-language pathologists affirm things that Wayne and I try to do that are solid, smart, and crucial. Speech-language pathologists repeatedly verify the importance of keeping active, connecting with other people, pursuing our own interests to the extent possible, and having fun. They do this without a hit-us-over-the-head lecture, or handing us a glossy "Staying Healthy" pamphlet, or directing us to a hollow wellness website or podcast. Instead, they "whisper" it ardently, arrange activities that promote it, and, best of all, live it themselves. Their affirmation is especially critical when my energy wanes or my knees tremble.

Postcrossing is a specific example of an affirming activity locally established and led by one of our aphasia group speech-language pathology leaders. "Postcrossing" is an online project begun by Paulo Magalhães in which members send and receive postcards from all over the world. Wayne and I meet monthly with other aphasia group postcrossers at a coffee shop, outdoors, or via Zoom to socialize, write postcards, and have fun. To date, we have written and sent 334 cards and received 328. In our latest project, we designed our own postcards using photos taken by individuals in the group. Again, led by the speech-language pathology leader, individuals with aphasia and family members selected some of our own photos, wrote a caption, created the layout, chose colors, and planned the back of the card. We designed 12 different postcards—all accomplished through group discussion. The final step awaits us: sending our personal postcards around the world and hearing from the recipients.

Another side of affirmation is seeing and hearing speech-language pathologists communicate with Wayne and other individuals living with aphasia. The speech-language pathologists' verbal and nonverbal techniques affirm my own attempts and encourage my confidence. In turn, I find myself sharing those techniques with friends and family. Examples include (1) writing out choices on Wayne's iPad whiteboard for him to circle, (2) speaking to him directly, using his name, and not speaking around him, (3) using his iPad calendar, (4) not speaking as if he is hard of hearing, and (5) practicing patience with being focused and purposeful. Knowing some basic techniques offers me an anchor in extremely stormy waters.

At the same time, it is also affirming when the speech-language pathologist with whom we've been meeting for several years admits, "We really don't know what works and what doesn't. It's a trial-and-error approach. Sometimes things work, and sometimes we just tank." And the many times I've "tanked," her comment picks me up, makes me feel a might stronger, and often coaxes a smile.

Again and again, this speech-language pathologist shapes her strategies to help manage the dailyness of our lives (e.g., traveling, training a puppy, exercising, and celebrating golf scores). In this Life Participation Approach to Aphasia (Chapey et al., 2000), she is so successful because she knows about our life. From the start, in many different ways, she skillfully learned who we are and what we do.

Thinking back, I still giggle as this speech-language pathologist role-modeled for Wayne how he might let Oreo (our small pet mutt) outside and then admit him back indoors. Except for his repetitive phrase, Wayne still does this without a word even though he learned and practiced this several years ago. Now he uses hand gestures with Oreo and strategically closes and opens doors as he fastens and later removes his remote training collar. He also feeds Oreo morning and evening and, naturally, provides a dog treat here and there (all accomplished with my minimal cueing). Oreo probably doesn't *think*—I suspect he just *feels* Wayne.

Because Wayne isn't able to describe any activities verbally, we continue to use a strategy we learned from our speech-language pathologist to help us share his life with others by using photos. He collects a few key photos of people and activities in our lives that I or others take. Each photo has a brief caption. Initially, Wayne was able to do much of this, and he's still able to save the photo and type the caption that I've written, with detailed cueing throughout the process. I am thrilled to see his joy when he shows these photos to others.

The captioned photos also serve as a way to help others communicate with Wayne (Figures 7-1 through 7-7). Someone asked me recently how she might best spend time with Wayne and engage with him. I appreciated her honest question and suggested she use the photos on his iPad, which he almost always has with him. "Just make a comment about the photo," I suggested. "You could say something like, 'Wow,

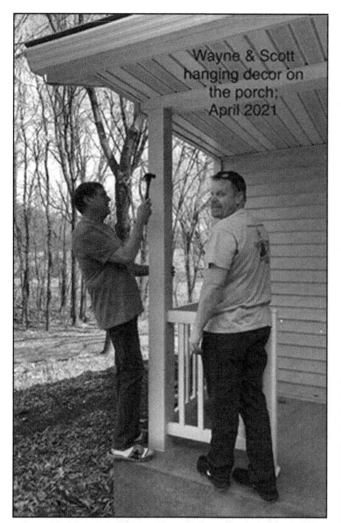

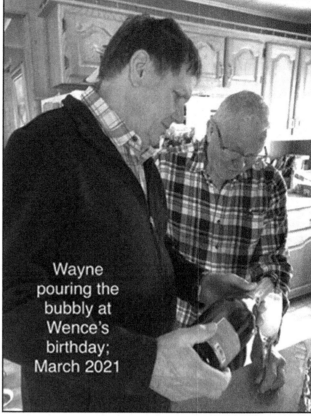

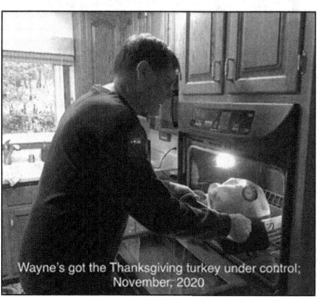

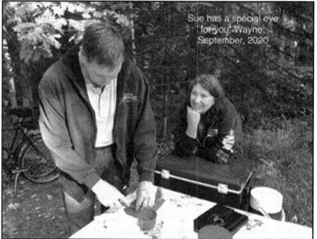

Figures 7-1 through 7-4. Captioned photos serve as communication supports.

looks like a beautiful place to canoe with a friend!'" Then I added, "That kind of comment would work much better than asking where he was canoeing, as he couldn't answer your questions." Now, as Wayne is becoming less focused,

he needs verbal or gentle physical cuing to show his photos slowly rather than rapidly swipe through them.

Finally, a major theme threading through our speech-language pathologist's practice with us is her ability to

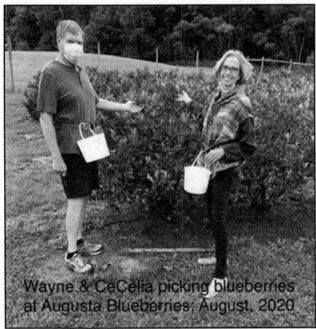

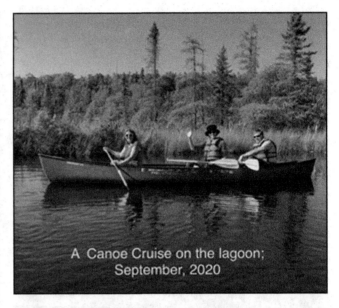

A Canoe Cruise on the lagoon;
September, 2020

Wayne & CeCelia picking blueberries
at Augusta Blueberries; August, 2020

Figures 7-5 through 7-7. Captioned photos used as communication supports.

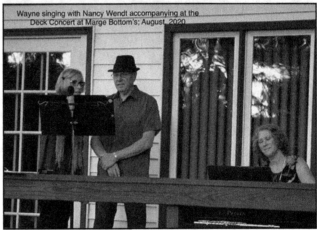

Wayne singing with Nancy Wendt accompanying at the
Deck Concert at Marge Bottom's; August, 2020

collaborate. Because the basis of collaboration is a two-way street, this approach helps us reach out to others, but it also helps others reach in to us. She, Wayne, and I have met with family members and friends (in person and using FaceTime) on several occasions to discuss communication techniques—achieving both a reaching out and a reaching in.

In another collaborative activity, this speech-language pathologist and I coauthored a peer-reviewed article in *The Journal of Humanities in Rehabilitation* titled "Three Voices at the Table." Throughout this months-long writing and publishing process, not only did I feel affirmed in what I could contribute, but I also learned more about PPA. Additionally, this collaboration helped me glimpse into speech-language pathology, as a science and practice-based profession. Understanding some foundation infuses meaning into the therapy that was becoming part of our lives.

More recently, in the depths of the COVID-19 restrictions, our speech-language pathologist suggested a group snail-mail monthly exchange. She and I invited a medley of our friends and family, most of whom did not know each other. Among its many benefits, the exchange provided Wayne

an opportunity to sign all our mailings, write addresses, and stamp and stuff envelopes, as well as open and display the mailings we receive from the group's other 10 members.

To help Wayne continue singing, over the past several years Wayne, our speech-language pathologist, and I have collaborated with our music-coach friend to develop specific strategies (e.g., preparing typed lyrics that integrate visual cueing and emphasizing certain vocal warm-ups). In addition, the speech-language pathologist created an 8-minute, aphasia-friendly video in which she demonstrated back, neck, and shoulder relaxation exercises particularly relevant for Wayne's singing. The positive effect of consistently using this video has been profound. We've learned this type of video is highly effective in communicating some how-to's. The speech-language pathologist previously created a strengthening-balancing exercise video that we've been using at least twice a week for nearly 2 years. Because of this collaboration and creative innovation, Wayne continues to sing in a community choir created for individuals with memory loss and their care partners, as well as in the International Aphasia Choir and other informal home gatherings.

We had the cherished opportunity to also collaborate with the speech-language pathologists in other roles in our community. Wayne, the speech-language pathologist in our individual therapy, and I were interviewed by a faculty member in the Department of Communication Sciences and Disorders at our local university (Box 7-1). He created a podcast offered through Aphasia Access, a national organization that emphasizes communication as a key to person-centered health care and a meaningful life. We also were key participants in a 20-minute video project led by another faculty member in that department. This video presented our living with PPA by including perspectives from friends, our individual speech-language pathologist, a speech-language pathology student, a speech-language pathologist aphasia group leader, and Wayne's music talents. Finally, at the national Aphasia Access conference, Wayne and I had the opportunity to collaborate with a speech-language pathologist faculty member and our individual speech-language pathologist to present a poster. All of these activities reflect collaboration at its finest.

The majority of speech-language pathology therapy work with us, both individually and in groups, seems related to central aspects of affirmation, Life Participation Approach to Aphasia, and collaboration. I've organized our activities into these three areas but, truthfully, most often these processes intuitively weave together. That is when success is strongest. That is also when Wayne and I feel most strengthened and have the most fun.

We Thank You!

Every night when I hold Wayne's head in both my hands, I think about what is happening in his brain, merely a centimeter under my hands. I wonder what is happening in those cells and, of course, I wish others or I could fix it. It's odd really, I couldn't hold a failing kidney or a heart or the lymph system so intimately in my hands, but I am able to hold Wayne's head. And when I kiss him good-night and

say, "I love you," he says, "I love you too." I shall always cherish that voice and be forever grateful. The speech-language pathology community has unfurled itself to us, one person, one group at a time. You wove us into your grid, poured your music into our ears. You kept us, and Wayne and I thank you!

Like in the life and work of seamen and their shanty-songs, as speech-language pathologists, you know there is forward motion, and you see a purpose to be learned. You appreciate a shore behind and a shore before.

References

Chapey, R., Duchan, J. F., Elman, R. J., Garcia, L. J., Kagan, A., Lyon, J. G., & Simmons Mackie, N. (2000). Life participation approach to aphasia: A statement of values for the future. *The ASHA Leader, 5*(3), 4-6.

Riske, T., & Zorn, C. R. (2018). Three voices at the table. *The Journal of Humanities in Rehabilitatio*n, 1-10. https://www.jhrehab.org/2018/11 /08/three-voices-at-the-table/

Wendy and Nick's Story
A Little Background About Wendy Allen and Her Son, Nick

Nicholas Carey Allen was born on March 31, 1981 to Wendy and Sandy Allen; their first child (Figure 7-8). He was older brother to two siblings, Nate and Ben; son to Wendy and Sandy; family to numerous personal care attendants. His 34 years of life far exceeded expectations given by doctors throughout his life, particularly in his early years. Nick helped teach numerous students and professionals throughout his life, providing crucial information about the etiology and pathology of Coffin-Siris Syndrome (CSS). Along with being Nick's mom, Wendy Allen was and continues to be a staunch advocate for Nick and for educating nurses and other health care providers about the importance of relationship-based care and listening to parents and families as experts. She continues to work as a nurse.

One in Several Million, in Every Way

Wendy and Nick Allen

The experience of being a parent of a child with severe speech/language deficits can often be a long journey. It requires parents and families to adapt as the child continues to grow. It often makes parents frustrated because they don't intuitively know what type of modalities are available. They struggle finding the resources and the guidance to purchase what might help their child. Often good and appropriate help is out of reach and unaffordable for families struggling

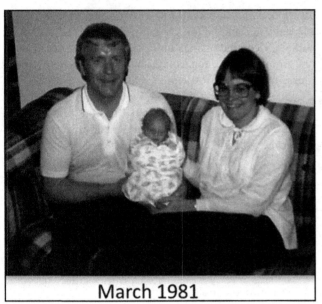

March 1981

Figure 7-8. Nick at birth.

to support a child with a disability. I don't remember hearing the words "counseling" from anyone. Most of our speech-language pathologists were empathetic with us, and some inquired about how we were coping but that's as far as it went.

The early days with Nick were filled with uncertainty. It would take 6 months before we had answers: learning that Nick had a rare genetic disorder, CSS. In fact, CSS is so rare that there are only about 80 to 200 confirmed cases in the world to date, depending upon clinical criteria. Drs. Coffin and Siris first identified CSS in 1970. Vergano and Deardorff (2014) provided a thorough description of clinical features and management. It is an autosomal dominant disorder, but it typically occurs in a family for the first time due to a new mutation. One hallmark is a tiny or absent fingernail on each of the fifth digits (i.e., pinkies and little toes). Other characteristics include coarse facial features, sparse scalp hair, hypertrichiosis (i.e., excessive hair growth on face, including forehead and body), feeding difficulties, failure to thrive, short stature, and severe intellectual disability. Other craniofacial features include bushy eyebrows, full lips, and a wide mouth with a mile-wide smile you cannot help but fall in love with. Organ-related issues include heart defects, spinal anomalies (e.g., severe scoliosis), renal anomalies, hearing loss, and dental anomalies. Did I mention that Nick is famous? Nick has been the subject of case study publications and descriptions of CSS clinical features (Vergano et al., 2018, p. 3). See Figures 7-9 through 7-13 for clinical features of CSS on Nick.

In our early experience, we were told that our son was most likely deaf and blind, and that due to the severity of his disability, he would most likely not speak. For the first 6 months, Nick was held 24/7. We wanted him to feel secure, if he couldn't see or hear. After 6 months, we had a child who was totally dependent on being held! We then needed to break him of this, and about this time in his development,

he would startle and track with his eyes (this tracking was marked by nystagmus—repetitive side-to-side movements of the eyes). Eventually, those two hurdles were taken care of, and he tolerated sitting without being held. He could cry but it was very weak—almost like a small kitten. We also noticed that his frenulum was attached to the very tip of his tongue, which limited his tongue movement for speech and swallowing. He had a very difficult time drinking from a bottle because his suck reflex was weak and often the milk would come out his nose. Feeding time totally exhausted him, and he would be drenched in sweat throughout it. We questioned his physicians about cutting the frenulum, but all refused and told us that it wouldn't make a difference with his eating, swallowing, or any eventual vocalizations. His vocalizations were basically "eeee..." and we learned what was a happy sound and a sad sound. He trained *us* to pay attention to these sounds. See Figure 7-14 for Nick walking at age 3 years, a milestone doctors predicted would never occur.

Encounters With Doctors: The Okay, the Bad, and the Worse

Our initial interactions with doctors included a variety of reactions. A common response was, "I don't know what's wrong with him." And "What should we do now?" As new parents, seeking answers, this was not the response we were hoping for. To be honest, these responses were better than many that followed. We were met by a forceful and accusatory response by our pediatrician, who suggested that we must have done something to make Nick this way. He accused us of hiding herpes infections and hiding hemophilia, blaming us for his disorder, which was still unknown at the time. This didn't move us any closer to answers and made us feel more defensive and frustrated than we already were. Next, he said, "We'd like to biopsy his liver," to which we responded, "Why? Because there might be something wrong with it? Did something show up?" The doctor responded, "No, but there might be something wrong with it." Keep in mind, doing a liver biopsy is not a simple, pain-free process. We fired that doctor. Another doctor advised, "He has no cerebellum, he'll never sit or walk. You should put him in an institution." And we never returned to him. When Nick had dental surgery, he was most comfortable getting drowsy with meds before the anesthesia mask was placed. One anesthesiologist refused to wait and was going to just put the mask on at the outset, which was really frightening for Nick. "I know how to handle these people," he assured me. Fired! Another doctor said, "I am the doctor and I know what's best, you're just the mom." Fired! Another doctor was going to open up Nick's tear ducts. He said it wouldn't hurt, so he probed them. You could hear the crunch of bone breaking over Nick's screaming. Fired! Late in his life, Nick had tumors that ruptured his spinal cord. When we initially brought him in, not knowing what was happening, I asked for a neurology consult. I

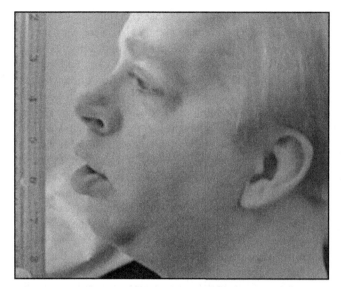

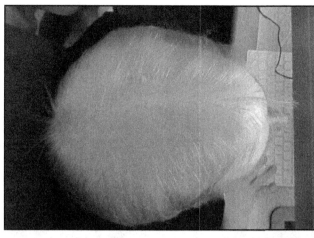

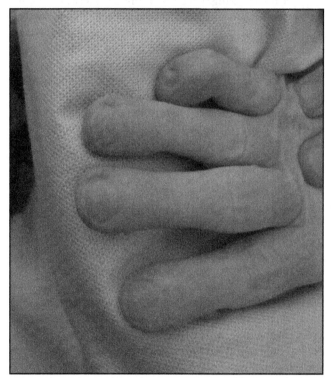

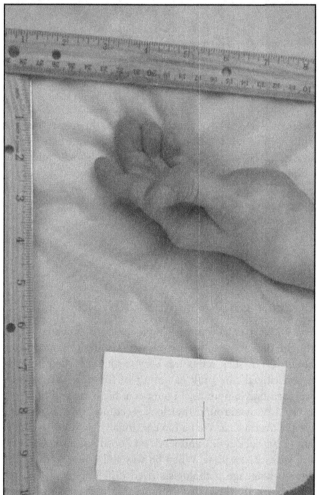

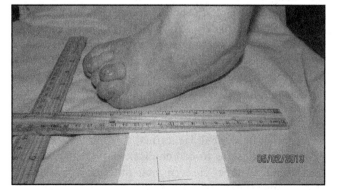

Figures 7-9 through 7-13. Clinical features of CSS.

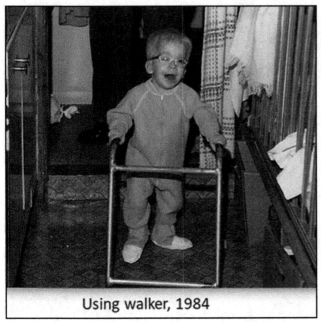

Using walker, 1984

Figure 7-14. Nick using a walker.

overheard one of Nick's doctors saying to the nurse, over the phone, "You tell that mom that I will decide when we call in neuro." He came to see Nick in the ER shortly after that phone call—Fired! Shortly after that, neurology was consulted, discovering multiple schwannomas. Dismissing family members' concerns and failure to recognize them as experts in their own care or care of loved ones is a costly mistake.

Feeding and Swallowing Speech-Language Pathologists

Nick's palate was very high, and he appeared to be tongue tied at birth, but no one was willing to do anything about it. His suck reflex was very weak, and when he tried to breastfeed, the milk came out of his nose. Because he weighed only 5 pounds, 14 ounces at birth, he had to be fed every 3 hours, around the clock. Feeding him was a struggle for over a year. We had to continually work on strengthening his suck reflex and work on coordinating his breathing with the swallow. When he was still bottle feeding, the speech-language pathologists tried different nipples to see what worked. They tried a nipple that is used for children with cleft palate but that was scary and only made him gag and throw up. Eventually, feeding and swallowing improved to the point where he could begin trying semisolid foods. Because he lacked lateral tongue movement, he was unable to move the food to the side of his mouth, between the teeth, to chew. This meant that any bolus of food went straight down without chewing. He also had severe texture aversions. One of our first experiences with speech-language pathology was when we started working on feeding textures at a

specialized pediatric hospital about 1.5 hours away from our home. The speech-language pathologists were very patient with us and with Nick and were very cognizant of when to stop because he had enough. We tried to work with feeding specialists but Nick was so unhappy and struggling with textures that we finally gave up. As much as the speech-language pathologists were helpful and knowledgeable about feeding and swallowing issues, they pushed us to continue solid textures at home that were a struggle in sessions, with the goal of Nick eventually eating solid foods. It is not clear if they did research on CSS kids or not, but this was very frustrating, as nearly all of them were tube fed for the same swallowing impairments Nick struggled with. We just could not see making him struggle for every feeding. Feeding should be a pleasure. One doctor explained that Nick experienced sensory inputs differently than we do. For example, when we smell a turkey cooking at Thanksgiving, it makes us salivate and anticipate the pleasure of eating. When Nick smelled those aromas, his response was pain and nausea. As parents, we eventually had to listen to our gut feelings and to Nick! We chose to focus on teaching him to eat and drink on his own, and to find pleasure in oral intake of foods. Nick loved minimarshmallows, which he eventually learned to seek out and bring to us to pour him a bowl. Who needs speech therapy for that? I'll just go get them and bring them to Mom and Dad—they know what I want!

Communication and Cognition Speech-Language Pathologists

Much of our initial interactions with speech-language pathologists were focused on feeding and swallowing. Once we reached an impasse on the goal of working toward eating solid foods, those interventions ceased. Eventually, we were referred back to the speech-language and hearing clinic at our local university (only a few miles away), a training program for speech-language pathology students. We took Nick there for a few years. The students and instructors at the university clinic were very kind, patient, and listened to our thoughts. They tried various modalities, including use of pictures and a language board, in case he never learned to speak. They even guided us through the process of getting an electronic speech-generating device for Nick. Unfortunately, it was very much a trial-and-error process. Meanwhile, Nick had already figured out how to get what he wanted through vocalizing for help. While he did not use words, he varied stress and intonation to call your attention, pointing or even holding your hand and physically bringing you along with him to what he wanted. He learned a handful of American Sign Language signs to communicate basic needs, such as "more" and "all done." He even got to the point he could sign, "Excuse me please Dad" when he was done at the table.

Early IEP (Individualized Education Program) meetings were tough. Because Nick didn't progress at the rate the other kids did, or they couldn't measure it anymore, IEPs were mostly focused on what he couldn't do. This was depressing and certainly not helpful. At some point, as Nick grew, I became increasingly vocal. Meetings were ridiculous. I would say, "You have a half an hour, summarize and move on." They would give us goal suggestions, many that were ridiculous—many tied to age-appropriate activities. For example, just because Nick is 21 years old doesn't mean he wants to sit in shop class with "the boys." From my perspective, he was developmentally at the level 2 to 5 years with receptive function closer to 9 or 10 years—he should have interests in this range. Since Nick didn't make progress with verbal communication (which happened early on in the schools), he did not receive speech services in the schools. As it turns out, CSS kids have far better receptive language than expressive. So, at some point, it would have been helpful for them to measure that receptive language instead of making the assumption that he wasn't communicating. An opportunity was also missed to try augmentative and alternative communication devices, such as the communication boards and speech-generating devices they tried at the university. Imagine if they had collaborated with the university and us, perhaps augmentative and alternative communication could have fostered more explicit, symbolic communication. Figure 7-15 shows Nick at 6 years old.

Making Things Worse?

When Nick was 9 years old, his brother got bacterial and viral pneumonia. Of course, Nick picked it up and spent 2 weeks in our local hospital before being transferred to a metropolitan children's hospital (1.5 hours away). Speech-language pathology and gastroenterology were consulted, and they insisted he be aspirated. I consented to having a tube inserted to inject contrast. Of course, they had difficulty inserting it through his nose and eventually had to insert it orally. Choanal atresia is a common consequence of CSS, where the nasal passages (chonae) are blocked or narrowed, something they should have researched prior to putting Nick through multiple, painful attempts. When I joined Nick in the X-ray room, they were injecting the contrast. His eyes were rolled back and his skin was blue. I was told, "Mom, it's okay," as if I didn't have a reason to be upset. Fortunately, an ICU doctor was walking by, so I grabbed him and brought him back to X-ray. They had inserted the tube into his lungs and injected the contrast there. Not only did he nearly die, but now he had bacterial, viral, and chemical pneumonia—and permanently scarred lungs. What we learned from this debacle:

- Listen to your gut. I knew he had pneumonia from Nate. I shouldn't have given in to the gastroenterologist and speech-language pathologist.

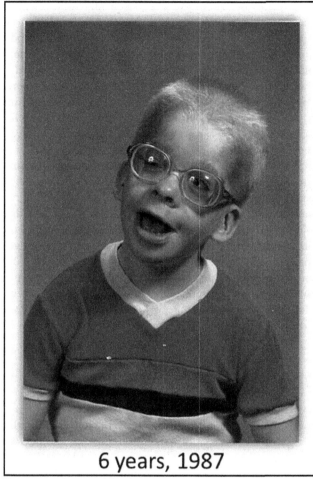

6 years, 1987

Figure 7-15. Six-year-old Nick.

- The nurse who inserted the tube was a new nurse and afterward, admitted that her "gut" told her that this was a bad idea.
- Make sure that they check the tube placement by X-ray (or perhaps insert it under fluoroscopy so they can see where they are guiding it).
- Hospital administrators show up pretty fast when they almost kill your child.
- This was the beginning of the need for Mom to be "the bitch"—as one doctor said when he walked in and asked me if I was "the bitch" listed in the chart.

I continue to mull over these things in my mind, years later. It leaves me with a lot of "what ifs." If only I had listened and said no . . . If the nurse listened to her gut and said no . . . If the speech-language pathologist listened to me about the family incident of pneumonia . . . If the doctor had listened . . . It would have avoided so much pain and suffering for Nick and he would not have had to live with scarred lungs.

In the last years of his life, when he struggled with multiple tumors and declining health, he would often get pneumonia, related to prolonged episodes of vomiting and subsequent aspiration. We were frequently confronted by speech-language pathologists saying that he needed more swallowing studies because "he might be aspirating food." One time, after a prolonged intubation at a university hospital, 1.5 hours from our home, we actually demanded a transfer to another facility. They did not listen to my experiences that extubating him, if done slowly, would cause him to aspirate. It needed to be fast, so he could manage his secretions. And yes, you can aspirate during extubation! However, they "knew better," slower is better, and they disregarded my input. Well this is Nick, I thought, and Nick does nothing the usual way. So, they didn't listen and within 24 hours, I could see the signs of pneumonia. I asked for a chest X-ray but was told "not unless he is running a fever," and we didn't want to expose him to more radiation. So, we checked him out, brought him home, bathed him, and by the time we got to our local hospital, his oxygen saturation was only 80% and guess what? Pneumonia! So, the speech-language pathologist shows up to talk to us about swallow studies, again. Honestly, I just about ate her alive. He aspirated on extubation, not while eating.

What Was the Impact on Us?

This is a question far too seldom asked. We tend to overfocus on the client, the patient, and overlook the family who is right in the thick of it, walking alongside of that person. Our goal for Nick was to help him survive and to make him happy. That meant devoting an unbalanced share of our time to Nick at home, in the hospital, at doctors' offices, at therapy, and simply providing the care he needed. While we tried to be intentional about balancing time with our two other children, some imbalance was unavoidable. Nathan, as the middle child, struggled with the inequity of our attention and even continues to have mental health issues to this day. Ben, the youngest, grew up as the protector, a deeply engrained identity that remains. When we were in the thick of it, for all of those years with Nick, just making it through, we had very little time as a couple. Now, we struggle to reconnect. It was hard to support Nick through all of this, make the best decisions we could, keep him happy and comfortable and not afraid of the medical community—and at the same time, trying to give our other two children a fairly normal life. In the end, there is really nothing normal about the family experience of raising a child with a disability. Unless you have been there, you just don't know. Figure 7-16 shows Nick in a standing device.

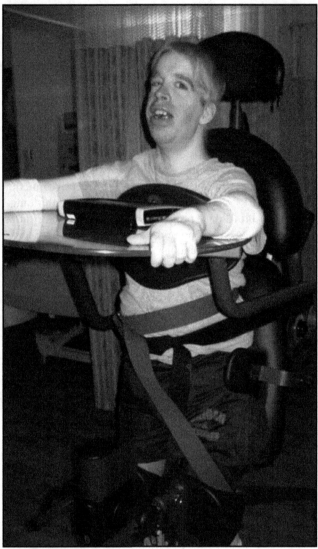

Figure 7-16. Nick in a standing device.

Advice for Speech-Language Pathologists and Other Disciplines

All practitioners must advocate for the patient. If that means disagreeing with the doctor, then so be it. Do the research, read the chart, talk to your colleagues before you see the patient and family. Sometimes I would say, "He had a swallow study done 2 days ago" and the speech-language pathologists didn't know. Several speech-language pathologists pushed so hard for repeated swallow studies, without doing their homework or listening to the patient or his mom. Above all, listen to the patient and their families, they are the experts on their lives.

Box 7-2

Formative Learning

Jerry K. Hoepner

One of the principles of sharing direct, lived experiences is that they stand alone and do not require our interpretation or shaping. It is because of this principle that I hesitated to comment on this case. You see, Nick and his family left an indelible mark on my life and the path it would take. I was one of those personal care attendants throughout my college years. I believe Nick was 9 to 12 years old during that time. The Allens were my second family. I spent weekday evenings with them, from supper to bedtime, caring for Nick, playing with Nick, taking him to playgrounds and parks, watching Disney movies together (*Pinocchio* and *Fantasia* were his favorites, but he liked them all), listening to Raffi songs ("Ducks Like Rain", "Baby Beluga"), helping with appointments at the children's hospital. I spent weekends with him, walking around the neighborhood, going to their family camper on the lake, playing together with Nick and his brothers. What I witnessed was a family that was close, who put their everything into making Nick's quality of life as good as it could possibly be, a family who was goofy and laughed together, parents who were intentional about spending quality time with Nick's brothers as much as they did with him, and a couple who did their best to carve out time for each other. I'm sure from the inside looking out, it felt as though they fell short of their aspirations for being the best family they could be, under the circumstances. From the outside with the privilege of looking inward, I saw a deeply caring and kind family who exceeded expectations of mere mortal human beings. I was witness to the ups and downs, the careless dismissals and ignorance of providers who overlooked the experts who were right in front of them. The Allen family was one of 80 families to live with a child with CSS and one of far fewer who lived well into adulthood. They had 24 hours of experience per day for 30-plus years to draw upon. Dr. Coffin himself could not boast such a résumé. I am forever indebted for the untranscripted learning I gained in 4-plus years with the Allens.

Supports

Along the way, aside from the challenges and missteps, we did receive some terrific supports that helped us. Early on, it was a social worker from the developmental achievement center who eventually became Nick's guardian. Throughout Nick's life, it was by far the personal care attendants who provided support. They gave us breaks, laughed with us, cried with us, and protected Nick with all of their being. Some even slept under his ICU bed. We taught them advocacy, and they ran with it. The local university speech-language pathology clinic really helped to give us ideas and support for many years. Nick and I spoke to classes of nursing and speech pathology students, which benefited us and the students. The metropolitan children's hospital specialized feeding and swallowing services were generally helpful. We received support directly from Dr. Coffin regarding what other CSS kids could and could not do. Mostly, we became the resource for other families, and we did a lot of research. In the years that have passed since Nick died, this remains a part of my identity and purpose.

References

Vergano, S. S., & Deardorff, M. A. (2014, September). Clinical features, diagnostic criteria, and management of Coffin-Siris syndrome. *American Journal of Medical Genetics Part C: Seminars in Medical Genetics, 166*(3), 252-256.

Vergano, S. S., Santen, G., Wieczorek, D., Wollnik, B., Matsumoto, N., & Deardorff, M. A. (2018). Coffin-Siris syndrome. *GeneReviews® [Internet].*

Where's Derek?: Finding Value in Myself as a Person Who Stutters

Derek E. Daniels, PhD, CCC-SLP

I begin my story with another story. As a college professor, I study many different topics. Two topics that are very important to me are how people define themselves, and what types of experiences they have. I once heard a clinical psychologist, Dr. Beverly Daniel Tatum, give a lecture on creating inclusive environments, and she gave an illustration that I now reference quite frequently. She said imagine if you were at an event, and there was a photographer assigned to take pictures of the event. After the event ends, and the pictures have been emailed to everyone, what would be the first thing you do as you scroll through the pictures? The answer is simple: you would first look for yourself in the picture. And if you find yourself in the picture, what is the next thing you would do? You would evaluate how you look in the picture: are you smiling, are your eyes closed, does your hair look right, and so forth. The bottom line is that we all want to be included in the picture of life, so to speak. We want to be affirmed for who we are. And not only do we want to be included, but we also want to look favorable in the picture.

Early Years of Growing Up

Growing up as a person who stutters, it was never easy to find myself in the picture. It was similar to the *Where's Waldo* book that many children love to read. You know that Waldo is there, but it's hard to find him. This is because Waldo is very good at hiding. He is very good at blending into the crowd. There are many scenes that catch your attention first, things that distract you from finding Waldo. But Waldo is also very distinct in how he appears, very different from others in the picture, so all you have to do is look for the outfit that no one else is wearing, and you find him. As a stutterer, much of my growing up years were all about hiding, blending, and doing whatever I could not to stutter—or in a sense, not being true to who I was. This was because stuttering had very little visibility. I heard all of the classic phrases that most stutterers hear: slow down, take your time, relax, take a breath, think hard about what you want to say. And none of those things were helpful, at least not in the long term. Since there were so few positive images of people who stutter in the media, and since stuttering was so poorly understood in society (all we had was Porky Pig), it was very difficult to "find myself in the picture." Sometimes, I just wasn't there. I can remember talking, and stuttering, usually on my name. And I can remember seeing frustration, disappointment, or amusement in the face of the person I was talking to. As a result, I went silent, lowered my volume, or changed what I wanted to say, all in an attempt to not stutter. No one ever said to me, "You're okay. I'm still listening." When you exhibit a difference that you don't understand, that you're penalized for, and that no one else around you shares, then you find ways of hiding yourself. After all, who wants to be constantly judged? I would describe my experience of stuttering in three ways: (1) I openly struggled through talking at the risk of judgment from others, (2) I concealed what I wanted to say, and (3) I changed what I wanted to say to appear fluent. In fact, my stuttering became a metaphor for my life in general: being open at the risk of judgment, concealment, and changing myself to appear normal. The early years of growing up laid a very important foundation for later years, so my first principle for clinicians working with people who stutter and families of people who stutter, is don't make stuttering the elephant in the room. In fact, don't make it an elephant at all. Yes, stuttering may be difficult and challenging, but communication is always the end result. You can talk about stuttering in healthy and helpful ways, and you can help children to understand that their way of talking may be different, but it is not wrong.

Grade School Years: Where Am I?

Sixth-grade reading class. There were approximately 30 students. I sat trembling in fear, knowing what was about to happen. It was reading time, and the teacher would require every student to read a paragraph in the story. She would start with the first person, and the routine would continue until everyone took a turn. I counted the number of people ahead of me, and then counted that same number of paragraphs in the story, to figure out which paragraph I would read. I practiced it over and over, wondering how I would navigate through the hard syllables, or slide through the soft sounds. I sweated. I trembled. My heartbeats increased. My mind raced with all kinds of self-defeating thoughts: What would my classmates think? What would the teacher say? Would I be able to get through this? Eventually, when my turn came, I started to read, only to discover that I was on the wrong paragraph. I had either miscalculated, or somewhere along the way, someone read an extra paragraph. Regardless, I now had to read a paragraph that I didn't prepare for. As I expected, I struggled through the reading much like a car on a road full of potholes. There were some periods of silence, where I was hoping that an angel would rescue me from the pit of being stuck. My classmates turned and looked. Some tried to hide their laughs. And my teacher looked at me with pity. The next go-round, I built up the same feared anticipation, and when my turn came around, she skipped over me. And I felt a sigh of relief.

Sixth-grade social studies class. We had a group presentation to complete, and I was assigned to work with two other classmates. As soon as the presentation was assigned, I knew right away that I would have trouble. My classmates and I went over our respective parts, and then we were all set. Or maybe they were. The day of the presentation, I was a bundle of nerves. When I opened my mouth to talk, the road once again filled with potholes, and I stumbled my way through it all. Afterwards, one of my groupmates annoyingly asked me, "What happened?" And I said something to the effect of, "I don't know. Sometimes I just get nervous. I'm sorry."

Seventh-grade computer literacy class. My teacher required each of us to read one boldfaced vocabulary word and its definition at the end of the chapter we were studying. And as usual, I took the most time when my turn came. My teacher overtly expressed his frustration toward me with audible sighs and a frowning face. I wrote a letter to three of my friends in that class, and expressed how I was feeling about the situation. After reading the letter, one of them said to me, "We read your letter. And the next time he does that, we are going to stand up and tell him how wrong that is." And I felt a sigh of relief, very taken care of. It felt great to know that someone was willing to stand in the space for me.

These experiences, among others not mentioned here, probably sum up most of what people who stutter have experienced in school. We try our best to hide stuttering, or we try our best to stutter as little as possible, because fluency is the normative expectation. And anything outside of fluency is considered deviant. The experience of stuttering, however, is more than how you hear someone talk. The physiological act of stuttering is only part of the experience. There is an element of physical anticipation, or the sensation of feeling like you might get stuck. When I started to read my paragraph in class, I could sense when my stuttering was about to happen. There's also a cognitive element of anticipation, meaning as soon as I knew it was reading time, I immediately expected that I would stutter. The experience of stuttering has emotional elements: feelings of shame, embarrassment, frustration, disappoint, anger, and guilt. There are psychological elements of self-defeating thoughts that we feed ourselves: "I'm never going to get through this. I am a terrible communicator." Stuttering might affect social relationships with teachers, peers, and family members. And finally, two very important elements to the experience of stuttering are public attitudes toward stuttering and built-in practices that work against people who stutter.

All of these experiences, both personal and social, affected my identity. How we eventually see ourselves is determined in large part by how others have reinforced us over the years. I often use the following quote by Beverly Daniel Tatum on identity:

> Who am I? The answer depends in large part on who the world around me says I am. Who do my parents say I am? Who do my peers say I am? What message is reflected back to me in the faces and voices of my teachers, my neighbors, store clerks? What do I learn from the media about myself? How am I represented in the cultural images around me? Or am I missing from the picture altogether? (p. 99)

Clinicians who work with stuttering should be mindful of the multidimensional experience of stuttering. Stuttering doesn't just exist at the level of the mouth. It includes perceptions and treatment of others toward stuttering; it includes practices that may work against people who stutter; and it includes the thoughts, feelings, and behaviors of the person who stutters. Every person will have a different experience of stuttering. This leads me to my second principle for clinicians: We can't only be concerned about the manner in which people stutter. We have to learn about how stuttering has affected the person, and target all of the roadblocks to effective communication for that person. These can include teaching people that stuttering is okay, that stuttering is not their fault, helping to reduce the struggle and adverse impact associated with stuttering, advocacy, correcting misinformed opinions, and connecting people who stutter to self-help groups and communities where their experiences can be normalized.

College Years: I Am Here, Now How Do I Look?

I went off to college, and began to see myself in new and different ways. I attended Grinnell College in Grinnell, Iowa, and I majored in sociology. Grinnell is a private, liberal arts college, and there, I was exposed to life where people were not afraid of being their authentic selves. As a sociology major, I was learning about racism, sexism, heterosexism, homophobia, classism, and disability rights. This new learning helped me place my experiences with stuttering in context. It helped me to see that I had an important place at the table. Talking was still difficult, and I still had a hard time in class. Sometimes, I would inform my professors that I stuttered, and sometimes I would struggle through oral presentations. It wasn't until the end of my undergraduate years that I learned about speech-language pathology and began to read more about the experiences of others who stutter. Reading about the experiences of others who stutter normalized stuttering for me. I decided to change my career to speech-language pathology, and use my past experiences to inform my work with people who stutter. I went to graduate school at the University of Houston. During my very first course in the program, Introduction to Communication Disorders, I met another classmate who was also a person who stutters. And from there, we talked all things stuttering. It was one of the first times I had ever experienced someone else who had very similar experiences. Moreover, when we discussed the unit on stuttering in my Introduction to Communication Disorders class, my classmate raised her hand and shared her story. This prompted me to nervously raise my hand and share my story. I received lots of positive feedback from my professor and classmates and felt very validated for who I was. I also learned about the National Stuttering Association, and attended a few local self-help groups.

My college years, and my studies in speech-language pathology, taught me that I was in the picture. Now, my task was to foster a favorable impression of myself in the picture. I didn't need to be silent. I could be in the picture as a person who stutters, and I could also smile while in the picture. I completed a project on the experiences of African American men who stutter, and later, during my PhD studies at Bowling Green State University, I completed a project on the school experiences of people who stutter. My college years taught me a third principle that I think is important for clinicians: We want to know that there are others like us, and there are others who care about our needs. Asking questions about what people experience and actively listening to the responses are critical skills for any clinician working with someone with a communication challenge. It is also important to foster connections (e.g., groups, websites, blogs) that emphasize they are not alone.

The Journey Still Continues, But I Am Here, and I Am Okay

I was on the airplane traveling to an annual conference of the National Stuttering Association, and the flight attendant came down the aisle to offer snacks. The choices were crackers, pretzels, and Biscoff cookies. When the flight attendant asked me what I wanted, I tried to say "cookies" but blocked on the "c." I tried again, and blocked again. Next, I tried to insert a carrier phrase, as in "I'll have the. . . ." and still blocked. So, I eventually said, "I'll have the Biscoff." I had a moment with myself, where I felt vulnerable and disappointed that I changed a word, given all that I now know about stuttering. But then I realized that it was okay that I felt vulnerable. And I didn't need to feel bad about changing a word. Part of what it means to be a person who stutters is that I will stutter, and that's okay, and there may be times when I want to switch a word here and there. I don't need to be perfect. I just need to be present. Ultimately, we all want to know that we will be okay. So, my final message to clinicians is to help the people they work with realize that they have value and purpose, and they add to the rich diversity of what it means to communicate. We don't just want to know that Waldo is there. We want to know how Waldo got there, how Waldo feels, and what we can do to make Waldo feel better. We don't want to change Waldo to look like everyone else. We want to bring out the best in the Waldo that we have.

Chapter Summary

You will all encounter Waynes, Nicks, and Dereks in your work as students and professionals. My advice is to seek to learn about their lived experience. Look beyond the standardized assessment measures and the daily data from your interventions. Build authentic relationships, therapeutic alliance, trust, and interactional capital that puts you in a position to motivate and foster participation in personally identified and meaningful activities. Remember those stories, as they are a strong guide to learning from the past and building off of successes. They are also a key connection to humanity and always seeing inherent competence and value in the people you serve. Thanks to excellent mentoring, I remember my first client at the university clinic and her favorite snack—ti kaekers (i.e., cheese crackers). I remember my first patient in the hospital, Emily, who had a right hemisphere stroke and didn't like the modified diet she was on. In my attempt to help her eat, she told me where I could put the spoonful of puréed food I held in my hand—it wasn't in her mouth. I remember one of my first clients with dementia in the nursing home, who had been a saxophone player in Lawrence Welk's band. They could tell me everything about that experience but never remembered to tuck their chin. I hold on to these memories because they ground me and remind me who the real experts are.

References

Campbell, P., Constantino, C., & Simpson, S. (2019). *Stammering pride and prejudice: Difference not defect.* J&R Press.

Jackson, E. S., Gerlach, H., Rodgers, N. H., & Zebrowski, P. M. (2018). My client knows that he's about to stutter: How can we address stuttering anticipation during therapy with young people who stutter. *Seminars in Speech and Language, 39*(4), 356-370.

Tatum, B. D. (2017). *Why are all the black kids sitting together in the cafeteria?: And other conversations about race.* Basic Books.

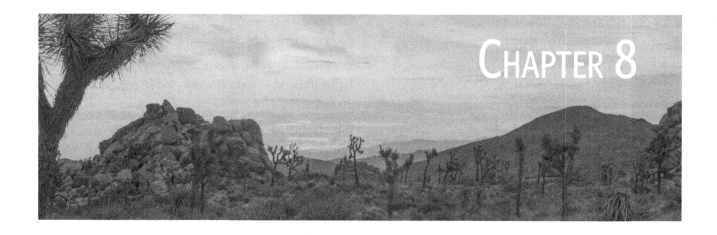

CHAPTER 8

Special Topics and Disorders

Jerry K. Hoepner, PhD, CCC-SLP

A wise man never knows all. Only fools know everything. ~ African Proverb
No one knows everything but together we know a whole lot. ~ Simon Sinek

Many of the techniques we have discussed throughout the text have been transferrable across the lifespan, disorders, and counseling contexts. That being said, there are unique needs and counseling challenges for each of the clients and disorders we encounter, as well as some special situations to consider. No one can be an expert in all of these areas or anticipate all of the potential counseling issues that may arise. Those who dedicate a large portion of their work with specific populations definitely have insights that the rest of us, as generalists, do not. With this in mind, I have gathered together a gifted group of experts in a number of topic areas that present unique challenges and needs. I have deep respect for these individuals because they are not only content or research experts on these areas (which many of them are) but first and foremost, they are master clinicians who are dedicated to serving the individuals in their caseload as effectively as possible. So, you can look at this chapter in two ways—(1) read it cover to cover because the insights of these master clinicians likely cross disorder or topic boundaries, or (2)

read the sections that apply to the clients you're seeing to get a more focused idea of what you may encounter and how to approach it. We will begin with the littles and work our way along the lifespan, recognizing that not everything fits neatly into that framework.

Obviously, there is substantial overlap between topic areas, and most topics don't fit solely in one section. As such, we have done our best to divide topics into manageable sections:

Chapter 8a—Special Topics and Disorders: Developmental

Rebecca Jarzynski, Charlotte Clark, Laura Arrington, Ryan Nelson, Holly Damico, Christine Weill, Jack Damico, Pamela Terrell, and Laura Plexico

Hoepner, J. K. (Ed.). *Counseling and Motivational Interviewing in Speech-Language Pathology* (pp. 133-134).
© 2024 Taylor& Francis Group.

Chapter 8b—Special Topics and
Disorders: Across the Lifespan
Jack Pickering, Eva Van Leer, and Dan Hudock

Chapter 8c—Special Topics and
Disorders: Acquired Medical
Rebecca Affoo, Miriam Carroll-Alfano, and Julia Fischer

Chapter 8d—Special Topics and
Disorders: Aphasia and Acquired
Cognitive-Communication
Deborah Hersh, Natalie Douglas, and Jerry K. Hoepner

Chapter 8e—Special Topics and
Disorders: Important Conversations
Robin Pollens, Nancy Petersen, Emma Power, Margaret
McGrath, and Sandra Lever

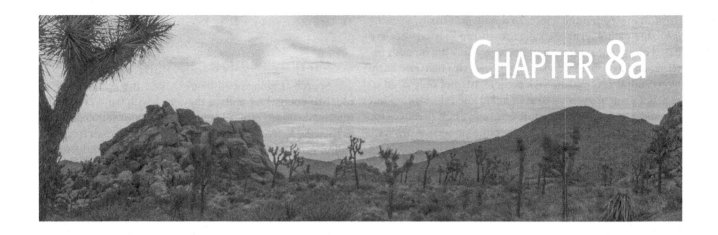

Special Topics and Disorders
Developmental

Rebecca Jarzynski, MS, CCC-SLP; Charlotte Clark, PhD, CCC-SLP;
Laura Arrington, PhD, CCC-SLP; Ryan Nelson, PhD, CCC-SLP;
Holly Damico, PhD, CCC-SLP; Christine Weill, PhD, CCC-SLP;
Jack Damico, PhD, CCC-SLP; Pamela Terrell, PhD, CCC-SLP; and Laura Plexico, PhD, CCC-SLP

Principles of Culturally Responsive Early Intervention Services

Rebecca L. Jarzynski, MS, CCC-SLP

Early intervention service speech-language pathologists are called to ground their work in five principles: services must be family-centered, culturally and linguistically responsive, supportive of children's natural environment, team-based, and based on the highest quality internal and external evidence (American Speech-Language-Hearing Association, n.d.).

Family-centered service provision requires speech-language pathologists to develop strong partnerships with families as they seek to build on family strengths and to understand and work within family priorities. The provision of culturally and linguistically responsive services relates closely to the principle of family-centered practices, as early intervention speech-language pathologists are expected to embed services within the culture of any given family system. Early

intervention speech-language pathologists will also work closely to embed strategy use within a child's natural environment, which not only includes the physical location in which a child spends most of their time, but also involves the use of family materials inside of family routines and preferred activities. The delivery of family-centered and culturally responsive practice requires strong counseling skills, as early intervention speech-language pathologists work to guide families in informed-decision making and to assist families in embedding strategies designed to support child development in the context of their life.

Speech-language pathologists must also work with team members to provide integrated, comprehensive team-based services. This is often accomplished through the use of a primary coach approach to teaming in which one member of the early intervention team develops a close relationship with the family and delivers integrated services through weekly visits while being supported through consultations with other team members. Speech-language pathologists will utilize their coaching skills as they guide their colleagues to support families in using natural opportunities

Hoepner, J. K. (Ed.). *Counseling and Motivational Interviewing in Speech-Language Pathology* (pp. 135-152).
© 2024 Taylor& Francis Group.

to promote communication development. Finally, speech-language pathologists are called to ensure that services are based on the most recent best practices, drawing on both internal and external evidence to guide service delivery. Early intervention speech-language pathologists not only need to seek out evidence related to assessment and intervention but also need to consume literature informing best practices for engaging caregivers from all backgrounds in service delivery.

Opportunities for Counseling

Diagnosis

Early intervention speech-language pathologists are frequently one of the first professionals to work closely with a child and a family. Therefore, they will often play a large role in the initial diagnostic process. Speech-language pathologists will diagnose children with speech, language, and feeding delays/disorders, will work with families whose children have just received life-altering diagnoses such as Down syndrome, and will walk beside families as they work with other medical professions to arrive at diagnoses such as autism spectrum disorder. Because early interventionists develop close partnerships with families, they are in a strong position to utilize counseling skills to help families work though the fear, grief, and confusion that frequently accompany these diagnoses. Speech-language pathologists are called to understand and support the process of grieving, to provide clear information across time that is grounded in a family's evolving needs, to help families interpret and apply information provided by other medical professionals, to listen carefully and deeply, to call attention to child strengths, to build on family strengths, and to validate a family's pain while also providing hope for the future.

As early interventionists use their counseling skills to support and guide families, they should be acutely aware of the ways in which culture may shape family perceptions of disability and help-seeking behavior. Families within some cultures may be more likely to view a disability as bringing shame to the family or may believe that they caused a disability by breaking cultural taboos (DuBay et al., 2018; Huang et al., 2010). Speech-language pathologists may also find that the use of diagnostic labels may not fit within a family's cultural expectations (Verdon et al., 2015) or that some families are more inclined to use informal supports as compared to formal supports (Magnusson et al., 2016). A strong understanding of cultural influences combined with deep listening skills will assist speech-language pathologists in the provision of effective counseling as families navigate the diagnostic process.

Selection of Intervention Strategies, Activity Contexts, and Communication Partners

Speech-language pathologists have the opportunity to use their counseling skills as they work with families to make informed choices around language facilitation strategies and as they guide families in the implementation of strategy use within activities that are preferred by the family, utilizing familiar communication partners.

Speech-language pathologists can begin the process of developing partnerships with families by using a routines-based interview (McWilliam et al., 2009), which is designed to elicit important information about a family's routines and priorities. Early intervention speech-language pathologists will also want to employ their ethnographic interviewing skills to understand family values, cultural parenting practices, and cultural expectations (Peredo, 2016). Speech-language pathologists will use their counseling skills as they implement routines-based and ethnographic interviews, tapping into their reflective listening skills to paraphrase the content they are hearing and to ask follow-up questions. Speech-language pathologists can also use the assessment process as a way to begin working with families to explore the use of everyday activities as contexts for facilitating communication (Wilson et al., 2004). Here again, speech-language pathologists will tap into their counseling skills as they use open-ended questions, listen to what is and is not being shared, reflect back what they are hearing, and share information in a way that supports family decision-making.

From an intervention standpoint, a coaching approach (Rush & Shelden, 2020) to early intervention is often used within early intervention service delivery. The coaching approach strongly parallels the principles of motivational interviewing, with speech-language pathologists utilizing joint plans, opportunities for observation and action/practice of strategies, reflective questions, and feedback to embed strategy use into a family's daily routines and activities. The use of a coaching approach leads to the development of a strong partnership with families, ensuring family-centered service delivery. See Box 8a-1 for an example of coaching in practice.

Culturally Responsive Service Delivery

Strong counseling skills become increasingly important when working to achieve culturally responsive service delivery within early intervention. The majority of naturalistic language interventions with high-quality external evidence have been developed within a European-American framework and have been predominantly researched with populations of Anglo-American decent (Cycyk & Huerta, 2020; Guiberson & Ferris, 2019a). Common strategies within early intervention include embedding techniques into play, following the child's lead, using wait time, and supporting the child's mother as the familiar communication partner. Culture, however, has a strong influence on parent-child interaction styles, use of child talk, expectations for child behavior, and parenting strategies. For example, depending on the culture and the individual family system, families may value activities other than play, may be more directive and less likely to follow the child's lead due to a focus on interdependent communication styles, and/or may highly value the involvement of siblings or extended family members as familiar communication partners (Cycyk & Heurta, 2020; Guiberson & Ferris, 2019b; Johnston & Wong, 2002).

Tensions may arise if speech-language pathologists are not flexible in their use of naturalistic language interventions with culturally and linguistically diverse families. Families may feel misunderstood and disempowered, impacting the speech-language pathologist's ability to build the partnership required to provide family-centered services built upon a family's values and priorities (De Gioia, 2013). This has the strong potential to impact treatment fidelity and child outcomes (Binger et al., 2018; Elder et al., 2003). Given the complexity that comes with balancing all five principles of early intervention, these tensions are not unexpected. However, early intervention speech-language pathologists can successfully work within these tensions by utilizing their counseling skills to ground their work intentionally and systematically in the culture of the families and children they serve. Because parent beliefs and values vary both between and within cultures (Dunst et al., 2017), strong counseling skills will provide the foundation for ensuring individualized, culturally responsive services. See Box 8a-1 for an example of culturally responsive and family-centered practice.

Supporting Families Who Live in Poverty

Speech-language pathologists deliver early intervention services in the context of family systems, making it is essential that they consider the influences of stress on the family systems of the children they serve. Poverty is not only a common issue, but a pervasive one, impacting nearly 15% of all children living in the United States and influencing many aspects of family functioning. Family routines, family responsiveness, and overall child development are adversely impacted when families do not have consistent access to housing, food, health care, or a stable income (Corr et al., 2016). Counseling skills are utilized when speech-language pathologists seek to understand these sources of stress, provide information and connection to resources to alleviate family stress, and work to ensure that they are not unintentionally placing additional stress on the family system. Wise early interventionists understand that supporting healthy families leads to better overall child development, including language development. Early intervention speech-language pathologists who work with families dealing with poverty will therefore need to ask more open-ended questions about the family as a whole, listen even more carefully to discover and find ways to support fluctuating family priorities, demonstrate consistent empathy and patience through reflective listening, and intentionally share information that is directly related to the whole family's priorities.

Support of a Child's Home Language

Early intervention speech-language pathologists serve an increasingly diverse population, with nearly 22 million children in America speaking more than one language (Santhanam & Parveen, 2018). A robust evidence base suggests that supporting a child's home language carries both social-emotional and linguistic benefits for the child (Chung et al., 2019; Hoff & Core, 2015). Families, however, may face tensions as they work to balance acculturation with preservation of their culture and language (Verdon et al., 2016; Yu, 2013). Despite evidence to the contrary, parents may also carry both overt and covert worries that exposure to multiple languages will cause or exacerbate a language delay or disorder (Yu, 2013). Effective counseling skills will allow speech-language pathologists to uncover parent viewpoints regarding dual language learning, provide relevant and evidenced-based information related to supporting dual language learning in children with language delays or disorders, and navigate potential tensions as they guide parents to make informed decisions about supporting their child's language development in multiple languages. See Box 8a-2 for an example of a speech-language pathologist using their counseling skills to support a family in decision making around supporting their dual language learner.

References

American Speech-Language-Hearing Association (n.d.). *Early Intervention*. ASHA practice portal—professional issues. https://www.asha.org/practice-portal/professional-issues/early-intervention/#collapse_1

Binger, C., Kent-Walsh, J., Berens, J., Del Campo, S., & Rivera, D. (2008). Teaching Latino parents to support the multi-symbol message productions of their children who require AAC. *Augmentative and Alternative Communication*, 24(4), 323-338. https://doi.org/10.1080/07434610802230978

Chung, S., Zhou, Q., Anicama, C., Rivera, C., & Uchikoshi, Y. (2019). Language proficiency, parenting styles, and socioemotional adjustment of young dual language learners. *Journal of Cross-Cultural Psychology*, 50(7), 896-914. https://doi.org/10.1177/0022022119867394

Corr, C., Santos, R., & Fowler, S. (2016). The components of early intervention services for families living in poverty: A review of the literature. *Topics in Early Childhood*, 36(1), 55-64.

Cycyk, L. M., & Huerta, L. (2020). Exploring the cultural validity of parent-implemented naturalistic language intervention procedures for families from Spanish-Speaking Latinx homes. *American Journal of Speech-Language Pathology*, 29(3), 1241-1259. https://doi.org/10.1044/2020_AJSLP-19-00038

De Gioia, K. (2013). Cultural negotiation: Moving beyond a cycle of misunderstanding in early childhood settings. *Journal of Early Childhood Research*, 11(2), 108-122. https://doi.org/10.1177/1476718X12466202

Box 8a-1
Angelina and Mai

Background: Angelina is mom to Mai, a 29-month-old girl being raised in a Hmong/English bilingual home. Mai presents with a language delay and has been receiving early intervention speech-language pathology services for 3 months. From the beginning, Angelina demonstrated naturally strong language facilitation skills and highly responsive interactions with her daughter. Speech-language pathology services initially focused on building up Angelina's confidence around her use of parallel talk and self-talk in the context of the "minischool" sessions she was already building into Mai's daily routine. Recent sessions have focused on the use of focused language stimulation provided in both Hmong and English in the context of book reading, songs, and puzzles. During the last session, the speech-language pathologist suggested using enhanced milieu training (EMT) procedures with time delay to increase Mai's use of independent word productions. The speech-language pathologist is now returning for her next visit with Angelina and Mai.

SLP: Great to see you both! How is the day going?

Angelina: (Appearing slightly flustered, as Mai is crying in the background.) It's going well I guess, although Mai has been crankier than usual over the past week or so.

SLP: Ah, yes—toddlers can be that way! [Affirmative Feedback]. What do you think might be leading to some of that crankiness? [Reflective Question].

Angelina: I've been trying to withhold things from her, like you suggested last visit. At first, she was OK with it, but now she just seems to get frustrated the minute I start to hold onto things.

SLP: OK, so you're feeling like the use of time delay is leading to her frustration. [Affirmative Feedback]. In what types of activities did you try out time delay? [Reflective Question].

Angelina: Mainly during our school time, when doing puzzles, like we tried last time you were here. I also tried just now during snack time and she was kind of OK then. But she still got mad and then just refused to eat snack, and now she's crying because I put snack away. ARGH. I'm thinking that we just need to take a break from withholding things for a while.

SLP: OK, so you're seeing the frustration in different activities. [Affirmative Feedback]. That can be frustrating for you, too. It's not uncommon for kids to respond this way at times, but it sounds like you'd like to steer away from this strategy for a while, to decrease her frustration levels overall.

Here, the speech-language pathologist might be thinking that they really need to work on independent word productions, that time delay would be the most effective strategy, and that they could explore different ways to implement time delay to make it less frustrating. However, Angelina is clearly stressed and has expressed a desire to take a break from using EMT + time delay. The speech-language pathologist recognizes and values the insights Angelina brings to the conversation as a parent with deep knowledge of her child. The speech-language pathologist also understands that high-quality relationships between a parent and child support child development and does not want to increase the tension between Angelina and Mai any further. The speech-language pathologist is also aware that Angelina tends to value strategies and activities that promote interdependence over independence. Understanding that this may reflect a cultural belief system and wanting to ensure culturally responsive, family-centered service delivery, the speech-language pathologist chooses to affirm the choice to move away from using time delay at this point, knowing that they can come back to this strategy at a different time if Angelina chooses.

SLP: I get that! She's been responding so well to your beautiful interactions with her as you surround her with language to hear without requiring that she say something [Evaluative Feedback]. So, what do you have in mind for today? [Reflective Question].

Angelina: I think I want to work on more action words. Like we talked about last time, she's using lots of nouns, but I know she needs to use more action words.

SLP: Sounds good to me—you're right that she needs different types of words to eventually start using phrases and sentences. [Evaluative Feedback]. What kinds of activities do you think would work best for action words?

(continued)

Box 8a-1 (continued)

Angelina and Mai

Angelina: I was thinking about that. Maybe not puzzles, because we mainly talk about the pictures on the puzzles. Although maybe I could just add action words and pretend the animals or letters on the puzzles are doing things?

SLP: Sure, you could try to use more action words while doing puzzles [Affirmative Feedback]. You're right, though, it's harder to see the actions happening with puzzle pieces [Evaluative Feedback]. I'm wondering if there are other activities where action words might be even more obvious? [Reflective Question].

Angelina: We could go outside and play—she's been loving being outside with the beautiful spring weather.

SLP: Sounds good! Let's head out.

The speech-language pathologist proceeds to observe Angelina and Mai playing outside [Observation]. She notices and points out how Angelina uses parallel talk to describe Mai's actions and proceeds to have a discussion with Angelina about how to choose action word for focused language stimulation. They discuss which words might be most frequently occurring during outside activities and think together about which words would contain early developing sounds from both a Hmong and English language perspective. The speech-language pathologist uses both reflective questions and informative feedback to guide Angelina's decision making as she chooses five words to be used in focused language stimulation over the week. The speech-language pathologist takes turns interacting with Mai, modeling repeated use of these words [Action/Practice] and at the end of the session, the speech-language pathologist uses reflective questions to elicit Angelina's insights about the feasibility of this strategy. Angelina discusses her plans to teach Mai's dad to model their selected action words during their gross motor/tickle games at night [Joint Plan].

A month later, when Angelina briefly mentions that she might like to try the time delay strategy again, the speech-language pathologist picks up on this, shares information about the value of this approach and discusses different methods for decreasing the intensity of the time delay. Because the speech-language pathologist has worked to build a solid partnership grounded in Angelina's priorities, values, and experiences with Mai, she is able to use her coaching skills to guide the implementation of EMT + time delay procedures that are more effective and well implemented inside of Mai's routines without causing frustration.

Box 8a-2

Carla and Julia

Background: Carla is mom to Julia, a 23-month-old little girl who isn't talking yet. Carla and her husband are Mexican American, having emigrated from Mexico 10 years ago. They are both bilingual language speakers with stronger skills in Spanish than in English. This is their first visit with the early intervention speech-language pathologist. Carla and the speech-language pathologist began the session by talking about potential strategies for building Julia's language and the topic of Julia being a bilingual language learner has come up.

Carla: I want all of us to mainly use English around her. She needs to learn English for school.

SLP: Oh, OK. Tell more me more about this. [Open-Ended Question].

Here the speech-language pathologist might be tempted to engage in a righting reflex response, as she knows that Julia will benefit from both a linguistic and a social-emotional development standpoint from continuing to hear and being encouraged to use her home language. But she withholds sharing this information for now, in order to better understand Carla's concerns and to listen for any potential change talk.

(continued)

Box 8a-2 (continued)
Carla and Julia

Carla: She's not talking. If she hears two languages, it will be harder for her to learn. I don't want her to be behind.

SLP: So, you're worried that hearing two languages will cause her to be even more behind. [Reflective listening]. You obviously want the very best for her! [Affirmation]. I'm wondering, how do you feel when you talk with her in English?

Carla: I feel good. She's hearing the language she will need for school.

SLP: You're working to make sure that she is ready for school, which is fantastic. [Affirmation]. How about when you talk to her in Spanish? [Open-Ended Question].

Carla: I don't know. I guess I feel bad because it might hold her back. But I love singing to her in Spanish. My mom sang to me the same way. And Spanish is easier for me, so I relax more. But I worry that it's not good for her.

SLP: So, you're feeling many emotions at the same time when you use Spanish: connected with her and relaxed, but also worried [Reflective Listening].

Carla nods.

SLP: That must be hard [Reflective Listening].

Carla nods.

SLP: I'm wondering, who else in your family speaks Spanish?

Carla: Oh, everyone. My husband, her siblings, her grandparents and everyone else in the family.

SLP: So, lots of people in your family speak Spanish [Reflective listening]. I'm wondering what will happen if she doesn't also speak Spanish? [Open-Ended Question].

Carla: Yeah, I'm worried that she won't be able to speak with her grandparents if she doesn't learn Spanish, too. I do want her to be able to talk to them. Maybe I should go back to using Spanish with her, too. But she's not talking at all. I just don't want to make it worse.

The speech-language pathologist, hearing the change talk among the ambivalence, choses to move into summarizing and then informing.

SLP: So, I hear you saying that you're just really conflicted about using two languages around her. On one hand, you want her to stay connected to you and your family and you feel most comfortable talking to her in Spanish. On the other hand, you worry that speaking two languages is causing her delay, and she won't be ready to use English in school. [Double-Sided Reflection].

Carla nods.

SLP: I do have some information I can share about how using Spanish with her will actually help with her language delay and will also help her get ready to use English in school. Would you like me to share that information with you now?

The speech-language pathologist shares information about both the linguistic and social-emotional benefits of supporting home language development alongside the development of English. Together, they then explore options for promoting both Spanish and English development at home while also continuing to expose Julia to English in other environments.

DuBay, M., Watson, L. R., & Zhang, W. (2018). In search of culturally appropriate autism interventions: Perspectives of Latino caregivers. *Journal of Autism and Developmental Disorders*, 48(5), 1623-1639. https://doi.org/10.1007/s10803-017-3394-8

Dunst, C. J., Hamby, D. W., Raab, M., & Bruder, M. B. (2017). Family socioeconomic status and ethnicity, acculturation and enculturation, and parent beliefs about child behavior, learning methods, and parenting roles. *Journal of Education and Culture Studies*, 1(2), 99. https://doi.org/10.22158/jecs.v1n2p99

Elder, J. H., Valcante, G., Won, D., & Zylis, R. (2003). Effects of in-home training for culturally diverse fathers of children with autism. *Issues in Mental Health Nursing*, 24(3), 273-295. https://doi.org/10.1080/01612840305276

Guiberson, M., & Ferris, K. P. (2019a). Early language interventions for young dual language learners: A scoping review. *American Journal of Speech-Language Pathology*, 28(3), 945-963. https://doi.org/10.1044/2019_AJSLP-IDLL-18-0251

Guiberson, M. M., & Ferris, K. P. (2019b). Identifying culturally consistent early interventions for Latino caregivers. *Communication Disorders Quarterly*, 40(4), 239-249. https://doi.org/10.1177/1525740118793858

Hoff, E., & Core, C. (2015). What clinicians need to know about bilingual development. *Seminars in Speech and Language*, 36(2), 089-099. https://doi.org/10.1055/s-0035-1549104

Huang, Y. P., Kellett, U., & St John, W. (2010). Cerebral palsy: Experiences of mothers after learning their child's diagnosis. *Journal of Advanced Nursing*, 66, 1213-1221. https://doi-org.proxy.uwec.edu/10.1111/j.1365-2648.2010.05270.x

Johnston, J. R., & Wong, M. Y. A. (2002). Cultural differences in beliefs and practices concerning talk to children. *Journal of Speech, Language, and Hearing Research*, 45(5), 916-926. https://doi.org/10.1044/1092-4388(2002/074)

Magnusson, D., Palta, M., McManus, B., Benedict, R. E., & Durkin, M. S. (2016). Capturing unmet therapy needs among young children with developmental delay using national survey data. *Academic Pediatrics*, 16(2), 145-153. https://doi.org/10.1016/j.acap.2015.05.005

McWilliam, R. A., Casey, A. M., & Sims, J. (2009). The routines-based interview: A method for gathering information and assessing needs. *Infants & Young Children*, 22(3), 224-233. https://doi.org/10.1097/IYC.0b013e3181abe1dd

Peredo, T. (2016). Supporting culturally and linguistically diverse families in early intervention. *Perspectives of the ASHA Special Interest Groups*, 1(4), 154-167.

Rush, D. D., & Shelden, M. L. (2020). *The early childhood coaching handbook* (2nd ed.). Paul H. Brookes Publishing Co.

Santhanam, S. P., & Parveen, S. (2018). Serving culturally and linguistically diverse clients: A review of changing trends in speech-language pathologists' self-efficacy and implications for stakeholders. *Clinical Archives of Communication Disorders*, 3(3), 165-177. https://doi.org/10.21849/cacd.2018.00395

Verdon, S., Wong, S., & McLeod, S. (2015). Shared knowledge and mutual respect: Enhancing culturally competent practice through collaboration with families and communities. *Child Language Teaching and Therapy*, 32(2), 205-221. https://doi.org/10.1177/0265659015620254

Wilson, L. L., Mott, D. W., & Batman, D. (2004). The asset-based context matrix: A tool for assessing children's learning opportunities and participation in natural environments. *Topics in Early Childhood Special Education*, 24(2), 110-120. https://doi.org/10.1177/02711214040240020601

Yu, B. (2013). Issues in bilingualism and heritage language maintenance: Perspectives of minority-language mothers of children with autism spectrum disorders. *American Journal of Speech-Language Pathology*, 22(1), 10-24.

Prioritizing Relationships in Servicing Pediatric Language Disorders

Charlotte Clark, PhD, CCC-SLP;
Laura Arrington, PhD, CCC-SLP;
Ryan Nelson, PhD, CCC-SLP;
Holly Damico, PhD, CCC-SLP;
Christine Weill, PhD, CCC-SLP; and
Jack Damico, PhD, CCC-SLP

As has been described through this textbook, there are a variety of approaches to counseling, each nuanced in ways well-suited to the client and reflective of the inclinations of the strengths practitioners bring to the therapeutic interactions. Relationships and relationship-building are the foundational ties binding these approaches. Irrespective of the framework a clinician adopts, each approach begins with the construction of relationships and alliances. At the beginning of this chapter, as authors, we feel it is important to disclose our counseling stance. A social-constructivist view of social action is the radiating lamp lighting our clinical decision-making and guiding our selection of counseling methods. In practice, this appears as a purposeful, eclectic selection of methods and strategies driven by our strengths as clinicians, the strengths and needs of the clients, and the context of intervention. Reflection on our practices suggests we most closely align with a strengths and wellness framework (Holland & Nelson, 2020). With this disclosure, we will now explore relationship-building in children with language disorders, their parents and the clinical relationships that emerge (Gergen, 2009). To begin, let's consider an example of a typical interaction between a mother and her son (Box 8a-3).

Relationship and the Co-Construction of Competence

At 3 years and 7 months old, Joey's utterances and gestures require a great deal of interpretation from his conversational partner. Fortunately, his mother draws upon her background knowledge and relationship with him to both impose and construct meaning from Joey's behaviors. It is their relationship that informs her responses. Demonstrated in her responses in Box 8a-3 is her assumption that Joey is purposeful in his contributions to the interaction. In the same interaction, another partner with a different relationship may have interpreted the same ambiguous double pointing gesture, to both his jeans pocket and his basket (see lines 10 and 11), as confusion on Joey's part. Consequently, his language challenges would have been made manifest and his lack of competence both emphasized and reinforced. In relationship with his mother, however, Joey's strengths as a jokester and an entertainer emerge. This simple interaction suggests to us that it is difficult to overemphasize the importance of relationships in the construction of communicative competence in pediatric language disorders.

Michelle, and her "silly" son were generous enough to share some memories with us. We first met Joey during an observation as he participated in a small preschool-age clinic group. We noted immediately that he was playing on his own and vocalizing to himself while most of the other children were playing a game together. His clinic files described a child with few words, including his name, "more," and "open." The clinicians were considering the introduction of an augmentative and alternative communication board to better help Joey communicate basic needs and wants. Such

---

Box 8a-3
Michelle and Joey

"You're silly. You're being silly!" says a mom to her son, as they both fall into laughter. Words likely to be uttered to any 3-year-old and on more than one occasion. Silliness in a 3-year-old is typical. However, children with language learning delays or disorders do not always demonstrate what is typical. The following conversation illustrates the challenges that arise with language disorders and the role relationships play in establishing competency. Notice in this example how few words the boy contributes.

Transcript 1: Michelle and her son, Joey, were seated on the floor interacting with cars and other small toys.

1. **Michelle:** (looking at her 3-year old son, Joey) Where did you put your
2. eggs when you went to the zoo and got eggs. Did you put them in your pockets? (smiles)
3. **Joey:** (looks at mom and whispers) yeah
4. **Michelle:** (shakes head and smiles) Nooo! Where did you put them?
5. **Joey:** uhh. Huuhh. (utters syllables with intonation similar to "right here" while pointing
6. to his pants pocket)
7. **Michelle:** They didn't go in your pocket. (points to basket) Did they go in your basket?
8. **Joey:** Ahhh (looking at mom, points in direction of basket)
9. **Michelle:** Yeah. They went in your basket. And did you—
10. **Joey:** Ahhh (looking at mom and slightly shakes his head, points to basket and his
11. pocket with each hand)
12. **Michelle:** They didn't go in your pockets (smiles and pokes his stomach). You're silly.
13. **Joey:** (laughs and rolls the toy car he had been holding)
14. **Michelle:** You're being silly. And did you see—What else? Was there a giraffe?

---

initial impressions of Joey naively led us to primarily concentrate on what he was not able to do. His interactional limitations seemed so pervasive. So, when we asked families in the preschool clinic if they would participate in a study of reminiscing conversations, we were surprised when Michelle volunteered. Michelle insisted that she and Joey talked about past events frequently, and so we set up the next observation. While theoretically we knew that a child's abilities will vary depending upon context, it was amazing to see how Joey's competency was enhanced through interactions with his mother. This child, who was alone in the corner during initial observations of his preschool group, was transformed into a storyteller when in co-constructed conversations with his mother. Having gained this deeper insight into the relationship between Joey and Michelle, it is easier to adopt a strengths-based approach to intervention. As counseling-oriented clinicians, our job in this or similar situations is to make explicit to Michelle her own strengths in this interaction. This counseling will require leading Michelle to recognize how her relationship with Joey and her stance of presuming competence in him contribute to his success. Further, as clinicians, we can model similar assumptions of competence and intentionality by reacting to children like

Joey with a mindset of attending to what they do well. When we make requests for clarification or attempts to provide re-mediating strategies, we must make these efforts through the lens of seeing Joey as a valued member in a relationship.

Another illustrative example of the importance of relationships is presented in Box 8a-4, in the segment of the transcription from the reminiscing of Michelle and Joey. Interestingly, we witnessed for the first time Joey's self-references as "Deedee," a term that only those who knew him would recognize as his name for himself.

Shared experience with Joey placed Michelle in a unique position to elaborate on Joey's references to their zoo trip. She was present for the zoo trip and could make inferences about the event. She recalled what animals he saw and what they did while at the park. She also had knowledge of all the unconventional means Joey used to communicate including his noises and word approximations. Joey had even constructed a way of marking the absence of a person when discussing memories with Michelle. In a post-observation interview, Michelle related how Joey would combine "Bye" with a name to signal that someone was not present at an event. It was within their relationship that Michelle and Joey constructed competencies not revealed or observed in Joey's interactions

---

Box 8a-4

Michelle and Joey

15. **Michelle:** Do you remember when we went to the zoo? What was at the zoo? When you

16. got the eggs? Did you see a snake at the zoo?

17. **Joey:** (looking at toy car makes a hissing noise)

18. **Michelle:** Yeah.

19. Joey: (looks up) Daddy hissss.

20. **Michelle:** Daddy saw the snake. Did mama see the snake?

21. Joey: (turns around to face Michelle) Maaa Hissss.

22. **Michelle:** Did mama see the snakes?

23. Joey: Deedee hissss.

24. **Michelle:** Deedee saw the snakes. What other animals? What where the animals in the

25. water

26. **Joey:** Fffuuusshhh

27. **Michelle:** Fishhh. Very good! And what were the animals in the trees?

28. **Joey:** (looks up from toy car) Muu eees/

29. **Michelle:** Mon-keys. Ooow eeees. Monkeys. What other animals did you see? What did

30. you ride on? (emphasis on ride) Did we go for a ride?

31. **Joey:** (looks at Michelle) shu

32. **Michelle:** (nods) On a chu. Was that/

33. **Joey:** xxxxxx Deedee. shuu. Deedee shuu (while rolling toy car)

34. **Michelle:** (nods) Joey went on a—Deedee went on a chu?

---

with anyone else. As counseling-minded clinicians, we need to be aware of the competency constructing potential in such relationships. These are relationships that we can encourage, support, and use to inform our interactions with children. Observation of the relationship in action provides us with data that could not be obtained through case history alone. We observed the strategies and abilities Michelle and Joey constructed for themselves and how they worked to mutually orient to one another's perspective within each conversational turn in the previous examples (Clark, 2018). Our privileging of information, obtained through observation of authentic interactions, illuminated these communicative and narrative-building strategies (DiLollo & Neimeyer,

2014). Our ability to recognize the complexity of Joey's contributions and to interpret these behaviors as strengths is informed by our counseling framework. Additionally, it was because of our relationship with Michelle and the trust associated with it, that she confidently provided information beneficial to our constructed understanding of Joey's abilities. Her disclosure demonstrates her belief in our view of Joey as competent and clever. Michelle trusts us to see the value and ability of Joey.

It is the relationship between Michelle and Joey and the assumption of proficiency and competence in interaction that enables both partners to invest the effort to reminisce. Characteristics of language disorder often confound the very interaction and communication that underlie the relating of shared experiences (Brinton & Fujiki, 2010; Damico, 1991). This has the potential to frustrate some relationships in a way that we need to be aware of as clinicians. Our conversations with another mother, Elaine, who was gracious enough to share her and her son George's stories, demonstrated the importance of resilience in relationships. George was a preschooler at the time; although his language challenges were relatively mild when compared to Joey, his communication abilities did create interactive challenges. We observed George and his mother discuss several shared memories about fishing trips, swimming lessons, and trips to the park. During a second observation, we asked Elaine what her experience had been with her son's communication challenges. She shared with us the difficulties faced in initially connecting with George. Having helped raise George's older half-sister, a precocious, early talking child, Elaine found herself overrelying on this relationship as she created expectations for George's development. She had connected with her daughter through language as related in this interview transcript:

> With his sister everything was verbal. And she would do the artwork. And you know, everything was make-believe—the stories we would tell. You know that magic.

However, Elaine and George did not bond with words in the same way, which was initially distressing.

> And with him, it's not as bad now, but when he was younger, especially before he got treated for the sensory stuff or the speech delay—it was like, I don't know. It was hard. It was bad. Because I went from one extreme to the other . . . I felt terrible that I didn't have that connection. And I wanted it. I mean, he is my own child.

Elaine then discovered she and George could bond by "doing" together, if not by talking together. She shifted her focus from what they weren't yet capable of to what they were.

> So that is how we built it [a relationship] by creating this life together . . . he loved to do . . . So beside the, well, we have always done the reading, but besides

that, we would do. We wouldn't hardly ever hang out at home. We would do the park. We would do whatever. I mean we just went everywhere (in town.) And I wasn't working, I was still in school. So, I mean we would go to Trampoline City literally every single week. We went to the Go-Cart Farm every week . . . And so what I did to compensate for that . . . because there couldn't be . . . that verbal connection that I had with [my daughter], that is when I started creating this life of activities for us.

In an effort to clarify understanding of Elaine's point, we asked, "Experience—going out and doing things—so that is how you felt like you could connect?" She elaborated, "And create a goodness together."

Counseling Interventions and the Fostering of Strengths From a Relational Lens

Frequently, deficits are a common focus of parents, clients, and clinicians; however, a more beneficial focus for Elaine was on George's strengths. Elaine's discovery that "doing" was a better means of connecting with George demonstrated a shift in her focus from deficits to strengths. Further, it is illustrative of the type of stance clinicians should both personally adopt and therapeutically develop within those we serve. That is, at times we may need to support our child clients by supporting their caregivers. As with children, we cannot bestow communicative competence on caregivers. But we can facilitate experiences that allow families to create together a competence unique to their relationship and shared experiences. Our efforts must assist those we work with in recognizing and valuing these relationships and experiences as strengths. Reconsidering the example of Elaine and George, her awareness and use of strengths in her son, herself, and their relationship should be fostered in our counseling and intervention sessions. Strengths should anchor our language intervention and counseling practices. Our role is to make explicit to clients and parents their individual and shared strengths, to purposefully include these strengths in therapy, and to use these strengths to address areas of concern. When ***ability over deficit*** is the primary focus, strengths become a lens for intervention. A strengths-based perspective, rooted in social work (Saleebey, 1992) and positive psychology (Seligman, 2011), has been applied to counseling in communication disorders (Holland & Nelson, 2020) and to pediatric language intervention (Arrington, 2019). Strengths-based intervention is a process in which clinicians continuously seek out ability over inability, use these abilities as a focus of intervention, and explore different relationships and interactions that foster growth.

It is from the lens of relationship that shared experiences foster the roots of later communicative proficiency (Brinton

& Fujiki, 2004). Viewing these interactions from a lens of ***relationship-building*** enables us to better understand how both mother-child examples were colored by the mother's underlying assumptions of competency and her unconditional valuation of her child's resilience and potential for growth.

As clinicians, prioritizing relationships in therapy helps us avoid the trap of viewing competence as a product we deliver to our clients. Competence is cocreated within the interactional relationship. The job of counseling-minded clinicians is to facilitate the type of interactions that construct and reveal competence—at whatever level necessary. Facilitating these interactions will require that we learn about and from the important relationships in a child's life. In building relationships, we create a space that allows children to create, discover, and demonstrate their own competence.

The stories and observations from Michelle and Joey and Elaine and George have highlighted the importance of relationship-building. We advocate a purposeful and mindful approach to counseling children with language disorders and their families. A counseling and clinical stance oriented to strengths enables the valuing of relationships. To begin the process of more fully valuing relationships, following are two recommendations for clinicians interested in developing a greater relationship-based focus.

Relationship-Building, Strengths-Based Counseling Approach

1. Demonstrate the importance of relationship-building in intervention (parent-child, child-clinician, parent-clinician). Ask questions and fashion opportunities that position both parent and child as competent communicators and equal partners in treatment.

   Questions for parents/clients:
   ° "What improvement would you like to see in the interaction and communication between you and Joey? Joey and others?" instead of, "What do you think Joey needs to work on?"
   ° "Joey, what should we play today?"

   Questions for self-reflection on my practice and interactions with clients:
   ° Are my interactions empowering the relationship between Joey and Michelle?
   ° How does my interpretation of the interactions contribute to relationship-building?
   ° How can I structure therapy to cede control to Joey and Michelle?
   ° Am I flexible and open to the potential of spontaneous interaction to reveal competence? Am I responding or prescribing?
   ° What expertise can I offer that will evoke expansions to these positive interactions or traits?

2. Ask parents and clients about their unique strengths and support them in identifying them. Use your questions to gain information and guide parent's reflection on strengths in their relationship.

Questions for parents/clients:

° "Tell me about how George communicates with you."

° "Describe something George does that impresses you (or makes you think he is smart or clever)."

° "Describe some interactions between you and George you felt good about."

° "How do George's strengths contribute to your relationship with him?"

Questions for self-reflection on my practice and interactions with clients:

° Am I focused on intent or competence rather than accuracy in performance?

° Am I looking for things that are working?

° Am I purposefully and overtly privileging client and parent strengths?

° What strengths in terms of knowledge and skills do I have as a clinician that I can lend to these relationships?

References

Arrington, L. (2019). *An investigation into speech language pathologists' understanding and use of students' strengths during intervention for students with language and learning impairment* [Doctoral dissertation, University of Louisiana at Lafayette]. ProQuest Dissertations Publishing.

Brinton, B., & Fujiki, M. (2010). Living with language impairment. *Journal of Interactional Research in Communication Disorders, 1*(1), 69-94. https://doi.org/10.1558/jircd.v1i1.69

Brinton, B., Robinson, L. A., & Fujiki, M. (2004). Description of a program for social language intervention: "if you can have a conversation, you can have a relationship". *Language, Speech, and Hearing Services in Schools, 35*(3), 283-290. https://doi.org/10.1044/0161-1461(2004/026)

Clark, C. (2018). *Joint-reminiscing between parents and their preschoolers with language impairment* (Publication No. 10844764) [Doctoral dissertation, University of Louisiana at Lafayette]. ProQuest Dissertations Publishing.

Damico, J. S. (1991). Clinical discourse analysis: A functional approach to language assessment. In C.S. Simon (Ed.), *Communication skills and classroom success*. Thinking Publications.

DiLollo, A., & Neimeyer, R. A. (2014). *Counseling in speech-language pathology and audiology: Reconstructing personal narratives*. Plural Publishing, Inc.

Gergen, K. J. (2009). *Relational being: Beyond self and community*. Oxford University Press.

Holland, A. L., & Nelson, R. L. (2020). *Counseling in communication disorders: A wellness perspective*. Plural Publishing, Inc.

Saleebey, D. (1992). *The strengths perspective in social work practice*. Longman.

Seligman, M. E. P. (2011). *Flourish: A visionary new understanding of happiness and well-being*. Free Press.

Counseling in Cleft Lip and Palate

Pamela Terrell, PhD, CCC-SLP

Counseling Concerns for Parents

Usually, the birth of a new baby is a time of excitement and joy for new parents. However, these emotions can be complicated when the baby is born with a cleft or craniofacial disorder. In the United States, cleft lip and/or palate (CL/P) occurs in approximately 1 out of every 600 newborns and is the most common birth defect (American Cleft Palate-Craniofacial Association, 2021b). Some parents find out via ultrasound that their baby will be born with a cleft lip and have time to prepare and process their emotional reaction (Sreejith et al., 2018). However, many parents are caught by surprise to find out that their baby has a CL/P. When the little one arrives, the parents may have conflicting emotions of joy, love, shock, disappointment, shame, or fear (Çinar et al., 2021). However, with education, good care, and a support system, parents tend to ultimately adjust well (Stock et al., 2020).

The parents may have never seen a baby with a cleft or known anyone with a cleft. A cleft lip can look alarming and even more so if the parents did not know about the cleft or if the cleft is bilateral or particularly wide. They may also be concerned about the infant's overall health or worry that the baby is in pain. At these initial stages of learning about and accepting the cleft, the parents need supportive, compassionate care by the medical and nursing staff, as well as a quick referral to a cleft palate team.

Depending on the size and location of the hospital or birthing center and preferences of the parents, a postpartum nurse, lactation consultant, or speech-language pathologist may be consulted to help with feeding. This is a time of significant counseling needs as the parents may still be in shock, be disappointed by their baby's appearance, and be scared to hold or feed their neonate for fear of hurting them. Motivational interviewing with reflective listening and normalization are very important counseling strategies at this time. Parents need to have an opportunity to share their feelings and concern with an empathetic, nonjudgmental listener who will validate their feelings. Connecting new parents to other parents who have a child with a cleft can also be beneficial, and the cleft palate team can be helpful in facilitating this.

If speech-language pathologists are involved in feeding assessment and intervention, it is important to remember that feeding a newborn is important for bonding, but can be a cause of distress, worry, or feelings of failure if it is difficult or not going well. When a mother desires to breastfeed her new baby, she can often be successful if the baby has only a cleft lip or an incomplete cleft palate. However, solely breastfeeding is not feasible for a baby with a complete cleft, and the new mother usually needs time to grieve the loss of that opportunity and her vision of what she thought motherhood would look like at this stage (Çinar et al., 2021). Practically, it will be important to give her time and space to talk about the loss of this bond opportunity, while gently reassuring her that complete bonding can still happen with "kangaroo care" and skin-to-skin contact, cuddles while bottle feeding, and allowing the baby to suckle at the breast when satiated. All of these will still benefit attachment, as well as increase milk production, if the mother is expressing breastmilk for bottle feeding. Gentle support for bottle feeding can empower the parents to feel confident that their infant is getting the necessary calories and nutrition and make them comfortable in the connection that feeding routines facilitate regardless of the method of delivery (American Cleft Palate-Craniofacial Association, 2021a). Bottle feeding also allows for the other parent to be more involved in this time of closeness as well.

As parents begin to feel confident in feeding, they must also prepare for upcoming surgeries at approximately 2 to 3 months of age for cleft lip and 10 to 15 months for cleft palate. Although most parents eagerly anticipate surgery so that their child will "look like everyone else," eat more efficiently, eliminate nasal regurgitation, and begin to speak more intelligibly, this anticipation may be tinged with worry about the surgery, anesthesia, pain, and recovery. Stress about insurance, finances, and time off work may add to feelings of being overwhelmed. After the initial lip closure surgery, parents may be surprised to discover that the lip repair surgery they had been looking forward to has left them with conflicting emotions. While they may be pleased to see the lip repaired, they may need time to adjust to their baby's new appearance and feel a little sad to see their baby's special wide smile gone.

As the child gets older, the counseling needs of the parents change. They have often come to a place of acceptance and love for their child after the initial shock, and perhaps disappointment (Stock et al., 2020). They have resolved feeding concerns and typically have a treatment plan in place for surgeries, therapy, and orthodontia. However, now the parents have concerns about time and money for treatments, their child being bullied by peers due to appearance or speech, and/or the child not being able to communicate as well as peers (Çinar et al., 2021). It is important for the cleft palate team members, as well as the local speech-language pathologist, to maintain an open supportive relationship with the parents and provide them with an opportunity to discuss their concerns without their child present. Additionally, as the child gets older, the parents should be encouraged to make the child a part of the decisions about surgery and interventions. Particularly with complex clefts or craniofacial conditions, teens and young adults may become more accepting of their differences and prefer not to have additional surgeries due to the pain, recovery time, or the "return on investment" (little change in appearance compared to the difficulty of surgery).

Counseling Concerns for Children

As children become elementary-aged and later go through puberty, they begin to be more aware of their scars, orthodontia, jaw and nose deformities, and residual speech and resonance problems. This can impact their psychosocial functioning and development. In particular, children and adolescents with repaired clefts need to be monitored for evidence of bullying, decreased self-esteem/self-confidence, poor coping strategies, and acceptance of their facial appearance. Additionally, they may feel that they are a burden on their families due to their medical care and frequent appointments, and they may sense their parents' anxiety as well (Al-Namankany & Alhubaishi, 2018).

Lorot-Marchand et al. (2015) found that over half of French children and young adults with CL/P had experienced teasing in school and wanted to change their facial appearance. Slightly less than half with cleft palate only also experienced taunting, but they were more satisfied with their facial appearance (likely due to lack of labial and nasal deformation). These participants, ranging from 12 to 29 years old, reported that the taunting made them sad, "depressed," or "scarred them for life," with some of the adults reporting that some verbal insults continued to occur in the workplace (Lorot-Marchand et al., 2015). Additionally, speech, language, hearing, and resonance difficulties might further impact children socially (Stock et al., 2020). Often, residual articulation and hypernasality persist among school-aged children, causing them to be embarrassed by their speech. With hypernasality in particular, Watterson et al. (2013) found that students had more difficulty making friends, "fitting in" with peers, and were more likely to be teased.

For the speech-language pathologist working with school-aged children with repaired CL/P, it is important to check in with the student about bullying, self-esteem, satisfaction with therapy, etc. A team-based approach with the school counselor or school psychologist, as well as open communication with the parents and cleft palate team, are important to make sure that the child is well adjusted, empowered, and can learn to self-advocate. The speech-language pathologist should have regular check-ins with the student to see how the child feels about social relationships, ensure that they are a partner in generating functional goals, and teach strategies for self-advocacy. Empathetic listening, normalization, and validation will be important techniques to use with these students. Additionally, some cognitive behavioral approaches may help to reframe cognitive distortions (e.g., "No one will ever want to date someone who looks like me" or "I'll always sound weird when I talk"), increase positive self-talk, and learn more flexible thinking. These skills and strategies will be especially important during the teenage years as peer acceptance, beauty standards, dating, and self-esteem coincide with treatment periods of orthodontia and additional surgeries to correct the nose, maxilla, and mandible.

Counseling Concerns for Adults With Cleft Lip and Palate

Generally, speech-language therapy is not needed into adulthood. Most people with CL/P end regular consultations with the cleft palate team in their late teens or early 20s. Although they are not receiving ongoing treatment, adults with CL/P may benefit from continued counseling by members of the cleft palate team. A study in the United Kingdom by Stock et al. (2015) found that the 52 participants had been discharged from the cleft team between the ages of 15 and 21 years old. Some felt that dismissal was positive and a means of closure, while others felt that termination of services was abrupt, with one expressing, "I know I'm supposed to be an adult now, but I will still need looking after, I still need to sit and ask questions" (p. 547). For those who might feel the need to "sit and ask questions," the counseling needs would likely fall to the cleft team's psychologist or social worker or the health professional providing ongoing services such as the orthodontist, plastic surgeon, or oral-maxillofacial surgeon.

However, there is one unique situation in which speech-language pathologists might need to counsel adults with CL/P, such as in the case of parents with CL/P who have a child with CL/P. Stock and Rumsey (2015) interviewed 24 parents with CL/P: 8 with children born with CL/P and 16 who had children without CL/P. The parents were interviewed about subjects such as heritability of clefts, reactions to their child's CL/P, adjustment to parenthood, and impacts of their personal experience with cleft on their parenting style. The researchers found that participants varied in their responses to having a child with CL/P, with some feeling like it was not a big issue, but others being distressed and "devastated" knowing the long road of treatment ahead. A few parents found that upsetting memories were triggered when their children had surgery, while others felt more at ease since they themselves had had a similar experience. In this study (Stock & Rumsey, 2015), as well as another study of adults in the United Kingdom with CL/P (Stock et al., 2016), results suggested that having open family discussion about the cleft, the treatments, and feelings about the cleft resulted in better psychosocial outcomes. Therefore, speech-language pathologists should encourage parents with and without clefts to create a nonjudgmental and encouraging environment for the child to talk about the cleft and for the parents to share openly about their experiences, too.

Studies of adults with CL/P provide an outlook into psychosocial issues and counseling needs in a retrospective manner. Stock et al. (2016) analyzed interviews collected from 52 adults with CL/P in the United Kingdom and noted recurrent themes. The researchers categorized the factors contributing to psychosocial adjustment into three primary areas: background (e.g., age, gender, socioeconomic status), external (e.g., treatment autonomy, family coping and support, psychological support), and internal psychological (e.g., confidence, acceptance, disposition, internalization of beauty ideals). Although background factors are not likely to change, they do need to be considered within the treatment context, with special consideration for how ethnicity, gender, etc. may impact treatment, self-perception, and outcomes. Also, additional impairments such as learning disabilities, hearing loss, and developmental delays often exacerbated or superseded the psychosocial impact of CL/P, so speech-language pathologists need to be cognizant of comorbid conditions and the additional counseling needs they present.

External factors can be addressed through training with families, health care providers, teachers, speech-language pathologists, audiologists, and others who may be called upon to provide psychological support to the child or adult with CL/P. Stock et al. (2016) noted that many adults with CL/P experienced a lack of autonomy related to the treatment they received, with one respondent stating, "When I was a child they talked amongst themselves in their own language and I didn't really know what was going on or what plans were being made for me . . . and I said yes to everything because I wanted to look better and I wanted to feel better . . . it was very disempowering" (p. 225). Speech-language pathologists can listen carefully to clients and become partners in developing therapy goals and assessing progress. Speech-language pathologists could also include teaching self-advocacy skills and vocabulary related to cleft conditions (e.g., resonance, maxilla, velopharyngeal insufficiency) as a means of empowering older children, adolescents, and young adults to be active partners on the cleft team. Additionally, speech-language pathologists may be involved in antibullying campaigns and programs at schools or in the community to address public perceptions and acceptance of those with facial differences (such as www.changingfaces.org.uk, www.wonderthebook.com/choose-kind). Finally, speech-language pathologists need to be aware of internal factors such as concepts of beauty ideals, disposition, social confidence, and client self-perceptions of issues such as teasing, "difference," and noticeability so that they can be open to honest discussion of such topics. As stated previously, active nonjudgmental listening, reflection, paraphrasing, normalization, and motivational interviewing skills are important. In addition to being open to exploring background, external, and internal psychosocial factors with clients as they relate to speech and language treatment, the speech-language pathologist needs to be in communication with the team and make sure that the team psychologist or social worker is providing additional counseling as needed.

Boxes 8a-5 and 8a-6 provide case illustrations of individuals with CL/P and their counseling needs. Both scenarios include thought-provoking questions about the case. Consider discussing these questions with colleagues or within your counseling course.

Box 8a-5
Jonathan

Jonathan, a fifth-grade student with a repaired CL/P, sees you for pull-out speech therapy in his elementary school twice a week for 20 minutes in individual sessions. He has a faint pink scar along his left philtral ridge, a mildly flattened left nostril, and a slightly retracted maxilla. Additional surgeries and orthodontia will resolve the nasal and maxillary defects, but not until his mid to late teens. Although he is a bit quiet, he seems well liked and included by his peers during class activities, field trips, recess, and lunch. Jonathan's teachers report that he rarely speaks up in class but participates well in small groups. He has appropriate resonance but has some persistent mild speech errors due to compensatory articulation. Jonathan seems a bit embarrassed about leaving the classroom, but he participates willingly in therapy sessions and jokes around once he is in the therapy room. One day during a therapy activity addressing affricates and using the mirror for feedback, he blurted out, "I hate looking like a freak" and was on the cusp of crying. This was very atypical behavior for Jonathan.

- What might have prompted this response and how could you gently find out?

- What might you say to both validate his feelings while also providing a framework for reframing?

References

Al-Namankany, A. & Alhubaishi, A. (2018). Effects of cleft and palate on children's psychological health: A systematic review. *Journal of Taibah University Medical Sciences, 13*(4), 311-318. https://doi.org/10.1016/j.jtumed.2018.04.007

American Cleft Palate-Craniofacial Association. (2021a). *Feeding your baby.* https://acpa-cpf.org/wp-content/uploads/2019/03/Feeding-Your-Baby-Online-2018.pdf

American Cleft Palate-Craniofacial Association. (2021b). *Introduction to cleft and craniofacial conditions.* https://acpa-cpf.org/acpa-family-services/family-resources/introduction-to-cleft-craniofacial-conditions/

Çinar, S., Ay, A., Boztepe, H., & Gürlen, E. (2021). "Unexpected events": Having an infant with cleft lip and/or palate. *Congenital Anomalies, 61*(2), 38-45. https://doi.org/10.1111/cga.12398

Lorat-Marchand, A., Guerrescgi, P., Pellerin, P., Martinot, V., Gbaguidi, C. C., Neiva, C., Devauchelle, B., Frochisse, C., Poli-Merol, M. L., & Francois-Fiquet, C. (2015). Frequency and socio-psychological impact of taunting in school-age patients with cleft lip-palate surgical repair. *International Journal of Pediatric Otorhinolaryngology, 79*, 1041-1048. https://doi.org/10.1016/j.ijporl.2015.04.024

Box 8a-6
Sarah, Marcus, and Anna

You are a speech-language pathologist at a children's hospital, and you have a feeding consultation with Sarah and Marcus Adams. Mr. and Mrs. Adams have a 2-week-old baby girl named Anna with a wide unilateral complete cleft lip and palate; she is their first child. Mr. Adams works as an insurance adjuster, and Mrs. Adams, an accountant, is home with Anna for 12 weeks of maternity leave. Mrs. Adams had planned to breastfeed but is unable to due to the size and severity of Anna's cleft. She has tried nursing as a means of non-nutritive sucking and bonding, but Anna becomes frustrated and cries.

Anna is not gaining weight as rapidly as desired, and it takes approximately 1 hour to feed her. The Adamses are using a Mead Johnson cleft palate nurser with a standard nipple. By the time Anna completes a feeding and takes a short break, it is time for her to eat again. Mrs. Adams is frustrated by the feeding difficulties, exhausted from round-the-clock feedings, mourning the loss of the breastfeeding relationship, and worried about her daughter's lack of weight gain. Mr. Adams does help with feedings when he is home in the evenings, but Mrs. Adams feeds Anna throughout the night since Mr. Adams must leave early for work. Mr. Adams is not concerned about Anna's weight or the time it takes to feed her and mentioned that Sarah is "probably having a hard time because of her hormones." You anticipate that trying some different bottles, nipples, and feeding positions would improve Anna's weight gain and the efficiency of her feedings.

- What would be some appropriate motivational interview questions or strategies to use in your consultation with Mr. and Mrs. Adams and Anna?

- Triangulation could happen in a situation such as this. What is triangulation, and what would it look like in this scenario? How can you prevent it?

Sreejith, V. P., Arun, V., Devarajan, A.P., Gopinath, A., & Sunil, M. (2018). Psychological effect of prenatal diagnosis of cleft lip and palate: A systematic review. *Contemporary Clinical Dentistry, 9*(2), 304-308. https://dx.doi.org/10.4103%2Fccd.ccd_673_17

Stock, N. M., Costa, B., White, P., & Rumsey, N. (2020). Risk and protective factors for psychological distress in families following a diagnosis of cleft lip and/or palate. *The Cleft Palate-Craniofacial Journal, 57*(1), 88-98. https://doi.org/10.1177%2F1055665619862457

Stock, N. M., Feragen, K. B., & Rumsey, N. (2015). "It doesn't all just stop at 18": Psychological adjustment and support needs of adults born with cleft lip and/or palate. *The Cleft Palate-Craniofacial Journal, 52*(5), 543-554. https://doi.org/10.1597%2F14-178

Stock, N. M., Feragen, K. B., & Rumsey, N. (2016). Adults' narratives of growing up with a cleft lip and/or plate: Factors associated with psychological adjustment. *The Cleft Palate-Craniofacial Journal, 53*(2), 222-239. https://doi.org/10.1597%2F14-269

Stock, N. M., & Rumsey, N. (2015). Starting a family: The experience of parents with cleft lip and/or palate. *The Cleft Palate-Craniofacial Journal, 52*(4), 425-436. https://doi.org/10.1597%2F13-314

Watterson, T., Mancini, M., Brancamp, T. U., & Lewis, K. E. (2013). Relationship between the perception of hypernasality and social judgments in school-aged children. *The Cleft Palate-Craniofacial Journal, 50*(4), 498-502. https://doi.org/10.1597%2F11-126

Counseling Autistic Children and Their Families

Laura Plexico, PhD, CCC-SLP

The families of autistic children can experience high levels of stress and feelings of distress that can affect their overall well-being and family system (Blacher & McIntyre, 2006; Craig et al., 2016; Hayes & Watson, 2013). Parental anxiety, marital tension, depression, and feelings that personal control have been lost are not uncommon (Bromley et al., 2004; Feldman et al., 2000; Hare et al., 2004; Higgins et al., 2005). The task of managing behaviors, communication barriers, and overwhelming emotions that can accompany having an autistic child can prove to be challenging for many families. Deficits in emotional expressiveness can also lower parental empathy between parent and child, creating another form of parental stress and guilt (Coyne et al., 2007; Meirsschaut et al., 2010). Often families can feel isolated, alienated, and stigmatized by the experience of having an autistic child (Galpin et al., 2018; Ludlow et al., 2012). The financial and logistical challenges associated with finding support and managing a treatment plan can also be complex, dynamic, and an added stress. Families are faced with the task of trying to manage and cope with the day-to-day challenges experienced in the home and outside environments while simultaneously being an advocate for the family unit and the child. Having an autistic child is a lifelong journey. Because autism is developmental, needs and barriers are ever changing and require continued attention.

As a speech-language pathologist, the opportunities for counseling autistic children and their families are numerous. Often, we play an early role in the identification of speech and language delays that can lead to the life-changing diagnosis of autism spectrum disorder. Parents experience feelings of grief, fear, anger, and confusion as they move through this diagnostic and service planning process. Following diagnosis, parents begin to rewrite the narrative they had imagined of their life with a nonautistic child and grieve the loss. As a speech-language pathologist, we need to take the time to appreciate where families and children are on their journey with autism spectrum disorder. To understand their journey and have context for their life experience, we must take the time to ask clients and families for their full story and be willing to patiently listen and suspend judgment. By listening to our clients' stories, we can learn a lot about how families are coping and whether the strategies chosen are a best fit and effective for the given situation. Coping with a situation that feels mostly outside of one's control is challenging and will require strategies that fit the specifics of individual situations. When listening to the parents' story we need to pay attention to their expectations for themselves and the child, thoughts about causation, quality of daily familial and child interactions, harmony within family unit, parents' views about the child's ability to make change, overall attitude and degree of optimism, and whether there is social support. Other factors that require attention are the family's beliefs, religion, treatment philosophies, and ideologies that guide the family unit's everyday life. While listening to the client's and/or parents' narratives, it is important to periodically check your understanding by paraphrasing back the narrative you are hearing. It is also important to ask follow-up questions and prompt the parent or client when clarity is needed or when portions of the narrative appear to be missing.

The narrative that is often told by families of autistic children is frequently problem-saturated and may describe a family structure that is overwhelmed and mired in a sea of negative emotions. As the speech-language pathologist, we can offer validation and reassurance that the difficult thoughts, feelings, and behaviors they are experiencing are understandable. We can also offer hope and belief that parenting an autistic child can be a rewarding experience and that there is a path forward. In addition to listening, validating, and providing hope, as speech-language pathologists, we are also in the position to provide counseling in the form of support, guidance, and advocacy. Limited access to support and concerns over the quality-of-service provision are not uncommon experiences for the families of autistic children. Support can come in different forms: social, professional, and respite. Social support is important and has been demonstrated to be a moderating factor for stress (Drogomyretska et al., 2020; Lu et al., 2018). For a family to cope effectively with stresses experienced and get the resources they need, professionals in the educational, medical, psychological, and therapeutic communities need to collaboratively work together and work with the families to make sure they have access to and are receiving the supports that they need. When professional support is perceived to be unavailable, inaccessible, unvaluable, unhelpful, and unaffordable, discontent and a distrust of professional services can ensue. Respite support is another form of support that families are often unaware of and has been demonstrated to be highly valued when the resource is available (Harper et al., 2013). Parents need the time and space to do something for themselves and to get routine tasks done.

Guiding Parents Through the Intervention Process

As speech-language pathologists we are also in the unique role to counsel and guide parents through the intervention process. Parents want to feel informed and involved in the decision-making process. The intervention process requires that the parents and speech-language pathologist form a collaborative relationship and work together toward outcomes that are meaningful within the context and routines of the family unit and autistic child's life. Developing a collaborative plan involves agreement on the intervention approach as well as the desired goals and outcomes. To keep the process collaborative and make sure sessions are going as expected for all parties, clearly outlined SMART (Specific, Measurable, Achievable, Realistic, and Time-based) goals as well as routine feedback about the sessions are important. SMART goals are helpful for creating a platform for communicating practical and attainable goals that can be measured within specified periods of time. It is important for parents and clients to be a part of the goal-making process as well as feel and see the progress they are making toward desired outcomes. When families and clients do not feel and see progress in a realistic time frame, they can become discouraged and motivation for the approach and strategies can diminish. Clinicians should also routinely check in and make sure the parents and client feel the therapeutic relationship, goals, and approach are commensurate with what is wanted and expected. Generating and maintaining this open dialogue can facilitate a more productive working relationship and trust with the client and family.

Facilitating Advocacy

When faced with feelings of isolation and potentially bureaucratic systems where parents feel that they have to push and fight for professional services to which they are entitled, advocacy and feeling someone is in your corner is important. Advocacy occurs when someone takes action on behalf of a child to ensure adequate support and care is provided. Fighting for services with no one in your corner is stressful and can result in feelings of helplessness and guilt. Parents report feeling misunderstood and as being labeled a problem parent when they fight for services (Fleischmann, 2005; McNerney et al., 2015; Preece, 2014; Tissot, 2011). The ability to fight for services often comes down to both the parents' personal and physical resources. Advocacy can be taxing, as it is often a daily undertaking requiring consistent attention. Often parents feel both worn down and let down by the system. They often feel that every time they are able to push one step forward they are quickly forced two steps back or stuck in a holding pattern. Being armed with knowledge about autism, having an understanding of the educational, social, and political systems as well as an understanding of their child's rights is paramount for advocacy. Further, parents need to be familiar with service delivery models and philosophies as well as legislative and budgetary issues that guide system-based decision making. Parents want to be a part of the team and feel a sense of relational togetherness with their providers (Galpin et al., 2018).

Box 8a-7 provides a case illustration of parental counseling.

References

Blacher, J., & McIntyre, L. L. (2006). Syndrome specificity and behavioural disorders in young adults with intellectual disability: Cultural differences in family impact. *Journal of Intellectual Disability Research, 50*(3), 184-198.

Bromley, J., Hare, D. J., Davison, K., & Emerson, E. (2004). Mothers supporting children with autistic spectrum disorders: Social support, mental health status and satisfaction with services. *Autism, 8*(4), 409-423. https://doi.org/10.1177/1362361304047224

Coyne, L. W., Low, C. M., Miller, A. L., Seifer, R., & Dickstein, S. (2007). Mothers' empathic understanding of their toddlers: Associations with maternal depression and sensitivity. *Journal of Child and Family Studies, 16*(4), 483-497.

Craig, F., Margari, F., Legrottaglie, A. R., Palumbi, R., de Giambattista, C., & Margari, L. (2016). A review of executive function deficits in autism spectrum disorder and attention-deficit/hyperactivity disorder. *Neuropsychiatric Disease and Treatment, 2016*(1), 1191-1202.

Drogomyretska, K., Fox, R., & Colbert, D. (2020). Brief report: Stress and perceived social support in parents of children with ASD. *Journal of Autism and Developmental Disorders, 50*(11), 4176-4182.

Feldman, M. A., Hancock, C. L., Rielly, N., Minnes, P., & Cairns, C. (2000). Behavior problems in young children with or at risk for developmental delay. *Journal of Child & Family Studies, 9*(2), 247-261. https://doi.org/10.1023/A:1009427306953

Fleischmann, A. (2005). The hero's story and autism. Grounded theory study of websites for parents of children with autism. *Autism: The International Journal of Research and Practice, 9*(3), 299-316.

Galpin, J., Barratt, P., Ashcroft, E., Greathead, S., Lorcan, K., & Pellicano, E. (2018). 'The dots just don't join up': Understanding the support needs of families of children on the autism spectrum. https://doi.org/10.25384/sage.c.4164812.v1

Hare, D. J., Pratt, C., Burton, M., Bromley, J., & Emerson, E. (2004). The health and social care needs of family carers supporting adults with autistic spectrum disorders. *Autism: The International Journal of Research and Practice, 8*(4), 425-444.

Harper, A., Dyches, T. T., Harper, J., Roper, S. O., & South, M. (2013). Respite care, marital quality, and stress in parents of children with autism spectrum disorders. *Journal of Autism and Developmental Disorders, 43*(11), 2604-2616.

Hayes, S. A., & Watson, S. L. (2013). The impact of parenting stress: A meta-analysis of studies comparing the experience of parenting stress in parents of children with and without autism spectrum disorder. *Journal of Autism and Developmental Disorders, 43*(3), 629-642.

Higgins, D. J., Bailey, S. R., & Pearce, J. C. (2005). Factors associated with functioning style and coping strategies of families with a child with an autism spectrum disorder. *Autism, 9*(2), 125-137. https://doi.org/10.1177/1362361305051403

Lu, M.-H., Wang, G.-H., Lei, H., Shi, M.-L., Zhu, R., & Jiang, F. (2018). Social support as mediator and moderator of the relationship between parenting stress and life satisfaction among the Chinese parents of children with ASD. *Journal of Autism and Developmental Disorders, 48*(4), 1181-1188.

Box 8a-7

Parental Counseling That Includes Storying, Cooperative Goal Setting, and Advocacy

Peter was a 12-year-old boy who came in for an evaluation for problems with reading, phonology, and auditory memory. Peter was diagnosed with pervasive developmental disorder—not otherwise specified at the age of 3. He received early intervention services from ages 3 to 7. He also received occupational therapy for several years to address fine and gross motor difficulties. At the time of evaluation, Peter was going to be entering the sixth grade and had spent his K-5 years in a special education classroom. Peter's mother indicated that he had difficulty concentrating, had a short attention span, was underactive, and that he preferred to play alone. He was described as schedule oriented and expressed unhappiness when his routines or schedule were broken. He also displayed sensitivities to loud noises. However, his mother also reported that he made friends easily and enjoyed swimming, books, and playing video games.

Peter had an Individualized Education Program (IEP) with goals focusing on written expression, reading, and mathematics. Weaknesses, based on the IEP, included difficulty remembering people's names, inability to write sentences with varied sentence structure, difficulty with reading comprehension, and inability to solve math word problems. Strengths included the ability to recognize two- and three-syllable words following oral reading and the ability to solve simple addition and subtraction problems using basic operations. The Wechsler Intelligence Scale for Children, Fourth Edition was given by the school psychometrist at the end of fifth grade. Peter's Full Scale IQ Score was 66 and was qualitatively categorized as extremely low.

During conversation at the onset of evaluation, I informally asked Peter's mother, "What's been going on?" and "What are your concerns, and what do you hope comes from this evaluation?" I asked for the story or the client's personal narrative as a mother of an autistic child. The mother indicated that it pained her to see how much Peter loved books but was unable to independently read age-appropriate material. She expressed that Peter really enjoyed being read to on a daily basis but could only read independently by sight or memorization after he had been repeatedly exposed to the same material. She stated that her goals for Peter were for him to be integrated into the regular classroom, receive a regular high school diploma, and attend college when he grows up. She expressed significant frustration with the school system and his classroom environment. She described how she believed he was not being taught or challenged in the classroom in a way that would facilitate him meeting his potential. She felt like the school saw their role as "babysitting" her child and that they just needed to get him through the day. She described the limited work she saw that he was doing at school generally included coloring and cut-and-paste activities in the classroom. She did not believe that he was being actively taught to read. She felt her son entered a one-way door into the contained classroom and that the system had already given up on her child. She asked me questions about how her child "could do things he had never been taught to do?" She believed he was capable of doing much more and that he could learn more with some direct instruction. She provided a story filled with worry, frustration, and sadness.

After testing Peter's nonverbal intelligence, receptive language, expressive language, phonology, and literacy, it was determined that Peter was performing more than two standard deviations below the mean and significantly below age and grade expectations with regards to language, phonology, and literacy. Academically, he was performing more like a kindergartner in all subject areas. However, his nonverbal language was age appropriate and within normal limits when compared to age- and sex-matched peers.

From the mother's story and the questions she asked, I recognized that she was drawing a line and trying to distinguish between performance and capability. She clearly felt the system was failing her son. The elephant in the room that needed to be addressed was whether her expectations were reasonable and whether she was denying the realities of her child's disability. I knew that in so many ways, she was asking me to confirm and provide evidence that her son was teachable. What I also needed to determine was whether she had expectations that I could make all of Peter's problems "go away." I also could tell that I was on the precipice of a litigious situation with the schools. Peter's mother wanted someone to listen and

(continued)

Box 8a-7 (continued)

Parental Counseling That Includes Storying, Cooperative Goal Setting, and Advocacy

give her son an opportunity. Simultaneously, she was looking for evidence that more could be done than currently was being done. She wanted hope and affirmation.

From my time with Peter and after hearing his mother's story, I was able to see great strength in his visual processing and could tell that he was motivated to learn to read. He talked about his love of books and how he enjoyed reading with his mother each evening. I felt connected and had great empathy for the situation. The mother had laid out some significant long-term goals and was struggling with and actively trying to work through how to best advocate for her child. After much listening and asking clarifying questions, it was clear that we needed to identify some SMART goals. From the mother's story, it appeared that many of the barriers were related to Peter's literacy. Therefore, we started to break down how we could approach teaching Peter to read, how we could assess progress, and whether this was an attainable goal. While I wanted to communicate optimism and did believe there was room for growth, I did not want to create false hope. I knew the time piece of the smart goal process was going to be particularly important. It gave myself, Peter, and his mother a clearly identifiable target date to gauge progress as well as a formal way to have a conversation about whether any adjustments were needed with regards to goal attainment or expectations.

After 12 weeks of therapy, it became increasingly evident that with instruction Peter was capable of doing much more than he was being asked to do. He had reached and exceeded his 12-week SMART goals. Both he and his mother were extremely motivated and excited to see the progress he was making. The sixth-grade school year had started, he was in the contained classroom, and she felt he, as in the previous year, was not receiving any meaningful instruction. His mother asked for an IEP meeting to revisit his goals and whether inclusion in the general classroom was a possibility. She asked that I also attend this meeting. This meeting will forever remain with me. I sat next to Peter's mother and across from the principal and teacher. Peter's mother began to ask whether more explicit reading goals could be established and whether a more programmatic approach could be taken to his reading instruction. She also asked what would need to happen for Peter to begin to receive instruction in the regular classroom environment. She explained that she was willing to do anything she needed to do on her end in the evenings to help him make progress and be successfully integrated. It was then that the principal leaned across the table and said, "In the sixth grade, kids don't learn to read. They read to learn." I was stunned and knew we had a problem on our hands.

Over the course of the next 2 years, I worked with Peter and his family to help Peter reach his full potential and get the services he needed to be successful. At the end of the day, Peter did learn to read and was fully integrated into the general classroom. He went from needing significant support to minimal support in the classroom. He graduated from high school and went to a junior college. His accomplishments have been many, and we are looking to see what great things he does next. Great things are possible when clients have the right resources and people in their corner. As a speech-language pathologist, it is important to remind ourselves that we are one of those people.

Ludlow, A., Skelly, C., & Rohleder, P. (2012). Challenges faced by parents of children diagnosed with autism spectrum disorder. *Journal of Health Psychology, 17*(5), 702-711. https://doi.org/10.1177/1359105311422955

McNerney, C., Hill, V., & Pellicano, E. (2015). Choosing a secondary school for young people on the autism spectrum: A multi-informant study. *International Journal of Inclusive Education, 19*(10), 1096-1116.

Meirsschaut, M., Roeyers, H., & Warreyn, P. (2010). Parenting in families with a child with autism spectrum disorder and a typically developing child: Mothers' experiences and cognitions. *Research in Autism Spectrum Disorders, 4*(4), 661-669. https://doi.org/10.1016/j.rasd.2010.01.002

Preece, D. (2014). A matter of perspective: The experience of daily life and support of mothers, fathers and siblings living with children on the autism spectrum with high support needs. *Good Autism Practice, 15*(1), 81-90.

Tissot, C. (2011). Working together? Parent and local authority views on the process of obtaining appropriate educational provision for children with autism spectrum disorders. *Educational Research, 53*(1), 1-15.

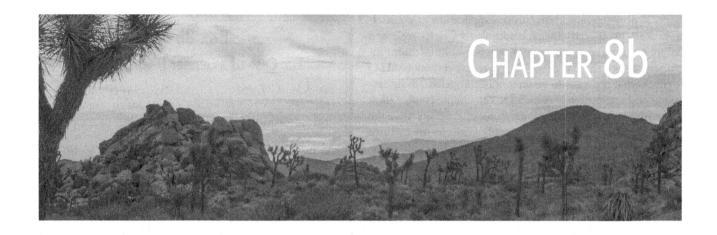

CHAPTER 8b

Special Topics and Disorders
Across the Lifespan

Jack Pickering, PhD, CCC-SLP; Eva van Leer, PhD, CCC-SLP; and Dan Hudock, PhD, CCC-SLP

Gender Affirming Voice and Communication Training for Transgender and Gender Nonbinary Individuals

Jack Pickering, PhD, CCC-SLP

Gender Affirming Voice and the Speech-Language Pathologist's Role in Counseling

People who are gender diverse may seek voice and communication training in order to produce a voice that is consistent with their gender identity (Adler et al., 2019). While the earliest work in this area focused on adult trans women, speech-language pathologists are seeing a wider variety of gender identities, including trans teens, trans men, and people who are gender nonbinary. Gender-affirming voice and communication training is most often a part of a broader transition process that includes mental health counseling, hormone therapy, gender-affirming surgery, and other services (Lev et al., 2019).

In the United States, people who are gender diverse are becoming more visible in social, educational, and occupational circles, but they also experience discrimination, hate crimes, and reduced access to health care, housing, and occupational protections more frequently than those who are not gender diverse. People who are gender diverse also attempt suicide more frequently than others (James et al., 2016). Trans and gender nonbinary teens experience an inordinate amount of bullying in school (Hirsch et al., 2019). Since many health care providers, including speech-language pathologists, do not feel competent to work with gender diverse individuals (Hancock & Haskin, 2015), it is essential to gain adequate training and be well-versed in counseling skills in order to facilitate an open, welcoming environment—one that can facilitate change.

Hoepner, J. K. (Ed.). *Counseling and Motivational Interviewing in Speech–Language Pathology* (pp. 153-173).

Of primary importance to the application of counseling skills by speech-language pathologists is to seek and apply cultural competence and practice cultural humility. American Speech-Language-Hearing Association (ASHA) defines what it means to be culturally competent, to understand and appropriately respond to the unique combination of cultural variables and dimensions of diversity that the professional and client/patient/family bring to interactions (ASHA, n.d.). Perhaps as important is a need for cultural humility, which refers to the process of learning how our own self affects the care we provide—demonstrating and promoting respect for all (Hancock & Siegfriedt, 2020).

If these represent two important underlying principles of intervention, there are also specific roles we need to attend to in our work, all of which are enhanced by the application of counseling skills:

- Creating a safe environment
- Applying unconditional positive regard
- Being an empathetic, reflective listener
- Facilitating the client's story
- Treating the whole person
- Addressing change
- Focusing on strengths to achieve authentic voice
- Providing peer support in a group setting

Box 8b-1 provides a case illustration of a gender diverse teen, which includes details about her psychosocial history, interests, and the intervention and counseling approaches taken.

Person-Centered Counseling

During the first session and throughout voice training, the clinician used a person-centered approach to develop a strong rapport and trusting relationship with Tia. The clinician was authentic and empathetic while listening, and practiced unconditional positive regard, listening without judgment. As she listened, the speech-language pathologist reflected and validated the client's feelings, summarizing and paraphrasing along the way, to make sure she understood what Tia said. The clinician attended using eye contact and body language and carefully observed Tia for signs of discomfort or distress. This was particularly important since Tia divulged some very personal, emotional life experiences (Rogers, 1995).

Identity Mapping

During the second and third sessions, Tia's mother was invited to sit in, so a plan could be developed that included mom and Tia's counselor. A plan was developed that included collaboration with the counselor and on-going interaction with mom in- and outside of sessions. A project was

---

Box 8b-1
Tia: Case of a Gender Diverse Teen

Tia was a 17-year-old trans teen who came to the College of Saint Rose Gender Affirming Voice and Communication Program in order to modify her voice so that it would be perceived as more female. When she came for group training, her voice was low in pitch, with limited use of inflections, and resonance that was focused back in her throat. While these areas were the primary focus of the voice training (Adler et al., 2019), there were also issues related to feelings and thinking that led to reduced confidence and a recent withdrawal from social conversation. Tia came to the sessions with her mom, but mom did not sit in on the initial session of the semester.

During the first session, Tia was initially quiet and shy. Fairly quickly in gathering intake information, Tia shared with the student clinician that she was being home schooled because her peers were bullying her. She also had suicidal ideations over the past 2 years. Tia began her gender transition 2 years before, when she was 15. Her voice deepened the year prior, which created significant distress. Tia has seen a mental health counselor "off and on" since beginning her transition, but was not seeing the counselor during the beginning of voice training.

One of the things that the student clinician noted in conversation with Tia was that she did not say anything positive about herself or mention any strengths when the clinician asked. However, Tia was a musician who loved to draw. She also enjoyed writing; Language Arts was her favorite subject in school. Tia's mom reported that Tia was a talented artist who was very compassionate to others. Given the intake information, planning started for gender-affirming voice and communication training.

---

implemented that involved identity mapping in order to increase confidence and facilitate a change in Tia's feelings and thinking toward herself and her voice (Bloom, 2010). The identity map was a visual representation of Tia's strengths and personal goals. She was able to explore her many talents and see herself in a new light. Interestingly, during the creation of her identity map, Tia commented that she did not realize all the things in her life that were strengths.

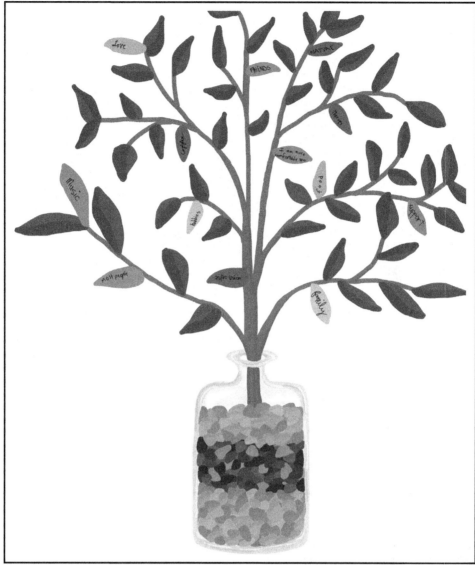

Figure 8b-1a. Gratitude tree.

Gratitude Visits

Another activity that Tia was engaged in during gender-affirming voice and communication intervention was to lead a gratitude activity at the end of the session, one of the group's traditions and a way of ending the session on a positive note. Ultimately, Tia did two gratitude visits with the group. In the first, she brought in a gratitude tree, a large vase filled with marbles that supported branches. On the branches, Tia taped leaves that contained expressions of gratitude written down by the clients and clinicians (Figure 8b-1a). Later in the treatment period, Tia brought in gratitude flowers that had petals containing expressions of gratitude created by the members of the group, clients, and clinicians (Figure 8b-1b). These two activities gave participants a chance to express gratitude for: (1) people in their lives, (2) places they have been, and importantly, (3) their strengths (Seligman, 2011).

A Word About the Program

Tia took part in the gender-affirming voice and communication program at The College of Saint Rose. The program utilizes both group and individual components, as described later (Kayajian & Pickering, 2017). The codirectors are joined by six to eight graduate student clinicians who serve as communication partners and coaches for the clients who attend. The program has been running weekly for over 13 years. There are five distinct components:

- **Mindfulness**—Each group starts with mindfulness, so everyone can begin in the same place: in the moment (Boyle, 2011). Early sessions focus on mindful breathing, but there is also an opportunity to focus on progressive relaxation, self-confidence, and self-compassion. The student clinician-coaches facilitate mindfulness activities early on in the semester, with clients invited to lead mindfulness as the semester progresses.

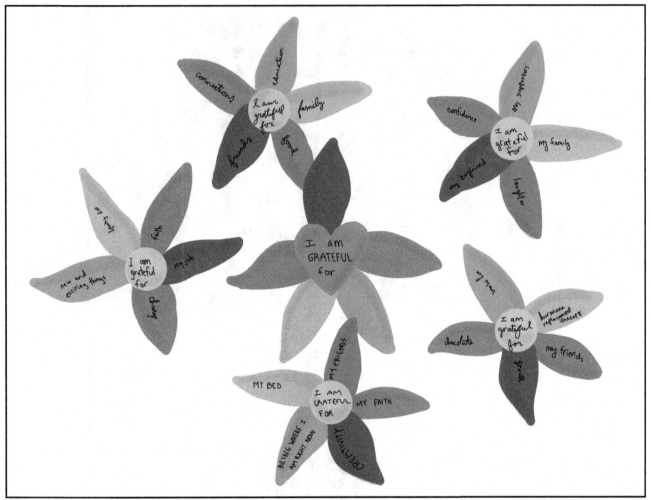

Figure 8b-1b. Gratitude flowers.

- **Vocal warm-up**—Components of vocal warm-up are initially introduced and practiced in the group context, so clients can be supported as they learn to balance their voice: respiration, phonation, and resonance. Aspects of vocal function exercises (Stemple et al., 2010) and resonant voice therapy (Verdolini-Marston et al., 1995) are applied. Over time, vocal warm up becomes individualized for each client during the next component.

- **Individual intervention**—Here each client works with their student clinician-coach to establish and address individual goals, practice an individualized warm-up program and work on important vocal characteristics, including but not limited to inflection, resonance, and projection. Intake information is gathered early on, providing an opportunity to practice active listening. Counseling skills can be utilized during individual intervention, when necessary.

- **Group discussion**—In the large group, the clinicians and the codirectors may focus on: (1) conversational activities to facilitate the use of voice in functional contexts, (2) a lesson on one aspect of communication, like nonverbal communication or articulation, or (3) feedback on the program and ways of improving services.

Occasionally a topic of interest to the gender diverse community, like the November 20th Transgender Day of Remembrance or legislation that may support or discriminate against gender diverse people may be discussed during this time. Peer support and feedback become an important part of group discussion time.

- **Gratitude**—At the end of each session, the members of the group take part in a gratitude activity, which was described previously and offers an opportunity to end the session in a positive way. Like mindfulness, gratitude is facilitated by the student clinician-coaches, and over time, by the clients.

Additional Scenarios

In addition to the examples provided for Tia, there are a number of circumstances when counseling skills can be applied to support change in our gender diverse clients. Some potential situations that may present themselves include:

- A trans woman feels frustrated and sad that she needs to express herself in a masculine way at work and has to rush to attend group after work.

- A trans client feels frustrated with the complexity of voice production, unsure about what they are doing early in their voice and communication training.

- A trans client is trying to manage depression because of their gender dysphoria. The sound of their voice contributes to their anxiety and feelings or distress.

- A trans man experiences vocal fatigue and a sore throat and is struggling with the relationship between his voice and his identity.

- An older adult trans woman feels like she cannot modify her voice characteristics because of her age and the vocal habits she has developed during her lifetime.

- A trans client does not feel comfortable using their voice in public, even with people who are supportive and will not judge them.

- A trans client is feeling a sense of loss because members of their family stopped interacting with them because they are transgender.

These situations and others may present themselves during gender-affirming voice and communication training. Under these circumstances, clinicians have the opportunity to utilize counseling skills to support change in the client's feelings and thinking (Adler & Pickering, 2019). Some of the skills that can be implemented include but are not limited to active listening, person-centered counseling, cognitive behavioral therapy, identity mapping, positive psychology, and counseling for grief and loss. This text provides valuable information on the application of these and other counseling approaches that would be appropriate for our work with gender diverse individuals. These scenarios also point out the importance of interprofessional collaboration between speech-language pathologists and mental health counselors.

Summary

Let me conclude with thoughts from David Azul, a trans man, speech-language pathologist, and university professor, who presented a paper with Adrienne Hancock during the 2017 ASHA Convention in Los Angeles (Hancock & Azul, 2017). It points out how important counseling skills are for this population (and certainly others, as well). Azul said that there are three things we should integrate into our training beyond voice and resonance techniques. These each require us to apply counseling skills in our work to support change in the people with whom we work:

1. Mindful awareness

2. Self-compassion

3. Assertiveness

As I think about it, these may be important attributes we should adopt for ourselves in our role as effective clinicians-counselors.

References

Adler, R. K., Hirsch, S., & Pickering, J. (Eds.). (2019). *Voice and communication therapy for the transgender/gender diverse patient: A comprehensive clinical guide* (3rd ed.). Plural Publishing.

Adler, R. K., & Pickering, J. (2019). The role of the SLP in counseling. In R. K. Adler, S. Hirsch, & J. Pickering (Eds.), *Voice and communication therapy for the transgender/gender diverse patient: A comprehensive clinical guide* (3rd ed.). Plural Publishing.

American Speech-Language-Hearing Association. (n.d.). *Cultural competence.* https://www.asha.org/practice-portal/professional-issues/cultural-competence/

Bloom, C. (2010). Finding the psychotherapeutic harmonies embedded within Mark Ylvisaker's holistic approach to executive function rehabilitation. *Journal of Behavioral and Neuroscience Research, 8(1),* 60-69.

Boyle, M. (2011). Mindfulness training in stuttering therapy: A tutorial for speech-language pathologists. *Journal of Fluency Disorders, 36,* 122-129.

Hancock, A. & Azul, D. (2017). Cultural and clinical considerations for EBP with transgender and gender non-conforming. A presentation at the 2017 Annual American Speech-Language-Hearing Association Convention.

Hancock, A., & Haskin, G. (2015). Speech-language pathologists' knowledge and attitudes regarding lesbian, gay, bisexual, transgender, and queer (LGBTQ) populations. *American Journal of Speech-Language Pathology, 24(2),* 206-221.

Hancock, A. B., & Siegfriedt, L. L. (2020). *Transforming voice and communication with transgender and gender diverse People: An evidence-based approach.* Plural Publishing.

Hirsch, S., Pickering, J., & Adler, R. K. (2019). Meeting the needs of trans and gender diverse youth: The varied, ubiquitous role of the SLP in voice and communication therapy/training. *SIG 3, Perspectives on Voice and Voice Disorders 4(1),* 111-117.

James, S. E., Herman, J. L., Rankin, S., Keisling, M., Mottet, L., & Anafi, M. (2016). *The report of the 2015 U.S. transgender survey.* National Center for Transgender Equality.

Kayajian, D., & Pickering, J. (2017). Connecting clinic and classroom to enhance group transgender voice and communication training in a college environment. *SIG 10, Issues in Higher Education, 2(2),* 116-122.

Lev, A., Cosgrove, D., & Crumley, T. S. (2019). Psychotherapy and support for transgender patients. In R. K. Adler, S. Hirsch, & J. Pickering (Eds.), *Voice and communication therapy for the transgender/gender diverse patient: A comprehensive clinical guide* (3rd ed.). Plural Publishing.

Rogers, C. (1995). *Patient-centered therapy: Its current practice, implications and theory.* Trans-Atlantic.

Seligman, M. (2011). *Flourish.* Free Press.

Stemple, J. C., Glaze, L. E., & Klaben, B. (2010). *Clinical voice pathology: Theory and management* (4th ed.). Plural Publishing.

Verdolini-Marston, K., Burke, M. K., Lessac, A., Glaze, L., & Caldwell, E. (1995). Preliminary study of two methods of treatment for laryngeal nodules. *Journal of Voice, 9,* 74-85.

Counseling Clients in Voice Therapy: Motivational Interviewing Strategies to Facilitate Adherence

Eva van Leer, PhD, CCC-SLP

Voice disorders comprise unfavorable changes in the pitch, loudness, quality, effort, or resilience of voice production (Stemple et al., 2018; Verdolini & Ramig, 2001). Voice therapy has documented efficacy for resolving or reducing the severity of various behavioral, organic, and neurogenic voice disorders (Ramig & Verdolini, 1998). However, clients can find voice therapy quite challenging and difficult to adhere to (Behrman, 2006; van Leer & Connor, 2010). Voice therapy protocols ask clients to replace their habitual voice production mechanics with optimal ones associated with particular techniques (e.g., resonant, breathy, loud voice) in all daily communication (Gartner-Schmidt et al., 2016; Ramig & Verdolini, 1998). To attain this goal, clients must typically practice their individualized technique multiple times every day as well as intentionally and consistently implement the technique when speaking. Per client report (van Leer & Connor, 2010), challenges include replicating, self-evaluating, and self-correcting the target technique independently (i.e., without clinician feedback) in both practice and generalization. Patients also report difficulty remembering to practice and implement the technique. Additionally, some clients experience self-consciousness when practicing (e.g., "Making these noises is weird") or perceive the target voice as inconsistent with their self-concept: "This doesn't sound like me," again resulting in barriers to practice and generalization. Thus, there are several motor learning, self-regulation, and self-concept challenges associated with voice therapy. Given these barriers to adherence, clients report that voice therapy is hard, that high motivation and commitment are necessary to adhere to voice therapy, and that the match with the therapist's approach matters (van Leer & Connor, 2010).

Although it is reasonable to believe that those who seek voice evaluation are inherently motivated to complete voice therapy, this is not necessarily the case. The factors that predict treatment adherence (van Leer & Connor, 2015)—client dedication to a vocal goal, confidence to attain this goal, and support received in pursuing the goal—differ from those that might lead a client to pursue initial evaluation. For example, clients may present to the clinic with substantial vocal complaints, but expect to resolve these through a course of medication. Their desire for vocal improvement may be great enough to take daily medications, but not to make daily changes in vocal behavior. Other clients may seek voice evaluation to rule out malignancy or to satisfy a concerned family member, but not to reduce their dysphonia in the absence of malignancy. In rare cases, clients may wish to maintain their disordered voice quality for primary or secondary gain. As such, one can neither assume that clients wish to resolve their voice disorder, nor that they wish to do so through behavioral means.

Motivational interviewing is a theory-driven, evidence-based, client-centered approach to discussing behavior change with patients: an interview about change! Since the goal of this interview is to uncover and support the patient's intrinsic motivation for change, the discussion is called a motivational interview. The sentence-level interview strategies are called counseling "microskills." The motivational interview can facilitate clients' dedication to a behavior change program by helping them discover the degree to which they are motivated to pursue behavior change goals. MI does not, however, attempt to persuade patients to pursue change, because doing so would encroach upon patients' autonomy and constitute a boundary violation that is inherently in conflict with MI's client-centered perspective.

While comprehensive training in MI requires coursework and workshops, the purpose of this entry is to discuss and exemplify how MI microskills can be applied to voice therapy in a straightforward manner. The reader can readily implement these microskills when speaking with their next voice client. Although doing so may at first feel unnatural to the clinician, it is important to remember that naturalness will increase with practice, and that MI microskills will have a positive therapeutic effect regardless of the clinician's comfort level. To increase naturalness and observe the therapeutic effect of microskills, the reader is encouraged to try them out in casual conversations with friends.

MI can be applied to any behavior health program, including voice therapy. In the area of voice disorders, a motivational interview can uncover patients' specific goals for their voice and their motivation to pursue these through voice therapy. If patients choose to participate in voice therapy after a motivational interview, MI microskills continue to hold utility over the course of therapy because they help ensure client-clinician agreement on the evolving goals and specific tasks of therapy. Since such goal and task agreement drives several predictors of adherence (van Leer & Connor, 2015), including the quality of the therapeutic alliance (i.e., the relationship) between client and clinician (Horvath & Greenberg, 1994), goal commitment (Klein et al., 1999), and self-efficacy (Bandura, 2010), such agreement is fundamental to the therapy process.

MI conceptualizes motivation for behavior change as "readiness" to take the behavioral action necessary to achieve a particular goal. This readiness is comprised of two factors: how important the goal is to the patient, and how confident they are to achieve it. When importance and confidence are both high, the client is likely to initiate therapy, to continue in the face of obstacles, and to ultimately achieve their goal with good outcomes. When both importance as well as

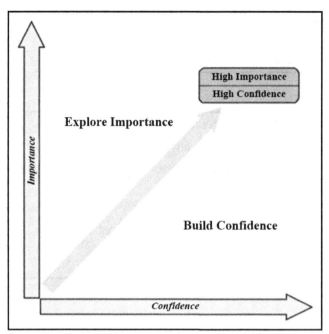

Figure 8b-2. Exploring importance and supporting confidence.

may never have been considered by many patients prior to the initial evaluation. These patients may benefit from exploration to know their own mind on the topic of voice change and voice therapy. In a motivational interview, the first step is to explore importance through open-ended, evocative questions about the client's values and goals in life, and what part their voice plays in these. Table 8b-1 lists open-ended questions that guide this exploration. Once the exploration has started, neutral open-ended questions (e.g., "What else?") can facilitate deeper introspection. The conversation can also be continued by restating the client's views with so-called simple reflections, such as "Your grandkids are important to you," "Voice is a large part of your identity," "Achieving tenure is your sole focus right now: everything else is on hold," or even, "Smoking is important to you" or "The voice exercises we tried today seem obnoxious." Simple reflections may seem unnecessary to the novice motivational interviewer, but they support the client-clinician bond by demonstrating that the clinician understands the client's perspective. Reflections also give the client the opportunity to clarify their perspective, for example, "No, it's not that my voice is not important. It's more like . . . I want to work on my voice, but I have too many other things going on right now."

If the client describes goals or behaviors that are in opposition to each other, this contradiction can be revealed through a so-called ***double-sided reflection*** (e.g., "On the one hand, you love going to bars with your friends. On the other, you don't like being hoarse when you teach the next day."). Double-sided reflections help the client develop discrepancy between their behaviors and their deeper personal values. When it comes to changing their voice production, it is common for patients to feel ambivalent—to feel two ways about the goal. Rather than attempting to choose which behavior or value is "best," the client must decide for themselves. Some clients may choose to prioritize their voice, while others choose not to. In addition to double-sided reflections, asking the client to look forward (e.g., "How do you see this playing out in the future?") can assist them in resolving ambivalence as well.

Once the client decides on a particular vocal goal, its importance can be quantified with the ***Readiness Ruler*** introduced earlier in Chapter 5. If importance is high, for example above a value of 7, confidence can be assessed next. However if importance is low, for example below a value of 6, perspectives that strengthen importance may be elicited by asking patients why they haven't chosen an even lower value, such as zero. The patient may state "Well, it does sometimes bother me that my voice isn't as clear as it used to be, and I do miss singing at church." When asked, "What would make it higher?" the patient may identify other aspects of importance, or alternately come to realize that this is simply not the right time for therapy. Next, the clinician can summarize the client's perspective and assess the client's confidence to attain their vocal goal.

confidence are very low, the client will not initiate therapy at all. In both these situations, the motivational interview is likely to be short because the former client will be excited to pursue therapy and the latter will quickly reject it. However, when either importance is high and confidence is low or vice versa, the motivational interview becomes a more essential part of the evaluation and may take more time, for example 5 to 10 minutes. The goal of the motivational interview is to *explore* importance and *support* confidence (Figure 8b-2).

Exploring Importance

MI is developed to "explore" importance because importance cannot be forced on the client. Rather, it can be revealed through exploration of the client's values and priorities. To initiate voice therapy, the client must perceive their vocal improvement goal as important enough to pursue with dedicated behavioral effort. The more important the goal, the more likely the client will be to pursue it. According to the theory underlying MI, importance tends to be high when a person's goal is closely tied to their personal values, daily priorities, and greater life purpose. For example, if a client's relationship with their grandchildren is a deeply valued priority in their life, maintaining a resilient voice for storytelling may be an important and meaningful goal to motivate voice therapy. Conversely, if verbal interaction is not a deeply rewarding emotional, social, or professional aspect of person's life, vocal improvement may hold very low importance.

Unlike physical therapy, voice therapy is not a commonly encountered treatment. Although vocal goals and their importance may be overtly obvious to some patients, they

Table 8b-1	
Motivational Interviewing Microskills and Potential Phrasing	
PURPOSE OF MICROSKILL	**EXAMPLE SENTENCES**
Evocative questions	• What kinds of things are the main priorities in your life right now? • What kinds of things do you value in your life at this time? • In what way does voice play a role in these? How does your voice help you do the things that are important to you? • What aspects of your voice are important to you? • We can improve your vocal _____ with voice therapy. Does that sound like something you're interested in? • Is that a goal for you?
Simple reflections	• You love _____ . • Right now, your life is about _____ . • _____ is important to you.
Neutral open-ended questions to continue the exploration	• What else? • In what way? • Tell me more about this . . .
Double-sided reflections	• On the one hand, you enjoy _____; on the other, you miss _____ . • You value _____, and on the other hand, you enjoy _____. • Both _____ and _____ are important to you at the same time. • It's hard to choose between _____ and _____ . • That sounds like a difficult choice. • Sounds like you have a dilemma!
Looking forward	• How do you see this playing out in the long run? • Where do you see this going? • Would you like a suggestion?

Confidence

After a goal has been selected and its importance assessed, it is time to assess and support the client's confidence to achieve it. Without adequate confidence, the client will not return for therapy, because people do not pursue goals they find unattainable (Bandura, 2001). Assessing self-efficacy can help shape the goal into one that appears realistic to the client (and the clinician). One can simply ask, "How confident are you that you can achieve this goal?" or "Does that sound like something you can do?" Alternately, in reference to stimulability probes (e.g., humming or clear speech), one may ask, "How confident are you that you could practice that twice a day?" or "The pursed lips breathing we practiced earlier to open your airway: could you practice that for 1 minute every hour?" If confidence is low, questions listed

in the Self-Efficacy section of Table 8b-2 might raise it, in particular, "What strengths do you have that can help you achieve your goal?" As with the exploration of importance, the Readiness Ruler can be used to facilitate this process. Asking the client why their confidence rating is not lower, and what they might do to increase it, can facilitate the patient's focus on strengths (e.g., "Well, I'm pretty organized, so I guess this is just something I have to add to my daily list. I brush my teeth every day, so I'm pretty sure can do this too.").

Two ways to adjust an unrealistic goal is to lower its difficulty level and to make the goal more concrete and proximal in time. For example, if stimulability testing reveals a strategy to reduce strain, a somewhat vague goal of "reducing strain when teaching, so that my voice isn't tired by the end of the day" can be replaced with a more operationalized and temporally proximal goal such as, "This week, I'll start

Table 8b-2

Motivational Interviewing Microskills and Potential Phrasing

PURPOSE OF MICROSKILL	EXAMPLE SENTENCES
Supporting self-efficacy for the overall goal of therapy	• What personal strengths can help you succeed in practicing your new voice technique? • What have you done in the past that can help you achieve this goal? • If you decided to work on this, what's the first thing you would do? • Who could offer you support in making this change? • What strategies do you currently use to remember daily tasks? • With whom would you feel comfortable trying this voice?
Supporting self-efficacy for weekly homework tasks	• If you had to make sure you'd do these every day, how would you go about that? • Let's try some different things. (Followed by) So, which one seems most doable? • Tell me what works for you. • What would be the easiest place to practice? What would be the easiest place to start? • What would be the easiest time to practice?

every lecture in my easy voice, and focus on that for just the first minute." The goal should be adjusted until the patient states, "Sure! I think I can do that!" or scores at least 7 on the Readiness Ruler. If no such goal can be identified, but the patient has high importance for vocal improvement, a trial therapy session can be scheduled to explore the matter further.

The MI construct of confidence is directly borrowed from social-cognitive theory's construct of self-efficacy. Self-efficacy is defined as an individual's belief in their ability to attain a specific goal or complete a particular task (Bandura, 2001). Self-efficacy has been shown to predict patient achievement for a wide variety of health and academic pursuits (Glanz et al., 2008), including voice therapy homework practice (van Leer & Connor, 2015). Since self-efficacy is task-specific, it doesn't generalize from one task to another. As such, a person may have high self-efficacy for dunking a basketball, but low self-efficacy for roller skating, or vice versa. Likewise, a patient may have poor self-efficacy for resonant voice production (Abbott, 2008) but good self-efficacy for confidential voice production (Verdolini-Marston et al., 1995) or for approaches that omit connected speech altogether such as straw phonation (Guzman et al., 2017) or vocal function exercises (Stemple et al., 1994). An approach should be chosen for which the patient has self-efficacy, not only during the session but also between sessions when practicing independently. If the patient consistently fails to adhere to a chosen approach between sessions and makes statements such as, "I can do it here, but I can't do it alone," "These

exercises are ridiculous," or "I don't see how this will ever help me cut through the noise while I'm waitressing," it is likely that another approach should be considered, for which the patient has more self-efficacy for independent practice and implementation. "Sounds like this may not be a good fit for you. Let's try something else," or "Let's try a couple of different things today and see which one feels right to you," are statements that can start this process. A good fit can typically be found if the objection to the technique is rooted in low self-efficacy rather than a lack of commitment to therapy as a whole.

Another way to increase self-efficacy for extraclinical practice is not to switch approach, but rather to provide more external support for the extant approach. The number of therapy sessions can be increased, for example, to three sessions per week until the patient is independent in performing the target therapy tasks. Short telehealth sessions have improved the feasibility for these sessions by eliminating the patient commute. External support can also be provided through standard apps located on the patient's mobile phone: a so-called "mHealth" approach to improving adherence. As part of the mobile support system, brief instructional videos can be recorded onto the patient's phone to guide independent practice, and reminders can be set to alert practice. Patients have reported that that clinician videos exemplifying technique, cues, and instructions improve adherence not only by clarifying treatment content but also by providing an emotional sense of support: "It felt like the clinician was always with me" (van Leer & Connor, 2015).

Box 8b-2

Case 1: Roger

Roger is a 70-year-old retired engineer who presents with mild to moderate dysphonia characterized by mild to moderate roughness, mildly reduced loudness, mild breathiness, and mild strain. Mean pitch in conversation is perceived as slightly elevated. Evaluation yields the diagnosis of presbyphonia resulting from age-related bilateral vocal fold atrophy and compensatory hyperfunction. During stroboscopy, reverse phonation on /i/ improves medial glottal closure that is maintained on the subsequent expiratory phase when the patient is asked to "keep everything the same as your gaspy /i/." After stroboscopy, the reverse phonation strategy is faded and a loud, twangy "beep beep" elicited. After 1 minute of producing sustained twangy /i/, voice quality in speaking is much improved. The clinician asks, "With some voice therapy, you can learn to produce this clear voice all the time. How does that sound to you?" The patient replies, "Well, honestly, I just came in to make sure I didn't have throat cancer. My uncle had that, so when my voice got hoarse a few years back, I was worried." The clinician responds by reflecting, "Your voice quality doesn't really bother you. You were concerned about cancer, and now you're relieved that it's just aging." The patient affirms, "Absolutely! I'm not a big talker so my voice being a little off isn't a problem for me. Anyway, now I can stop worrying about this and focus on my garden." The patient and clinician discuss his health goals, none of which relate to his voice. The clinician assures the patient that, "Well, if you ever change your mind and want a voice tune-up, we're here for you!" She wishes him well with his garden, and the evaluation is over.

Box 8b-3

Case 2: Vernon

As in Case 1, Vernon is a 70-year-old retired engineer with the same vocal presentation, diagnosis, and stimulability for vocal improvement as Roger. As in Case 1, the clinician offers voice therapy. However, in this case, Vernon responds, "I'd like to improve my voice, but when I do what you say, I think I sound like I'm yelling. I can't stand loud people. Never have. You can hear them from the other side of a restaurant." The clinician reflects, "You want your voice to be clearer, but not obnoxiously loud." to which the patient agrees. The clinician reflects, "I take it your voice is important to you." Vernon replies, "Although I'm not a big talker, I like to read my grandkids stories, and I like to do funny voices with them. I can't just lose the ability to do that." The clinician reflects, "Your voice plays such an important role in your relationship with them" to which the Vernon agrees. As a strategy to improve self-efficacy for the approach, the clinician uses a mobile device to video record the patient as he demonstrates both his habitual voice and his louder, clearer voice achieved via the twangy /i/ strategy. Upon viewing the video, the patient responds that, "Well, that doesn't sound quite as bad as I thought. Sure sounds better that my regular voice!" Thus, the patient realizes that he does not have to alter his vocal self-concept drastically to achieve a better quality. The clinician states that, "It'll probably start to feel more natural with practice. We can also try some other approaches in therapy as well. Would you have time to practice every day?" The patient responds, "Yes, I'd be up for that!" indicating good importance and self-efficacy. Therapy is scheduled and completed with good outcomes.

In addition to clinician recordings, patients can be provided with video examples of their own successful practice during the therapy session: the so-called "self as model." Watching oneself succeed has demonstrated positive effects across areas of speech-language intervention and health behavior including voice therapy (Bellini & Akullian, 2007; van Leer & Connor, 2015). These recordings can be made during the session (e.g., "That went well: let's repeat that and record it!" or at the end: "OK, let's record your examples for the week. Also make sure to say what you're feeling and what to remember when you do this!"). Box 8b-2 provides a case illustration of Roger, while Box 8b-3 is a case illustration of Vernon. Both cases are illustrations of a gentleman with mild to moderate dysphonia but with very different perspectives on change and motivation. Likewise, Box 8b-4 is a case illustration for Bridget and Box 8b-5 a case description of Nia. Both cases

Box 8b-4

Case 3: Bridget

Bridget, a 24-year-old female graduate student, presents with moderate phonotraumatic adducted hyperfunction, vocal nodules, and a perceptual voice quality characterized by moderate roughness and strain. Resonant voice stimulability probes reduce the severity of dysphonia to mild across all characteristics. The clinician explains, "With voice therapy, you could learn to speak this way consistently. Over time, this could resolve the nodules as well, or simply give you a more resilient clearer voice in spite of them. Is clearing up your voice quality a goal for you?" Bridget responds, "My voice doesn't really bother me. I can hear that it sounds better when we do the humming, but I don't really care. It bothers my mom, but it doesn't bother me." The clinician asks the patient what kinds of things are a priority in her life right now, to which she replies, "I'm going through grad school, so when I'm not studying, I like to go out with my friends. We're all pretty loud and we like live music. I am hoarse after I go out, but it's not something I want to give up right now. Maybe one day when I'm working full time." The clinician reflects, "At this time, blowing off steam with your friends plays a much bigger role in your life than clearing up your voice," to which Bridget emphatically agrees. As in Case 1, the clinician ensures the patient that, "Should things change, you know where to find us," and the evaluation is concluded.

Box 8b-5

Case 4: Nia

A very similar patient to Case 2 presents to the voice clinic. When voice therapy is offered, Nia states, "When I speak this way (i.e., in resonant voice), I don't feel any strain in my throat. Right here (points to thyroid cartilage). I didn't realize how much I strain when I speak. I wonder how long I've been doing that." The clinician reflects, "You've been using your voice with a lot of effort, and you weren't aware of that." The patient nods and adds, "I wonder how hard I'm pushing when I'm out with friends. It's great, but now I'm worried." The clinician reflects, "The strain concerns you." When Nia agrees, the clinician asks if the voice is worse after going out, to which the patient responds, "Yeah, it always used to be worse just the next day, but now it's getting hoarse for several days after." The clinician asks, "How do you see this playing out in the long run?" After a long silence, Nia reflects, "I guess it's going to get worse." The clinician asks if this is a concern for the patient, to which the patient replies, "Well, I'm going to student teach next semester, and I can't have my voice be like this. I also don't like this feeling of strain now." The clinician responds with a double-sided reflection, "On the one hand, you enjoy hanging out with friends in some pretty loud places. On the other, your voice is becoming more important to you," which the patient affirms. On the Readiness Ruler, the patient rates the importance of reducing vocal effort and improving voice quality a 7.5 on the Readiness Ruler, and confidence a 6 because, "I'm not quite sure if I can change my lifestyle." The two make a plan to initiate voice therapy with the goal to reduce vocal effort and develop some strategies for socializing without phonotrauma.

A week into therapy, the patient expresses, "This is really hard. It's not so much remembering to practice as knowing if you're doing it right. It's really clear when I'm here with you, but not when I practice by myself." Therefore, the clinician reviews the resonant voice work and provides the patient with video clinician and self-as-model recordings on her phone. Nia expresses that "OK, I think I should be able to figure it out with these examples." Next, the patient expresses concern about going to a concert later that week. The clinician teaches the patient the approach of "twang" specifically for use in loud environments. The patient is immediately good at this approach because she can imitate the TV character of "The Nanny." Although the patient is hesitant to use twang because "it just sounds way too nasal," she decides to try out her twang at the next concert. When her friends do not notice the twang in this setting, she returns with high self-efficacy for managing her various vocal environments. "I was still hoarse afterward, but it was less. I think I need to lay low on the loud concerts until I'm a little better at this." Over the course of therapy, the nodules do not fully resolve, but the patient's voice is much improved in quality and resilience. Although the patient is discharged, she returns every 6 weeks for "tune-ups" in voice technique.

are illustrations of college-aged women with hyperfunction and vocal nodules but with very different perspectives on change and motivation.

Summary

MI provides the clinician with tools to assess patient readiness for vocal behavior change, and direct a conversation about vocal behavior change. A motivational interview addresses both the patient's perceived importance to change a vocal behavior and their confidence to do so. In addition, other strategies to improve self-efficacy are available to the clinician and were briefly exemplified in this set of case studies.

References

Bandura, A. (2001). Social cognitive theory: An agentic perspective. *Annual Review of Psychology, 52*(1), 1-26.

Bandura, A. (2010). Self-efficacy. *The Corsini Encyclopedia of Psychology*, 1-3.

Behrman, A. (2006). Facilitating behavioral change in voice therapy: The relevance of motivational interviewing. *American Journal of Speech-Language Pathology, 15*(3), 215-225.

Bellini, S., & Akullian, J. (2007). A meta-analysis of video modeling and video self-modeling interventions for children and adolescents with autism spectrum disorders. *Exceptional Children, 73*(3), 264-287.

Gartner-Schmidt, J., Gherson, S., Hapner, E. R., Muckala, J., Roth, D., Schneider, S., & Gillespie, A. I. (2016). The development of conversation training therapy: A concept paper. *Journal of Voice, 30*(5), 563-573.

Glanz, K., Rimer, B. K., & Viswanath, K. (2008). *Health behavior and health education: Theory, research, and practice.* John Wiley & Sons.

Guzman, M., Jara, R., Olavarria, C., Caceres, P., Escuti, G., Medina, F., Medina, L., Madrid, S., Muñoz, D., & Laukkanen, A. -M. (2017). Efficacy of water resistance therapy in subjects diagnosed with behavioral dysphonia: A randomized controlled trial. *Journal of Voice, 31*(3), 385.e1-385.e10. https://doi.org/10.1016/j.jvoice.2016.09.005

Horvath, A. O., & Greenberg, L. S. (1994). *The working alliance: Theory, research, and practice* (Vol. 173). John Wiley & Sons.

Klein, H. J., Wesson, M. J., Hollenbeck, J. R., & Alge, B. J. (1999). Goal commitment and the goal-setting process: Conceptual clarification and empirical synthesis. *Journal of Applied Psychology, 84*(6), 885.

Ramig, L. O., & Verdolini, K. (1998). Treatment efficacy voice disorders. *Journal of Speech, Language, and Hearing Research, 41*(1), S101-S116.

Stemple, J. C., Lee, L., D'Amico, B., & Pickup, B. (1994). Efficacy of vocal function exercises as a method of improving voice production. *Journal of Voice, 8*(3), 271-278.

Stemple, J. C., Roy, N., & Klaben, B. K. (2018). *Clinical voice pathology: Theory and Management.* Plural Publishing.

van Leer, E., & Connor, N. P. (2010). Client perceptions of voice therapy adherence. *Journal of Voice, 24*(4), 458-469.

van Leer, E., & Connor, N. P. (2015). Predicting and influencing voice therapy adherence using social-cognitive factors and mobile video. *American Journal of Speech-Language Pathology, 24*(2), 164-176.

Verdolini, K., & Ramig, L. O. (2001). Occupational risks for voice problems. *Logopedics Phoniatrics Vocology, 26*(1), 37-46.

Counseling in Fluency Disorders

Dan Hudock, PhD, CCC-SLP

Speech and communication may inherently appear to be a simple effortless process where senders and receivers efficiently convey information to one another, which may be taken for granted by some typically fluent speakers. However, as you already likely know, it's far more complicated than one might initially believe. Human communication involves senders and receivers formulating, encoding, organizing, transmitting, decoding, interpreting, and inferring verbal and nonverbal information in an attempt to conceptually understand the sender's intent and emotional state. While engaging in verbal communication, both senders and receivers cognitively and emotionally evaluate the words used, the sequence they are presented in, the rate, rhythm, prosody, fluency, continuity, effort, and emotion that they are presented with, and evaluate, make judgments, and form opinions about the individuals and their intended messages. This only starts to illustrate the depth of the complexity and the cognitive, emotional, behavioral, social, and functional aspects along with the interplay between and within them, especially when taking into account intra- and interpersonal dynamics.

Establishing the Complexity of Fluency Disorders

The ability to communicate broadly allows us to fulfill some of our basic needs for safety and security, while efficient, effective, and effortless communication evolutionarily allows us to feel connected to one another, and form and maintain various relationships and societal standing. Not surprising then, when atypical communication is presented, as is the case with clients who have fluency disorders, it can impart profound consequences on the intrapersonal and interpersonal well-being and functioning of the individual. Although the terms fluency and fluency disorders have a wide range of meanings, based on the context and background or purpose of the person using them, for students majoring in communication sciences and disorders, or other closely related fields, speech-language pathologist assistants, speech-language pathologists, and people who stutter (PWS) themselves, along with their loved ones, the term *fluency disorders* is most often intended to represent a broader category of communication disorders including stuttering, cluttering, and other less common disorders that affect verbal fluency. Stuttering, being arguably the most prevalent fluency disorder, can be further classified as developmental or acquired, having some counseling-related differences between them; however in this section, I am just going to focus on developmental stuttering (DS).

Between the ages of 2.5 and 7 years old, with a median age of 3.5 years, DS affects roughly 4% of the world's population for some degree of prolonged period of time; however, approximately 70% to 80% of children will recover, usually within 1 to 1.5 years post onset, thus resulting in approximately 1% of the world's population who chronically stutter, or **persist**, throughout their lives. DS has a multifactorial epigenesis likely rooted in genetic predispositions that, when expressed, affect neural sensorimotor functioning for speech and other related behaviors. However, the influence of various factors on recovery or persistence, such as therapy vs. no therapy, effects from various types of therapy, and other predictive or prognostic indicators for not only recovery or persistence but also for treatment efficacy, are still under investigation without consensus agreement.

Speech disruptions, or disfluencies, are usually classified as typical disfluencies or stuttering-like disfluencies (SLDs). Typical disfluencies include between-word events such as whole-word and or phrase repetitions/revisions, hesitations, pauses, and or interjections. Typically, fluent speakers do experience these types of disfluencies to varying degrees, but it should be noted that this is not stuttering. Children who stutter (CWS) and adults who stutter, on average, present significantly more typical disfluencies and nonspeech behaviors than their fluent counterparts. SLDs, typically within-word, such as syllable and part-word repetitions, phoneme prolongations, and postural fixations/blocks, are usually progressively accompanied by increased effort, struggle, awareness/impact, avoidance, and secondary or concomitant behaviors lasting anywhere from a fraction of a second to several minutes per stuttered word or syllable. DS is an intermittent and involuntary disorder with a majority of the disfluencies occurring during moments of speech initiation, which coincidentally is when snap judgments occur during communication exchanges. This unfortunately creates the perfect storm of negative reinforcements of anticipation, avoidance, and perceived or actualized consequences of stuttering. Other internal and external factors may also impose dramatic and consequential effects on the psychological, emotional, social, and functional states of the individual along with their choices, willingness, motivation, expressed behaviors, beliefs, judgments, and perceptions of self, other, communication, and limitations.

The Iceberg Analogy

Joseph Sheehan (1970) is credited with first describing the iceberg analogy of stuttering (Figure 8b-3). As illustrated in the image, overt stuttering, or what can be outwardly observed (e.g., disfluencies, secondary behaviors, and other features, some of which may be difficult to operationally differentiate from covert symptoms/impact experienced by those who stutter) is portrayed as the top of the iceberg, floating above the surface of the water, contributing only about 10% to 20% to the overall mass of the iceberg. Covert

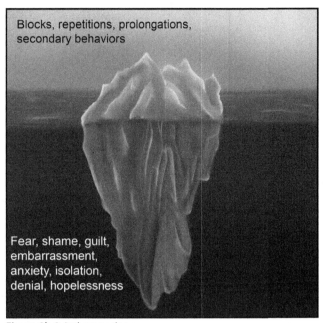

Figure 8b-3. Iceberg analogy.

features, or consequential impacts and functional limitations experienced by individuals who stutter reside below the surface and make up 80% to 90% of the mass of the iceberg. These are the psychological, emotional, social, and functional impacts and internal states that are frequently seen as the majority, or crux, of the disorder. Yaruss et al. (2002, 2004, 2019) have progressively represented the experience(s) of PWS, both overt and covert, through the World Health Organization's International Classification of Functioning Disability (Figure 8b-4; Yaruss & Quesal, 2004). The WHO-ICF (World Health Organization, 2001), and other similar frameworks, clearly depict the multifaceted dynamic interrelationship and influence of various domains, elements, and interactions upon one another within the context of constructivist lived experiences with stuttering, and how one event or therapeutic strategy may express multifaceted influence. Therefore, when treating clients with fluency disorders, it's very beneficial to have an understanding of and practice with counseling-based theories and approaches.

Acceptance-Based, Holistically Focused Approach

When communication and personhood are the primary goals of an acceptance-based, holistically focused therapeutic approach rooted in counseling theories and practice, a wealth of opportunities open up for treatment, short- and long-term outcomes, and improved client and clinician satisfaction and perception of quality of care. Through counseling-based speech-language pathology procedures and such types of approaches, you can help the client who stutters find the value and worth of their voice and opinion,

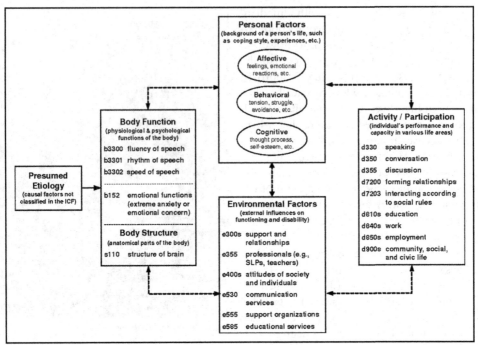

Figure 8b-4. Stuttering behaviors mapped onto WHO-ICF framework.

along with the confidence and strategies to use it. Then they can consciously and intentionally make different choices to live their life as they would like, rather than being controlled by their fluency disorder. Although there is so much more complexity, context, and depth to these topics than has been initially presented here, the primary purpose of these supplemental sections is the provision of illustrative contextual case examples portraying what's below the surface for clients and within real-life therapeutic environments, which speech-language pathologists should and can be targeting through the holistic, person-centered, evidence-based practice counseling skills and procedures presented throughout this text. With that being said, I am making an assumption of your knowledge regarding counseling within speech-language pathology that has been presented to you thus far in the text. Therefore, terms, approaches, and practices will be included in this section without further expansion; however, while reading this section, please take note of the citations and included references, as I have tried to thoughtfully include clinically relevant and oriented ones that may help your understanding and practice if you go back and read the cited articles.

Case Example of Early Childhood Stuttering

Box 8b-6 provides a case illustration for Charlie, a young CWS, followed by a summary of the approach to the case. Box 8b-7 provides an illustration of Charlie's case if the approach was different.

Approach to the Case

As depicted in the previous example, and as you may be able to imagine for yourself, either through your past personal pseudostuttering experiences, or through open, nonjudgmental and vulnerable conversations with your clients, experiences during support group attendance, listening to podcasts about stuttering, watching documentary films representing stuttering, and/or other multimedia-type exposures to real lived experiences with and depictions of stuttering, there is a lot going on in the case example. It should also be noted that nearly all of the elements from the case are frequent real experiences for clients who stutter and their families, which I can personally attest to.

Initially the case portrays how stuttering does have a strong familial representation, especially with males, and that experiences with stuttering and therapy can influence, for better or worse, perceptions and practices (Ambrose et al., 1997; de Oliveira et al., 2012, 2013). The taboo surrounding the topic of stuttering and the foreshadowing of the potential consequential impacts are then presented, which affect the child, siblings, and caregivers (Berquez & Kelman, 2018). Behaviors of increased anxiety are then portrayed and expanded upon by broadly including some internalized representations. The server's, siblings', and parents' reactions and responses are then portrayed. Such, unfortunately common, experiences act as intermittent reinforcers for self-doubts, judgments, criticality, and an overall sense of devaluation and reduced worth. This not only comes from the outward mocking behaviors and obvious misunderstandings, but also from the altered power dynamics, which may result from the child having their "*voice*" taken away from them in a number of ways, let alone opinion/value/worth. Furthermore, the

Box 8b-6
Charlie

Charlie, a young CWS recently assessed for therapy, went out to eat at a restaurant with his family. The maternal grandfather has stuttered throughout his life and is very resistant to his grandson attending speech therapy, due to his own negative personal experiences with stuttering therapy. Within this family, stuttering is a very taboo topic and is not directly talked about with the exception of the frequent statements of "Stop, take a breath, think about what you're going to say."

A server comes to the table to take the family's order. The adults and older children place their orders, and then it's time for Charlie to do so. Charlie is noticeably nervous, anxious, appearing shy/withdrawn with a closed-off reduced-size posturing, no eye contact, and is in close proximity to his parent (hiding face and clinging). Then Charlie quietly and quickly mumbles his order, which the server doesn't understand and then asks him to repeat. At this point, Charlie becomes even more nervous and starts to perceive the increased attention is on him, like a magnifying glass of judgment from the server and everyone else. Charlie experiences a very high degree of anxiety, time stops, judgment, criticality, feelings of inadequacy, worthlessness, very low value and power, he feels stuck/frozen in that exposed and vulnerable place with a complete sense of loss of control, that this terrible thing is happening to him. He begins to feel like he's inconveniencing the server and his family, wasting valuable time. While Charlie attempts to place his order for the second time, he has SLDs, which puts him in an even more escalated state of anxiety and causes him to just blank out, cognitively dissociating from the moment. The server then giggles, briefly imitating Charlie's stuttering behavior and proceeds to interrupt him by making a joke of it by saying that the restaurant has a lot of great, tasty options and they'd be stuck too. The server then proceeds to verbally and gesturally offer suggestions and guesses at what Charlie might be trying to order. Charlie just wants to get through this moment and survive, so he agrees to a suggestion, changing his order. One of the parents then requests a side substitution for the child, not addressing the situation or letting Charlie finish. Charlie already feels hugely embarrassed, defeated, shameful, and guilty. Then after the server walks away, a sibling briefly mocks Charlie and a parent asks Charlie, "Why didn't you use the techniques you were taught (possibly also asking them to stop and say it again with them)?"

child may feel judged, criticized, and shame from the parent for not using their techniques. Of course, this was not the parent's intention at all. The parent's seemingly harmless question in addition to their enabling actions sends the message that stuttering is not OK and that fluency should be the goal. This is further reinforced by not talking about the lived experience of stuttering, but rather focusing on the use or lack of use of techniques. Children, and people in general, pick up on and inherently understand not only what was said but also what's unsaid but implied or interpreted (accurately or otherwise), so it's very important to focus on what message/intent you mean to convey is *and* how that message may be received/understood.

Case Example of Elementary School-Aged Stuttering

Box 8b-8 is a case illustration of Avery, an elementary school-aged CWS. It is followed by a description of the approach taken for this case.

Approach to the Case

There's again a lot to unpack here and given space, we won't be able to get to everything. Some of the elements sequentially presented in the case are avoidance and social withdrawal, stereotyping leading to self-stigmatization, bullying, narrowing of the perspective, distorted patterns of thinking, deterministic thoughts, externalized locus of control, and overarching power dynamics that led to decreased self-worth/value/confidence/efficacy embodiment of self-stigmatization, shame, guilt, failure, etc. Again, much of the case is based on many real experiences that I've encountered either personally or clinically. When actively engaging in a change process, awareness is nearly always the first item to focus on. Without truly being aware of the item(s), or unintended consequences surrounding them or avoidance of them, there tends to be low motivation and drive for change. Therefore, understanding and then assessing awareness and motivation is crucial. Using a conceptual framework, along with gaining an understanding of the stages, progression, and processes involved with grief and bereavement and how to navigate them as a speech-language pathologist staying within our scope of practice, is paramount when working with clients.

> # Box 8b-7
> ## Charlie: What if Things Had Been Done Differently . . . ?
>
> During and after the speech-language pathologist's assessment of Charlie's stuttering, the speech-language pathologist openly talked about stuttering and the child's, siblings', and parents' lived experiences with and reactions to stuttering. The speech-language pathologist briefly provided psychoeducation counseling to the client and their family by describing stuttering; presenting both the overt and covert aspects; talking about the incidence, prevalence, etiological factors, famous people who stutter, recovery, and persistence; and then facilitated a communication interaction between the child and their family regarding what people do, and want to have done, during stuttering and communication. Especially when in that state of survival and dramatically heightened anxiety, our perspective often narrows, if not becomes completely monocular, not being able to envision or even take in alternative options. What if during the assessment, the speech-language pathologist presented ideas and practices of disclosure statements, advocacy and communication confidence–building activities, pseudostuttering (not only for the client, but also for the siblings and caregivers etc.), and interpersonal relational counseling (i.e., basic counseling skills and requisites such as empathy, nonjudgmental positive regard, feeling reflections, and paraphrasing) were described and then practiced? Take a few minutes to think through and reflect upon how the described case may have played out differently.
>
> Taking a family/community-centered approach to therapy is crucial. In addition to understanding and influencing caregiver and sibling perspectives and behaviors to more open and supportive ones (Coleman, 2018a, 2018b), it's important to help normalize stuttering and the related experiences and challenges while prioritizing and emphasizing communication and communication attempts.

Clients at this age, as well as clients who are older, frequently have years, if not decades, of compounded negative communicative, and sometimes therapeutic, experiences and consequences from living with stuttering. So, depending on the age, or likely more accurately exposure and openness, of the client to stuttering, they may still have hope and an expectation of being fixed, and becoming fluent. Hope is very important and may be used to increase motivation, but it's also our job as speech-language pathologists to help the client reframe what success can entail. How might you prepare for or approach the conversation of likelihood of persistence with a client and or their families? What considerations would you take into account?

Pseudostuttering and Video or Audio Review

As speech-language pathologists, you will have to increase awareness of not only the overt behaviors but also for the covert features, attitudes, beliefs, thoughts, emotions, and impacts. Having open and nonjudgmental conversations regarding lived experiences with stuttering and communally sharing experiences of others discussing their stuttering, either through support groups or multimedia productions and documentaries, will decrease the sense of isolation in the client and should prime them for more openness and cognitive flexibility. As you progress with resilience building and exposure, it's often helpful to use some type of contextual

theoretical sociological framing, such as Bandura's (1986) social-cognitive theory, which presents the interaction and influence of self, behavior, and environment. Additionally, incorporate elements that increase a client's self-efficacy. The four sources of self-efficacy include personal experiences with success, vicarious experience, verbal persuasion, and physiological state. For example, vicarious experiences may include demystifying stuttering by presenting others who stutter, their success stories, through story books with characters who stutter, online TEDx talks from PWS, documentaries about stuttering, podcasts about stuttering, attending support groups or conferences, and pseudostuttering. These all have normalizing effects on stuttering, decrease senses of isolation and withdrawal, and increase perception of membership within a community. Experiencing the exposure to stuttering communally and then discussing and reflecting on the meaning brought by it will further help to broaden the client's perspective. One very powerful way to create vicarious experience templates for client(s) to remember and call upon later are for you, the speech-language pathologist, to pseudostutter in generalized situations and then to discuss the pre-, peri-, and post-cognitive, emotional, social, behavioral, and functional impressions. However, as a note of caution with this, you should always start by describing what pseudostuttering is to the client, clearly explain why you want to do it, what you hope to accomplish by it, and then ask for permission. As research demonstrates, clients may have a high degree of resistance to this for a number of reasons, but through exposure and practice they, and you, become much more comfortable with it and the potential benefits cannot

Box 8b-8

Avery

Teachers informed you, the new school-based speech-language pathologist, that an elementary school-aged client who stutters on your caseload, whom the previous speech-language pathologist was about to discharge from therapy, was appearing to become shyer and more withdrawn, and rarely participated in class or group discussions. Some teachers have made comments to you about how people who stutter are just more anxious, tense, nervous, shy, and withdrawn. During a recent session with Avery, they indicated that they just played games in the therapy room with the previous speech-language pathologist and that they were told that they would be discharged from therapy because they didn't stutter enough. Avery couldn't describe what they were doing, why they were doing it, or what the long-term goal was, and Avery reported to you that they rarely used the techniques out of the clinic room as they sounded and felt weird, people looked at them oddly when they used them, they were very exhausting to use, and mostly because they expressed feeling disingenuous while using them, almost like they were putting on a show or an act. Also, Avery mentioned that the previous speech-language pathologist had never asked them what they wanted or expected from therapy. In talking with others, including calling the previous speech-language pathologist, you learned that they had been taking a fluency shaping approach, trying to make the client as fluent as possible and rarely talked about the client's lived experiences with stuttering, the psychological, emotional, social, or functional aspects, and that the clinician pretty much only modeled the techniques in the clinic room. When you openly and nonjudgmentally talk with the client about their past experiences with stuttering and stuttering therapy (e.g., what was helpful and not, what the long-term goal was, why, and how you and the client may get there, along with what the client's goals are), it becomes apparent that they have pretty much only been exposed to a fluency-at-all-costs framing and didn't know that there were other options. So, there's much resistance from them and their parents/caregivers when you mention alternative approaches to them. Avery also reluctantly indicates some negatives from their previous therapeutic experiences, such as never having openly talked about their lived experiences with stuttering; not discussing the long-term goal, rationales, or approaches; and the speech-language pathologist laughing at them when they described an experience of relational bullying. As the client described it, they were talking in a small group of peers and got stuck on a word when a peer said, "s-s-s-s-spit it out, waterboy." As recounted, Avery described the previous therapist laughing out loud and saying that's funny, can't you see why that's funny, to which Avery sadly reported going along with and then internalizing not bringing up any experiences of bullying or emotions related to stuttering again. In continuing the discussion, Avery also made similar comments about their personality as the previous teachers and mentioned that it's just them, not because of their stuttering. When talking with Avery about specific instances when they communicated with others, rather than framing it through stuttering specifically, the client was superficial and stated that everything was OK, that they aren't bothered by their stuttering and that the other kids don't even seem to notice or care about it. Having a good degree of concern and inferring that there's more under the surface that Avery doesn't know or isn't presenting, you probe by asking more direct questions about the specific communication interactions (e.g., who initiates, turn-taking, relational connections, reactions [if the child is old enough you may even be able to be more process oriented with theory of mind type questions]). You pick up on some of Avery's statements that indicate that relational bullying has been happening and has been getting progressively worse. When again framing and asking Avery about overall communication, not stuttering specifically, and discussing objective features from interactions, you start picking up on more and more contradictions and or points of misalignment between the words that Avery speaks and the nonverbal communication that is conveyed. Through the interaction(s) you come to the conclusion that Avery isn't comfortable with or accepting of their stuttering and that they are actively trying to hide or conceal it at some pretty significant costs to their psycho-emotional-social well-being. Avery reports never having seen, heard, or met anyone else who stutters and that they feel alone and isolated, and that no one understands them. When discussing their lived experiences with stuttering and self-concepts/identities and barriers, you notice a lot of deterministic language, verbalization of externalization of control, and fairly signature cognitive distortion-like phrasings (e.g., all-or-none thinking, mental filters, discounting the positives, jumping to conclusions. In trying to

(continued)

Box 8b-8 (continued)

Avery

broaden Avery's perspective, you start encountering a large degree of resistance, especially when you bring up the ideas of talking more openly about stuttering, pseudostuttering, and recording/analyzing a video of them speaking. To add further challenges, during an IEP meeting, Avery asks you when you are going to fix them.

---

be overstated. For PWS engaging in pseudostuttering, they frequently experience it in a very deescalated state, similar to projecting the ease of speaking experience that may occur with typically fluent speakers. Unlike even when using other behaviorally oriented speech motor control techniques to influence stuttering, which may still result in increased anxiety, judgment, tension, effort, and imposter-like feelings, pseudostuttering has a greatly reduced effort and tension, albeit some of the covert features may still be present to varying degrees. Pseudostuttering alters the perception of the locus of control from external to internal. Instead of stuttering being something that happens to the client, they become exposed to the influence that they can have over it and communication, also setting the foundation for choice engagement with emotions and thoughts down the road.

There are also a number of other ways to demonstrate shifting of locus of control with speech and stuttering and some of those have previously been presented throughout the text. Vicarious exposure to other forms of stuttering and those talking about stuttering with verbal persuasion can also often help to set the stage for the client to become open with reframing what success is or can be. Through reframing, you and the client can then set your own benchmarks and criteria for what success is and may look like. Again, bridging the gap between what's observed in you/your pseudostuttering and what's viewed, listened to, or experienced while deconstructing the various features and dedicating adequate time to discussing it, clients gain personalized experiences with success that may be more meaningful to them. Lastly, the physiological state source of self-efficacy, including emotional valence, pre/peri/post reactions, elements of attribution, identification of physical representation of emotion(s), and desensitization may be engaged with a number of ways for an array of reasons.

To start, let's revisit awareness and the locus of control in the context of our previous discussion of resilience. Increasing awareness of emotions, emotional vocabulary, and the physical representations of emotion will help the client to more quickly and effectively identify what is happening and what influenced it to happen along with why it's meaningful. In other words, being able to identify and describe these features allows clients to go below the surface and explore what is motivating them, and it allows detachment from more concrete embedded beliefs, thus enabling them to increase their psychological flexibility and perspective. Ways to do

this include mindfulness, meditation, progressive relaxation, and tension/relaxation techniques. Integrating these practices also have the added benefit of helping clients increase tolerance and self-regulate their emotions much more effectively. Other frequently used strategies to build conscious and objective awareness are through alignment discussions of stuttering and communication from you, the speech-language pathologist, and the client defining and describing the overt and covert aspects of stuttering *and* communication, including nonverbal ways to increase engagement, acceptance, and confidence and through exposure to and then analysis of stuttering, which come with some cautions. PWS, especially CWS, have very seldom seen or heard recordings of themselves speaking/stuttering, so it's not surprising that they frequently have an inaccurate perception of what's actually going on. This is true for both the overt and covert elements. Remember again that prior to exposure to more person-centered holistic approaches, PWS frequently report experiencing the moment of stuttering as analogous to drowning, where they are frozen, terrified, disconnected, overwhelmed by the tidal wave of anxiety and self, along with projection of others' judgments, and are just trying to survive that moment. Now imagine having that very vulnerable and exposed moment right there in front of you for the first time and having someone scrutinize it, while also being asked to impart your own judgments to your self-execution! This is where some resilience and tolerance building, mindfulness, and active and intentional engagement with emotions will come in handy. Awareness, exposure, and in vitro desensitization are necessary and beneficial elements. Again, we aren't motivated or typically cannot change what we aren't aware of, but ensure that the client is ready for and appropriately supported throughout such activities. It's often best to proceed from temporally and personally distant to more proximally close, such as real-time self-scans during communication. What I mean by this is that it's often best to start with you and the client analyzing and discussing still characters in books (or stories that the clients create illustrations or narratives from), which don't directly depict all of the sender and receiver dynamics of communication unfolding in real time. Then watch, analyze, and discuss videos of others who stutter, such as stuttering for kids by kids that has positive vicarious exposures as well. After this progressing to more temporal proximal, real time instead of video that can be stopped and played back by you, the speech-language pathologist, pseudostuttering and having the client stop and freeze you and then analyzing your "stuttering" and communication. Eventually you want to support the child in analyzing their own stuttering, and communication, and then to be able to do this in real time during conversations.

Throughout most of these progressive descriptions I have been focused on the sequence and procedures, but I've omitted the content. This was done intentionally to set the appropriate scaffolding. When progressing through these activities, remember to also discuss cognitive, emotional, behavioral, social, and functional elements from pre/peri/post frames, while also including positives that will help lay additional groundwork for later reframing procedures. Awareness building in a supported nonjudgmental fashion also has the added benefit of reducing avoidance and secondary stuttering behaviors. Focus on these areas, as well as "good" communication, including nonverbal aspects, engagement through openness and vulnerability, and openly discussing and training communication and small talk practices will also provide broader holistic avenues for success. I often include TED or TEDx videos and content such as Brené Brown and open discussions and analysis with my clients who stutter. This is very important when taking a more person-centered approach that does not just focus on fluency, because communication and relational elements are so much more than how the message is sent. When clients start to report joy with communication, especially to strangers, regardless of categorical presence or absence of SLDs, that is success! Through therapy, and life, duration of stuttering, use of secondary avoidance behaviors, and degree of effort or struggle (again both overtly and covertly represented) can drastically change if the right approach and support are given. Lastly, once you've successfully progressed through these activities and the client is able to use the strategies, including mindfulness, grounding, and defusion in real time, the client can be fully present when communicating and stuttering. This will enable greater degrees of success when implementing speech management strategies (e.g., prolongations). A representative analogy to this is that when the client is taught about emotions and how to engage with them in more productive ways, they are then learning to swim in the shallow end of the pool vs. when overt stuttering and fluency are the primary goals and emotions or emotional regulation are not adequately addressed, the speech-language pathologist is trying to teaching the client to swim in open water while they are standing on the boat and the client is drowning. This may be an exaggerated analogy, but I hope you understand my point.

As noted earlier, some of the intent behind the procedural sequences that have been described are *awareness building*, creating *objective experiential templates*, *expanding the discussions regarding successes* and *various other influential factors* so clients can recall them more easily and for longer durations, increasing psychological flexibility, reframing, desensitization, and emotional regulation, but also confidence building, increased self-efficacy/worth/value,

being understood and part of a community, *and* the foundations for advocacy, which we will see later through more disclosure statements, actions of transparency and immediacy (e.g., directly addressing inappropriate reactions to their stuttering and or bullying), and continuing to talk over and finishing their sentences when others try to interrupt them or finish their sentences. Teaching the client to be knowledgeable about speech, communication, and stuttering processes, as well as being able to present to others about them either in formal or informal ways, also helps with confidence, agency, and shifting the locus of control.

One very beneficial activity for clients who stutter, especially school-aged ones, is to cooperatively do a classroom presentation as well as possibly an in-service. Flynn and St. Louis (2011) even revealed that one classroom presentation about stuttering increases peers' positive attitudes and perspectives about stuttering and their peers who stutter for up to 7 years after the fact. More anecdotally, I have also noticed this in addition to increased inclusion and engagement from students who stutter after such exposure and activities. Creating a stutter-friendly and more knowledgeable environment is beneficial for so many reasons. Similarly, disclosure statements and openness have similar benefits. As the saying goes, if something doesn't seem to bother the person with it, why should it bother others? This is to say that, as much current research is demonstrating, when PWS are more open and accepting of their stuttering, speech, and themselves, their quality of life dramatically improves and their overt severity decreases.

Case Example of Adolescent School-Aged Stuttering

Box 8b-9 is a case illustration for Jordan, a teenage client who stutters. It is followed by the approach to the case.

Approach to the Case

Let's be honest; for most people, going through adolescence is tough. Children are trying to transition into adulthood forming a new identity with increased agency, possibly autonomy and decision-making capabilities; however, they likely don't fully possess the cognitive, emotional, or social capacities or experiences to rationally understand certain aspects. Life may become much more real, as may emotions. If the client doesn't understand their emotions, the physical representation of them to understand what they are, ability to introspect about them why they are so strong and what has motivated them; how to regulate them; or doesn't possess a decent emotional vocabulary, they can become overwhelming very quickly. By this time, the client may have been therapized to excess. They may be emotionally done with therapy, may not see the point in it, or they may have other priorities. There may also still be a real disconnect between what the

---

Box 8b-9

Jordan

Jordan, a teenage client who stutters on your caseload, has recently become very disinterested in therapy, misses if you don't specifically go to get them from their class (which they hate), is disconnected, clock watching while in therapy, and through their statements and actions you infer that they are disengaged from life, possibly depressed. When assessing what to do in therapy in terms of continuation with the IEP, shifting to a 504 check-in and consultation plan, or exiting/discharge from therapy, you ask Jordan about what impact stuttering has on them and how often they think about it. Jordan states that it doesn't bother them or hold them back, and that they don't think about it often. You ask Jordan what they want to do, in terms of continuing with therapy or not. Jordan initially gives a nonverbal fear/shock response, but then says that they want to be done. Taking this at face value, you agree and work toward discharging Jordan. However, when discussing this with the parents, they express major concern and want therapy to continue. They reveal to you that Jordan doesn't seem to have many friends, is lethargic, disinterested, disengaged, and has even been doing self-harm behaviors. Now knowing this, you contact the school's counselor in hopes of getting them involved. Either not understanding your request or the situation, the school counselor initially expresses that they shouldn't be involved because it's stuttering and that's your area. The next time Jordan comes to therapy, instead of asking about stuttering specifically, you take the approach of asking about specific communication situations and interactions, to which the same client who had just previously stated that stuttering doesn't bother them and they don't think about it often, replies by stating that they don't talk in class or in groups, that they don't have any friends because they stutter, that sometimes it seems like it would be easier without all the hassle. Being concerned about the client's mental/emotional state you perform a suicide screening, as previously described in the text. It doesn't appear as if Jordan has plans or intentions to act on the thoughts, but they do express suicidal ideation, which is more common in PWS (Ardila et al., 1994; Briley et al., 2021; Rezaeian et al., 2020). You then go with Jordan to the counselor's office and talk through the lived experiences of stuttering, the self-doubt, judgment, overall impact that it has on their life, along with the very real anxiety, feeling isolated, like an imposter, and how Jordan has stated feeling less than human. As the speech-language pathologist, you help to normalize some of Jordan's experiences and statements through knowledge from your past experiences and documentary portrayals, and then you frame what you have recently started to work on, being a new speech-language pathologist to the school and how you're focusing on communication, openness, acceptance, confidence, and then toss the metaphorical ball to the counselor. Many of these elements are directly in the counselor's area of expertise and training, so they now understand how they can be helpfully involved with Jordan, and they work to create inclusionary groups, as well as work with Jordan on the various other aspects. It should be noted that this was presented in a very accelerated fashion that invariably missed some good professional steps to take, but my intent is to present something more standout-ish. Again, as is true with the other cases that have been presented, nearly all of this case and statements come from real examples.

---

parents or guardians want (the client to still attend therapy regularly and possibly for a fluency focus) and the client's desires (likely to be done with therapy), so you may be up against a formidable amount of resistance, if not outright teenage angst.

As is true with life in general, there is much complexity presented in this brief case example. We again see contradictions in statements and actions compared to intent and what may be taken from inference. There are some real telltale signs indicating concern and some blurry lines regarding scope of practice. The point of bringing this up isn't to instruct you where the scope of practice or ethical lines are, as those inevitability vary from individual to individual due to a number of factors. Instead, the point was to present a

real-life depiction of the possible intersection of the lines, scopes, and opportunities. As has been emphasized throughout this text, elements of counseling are within our scope of practice, but there's not always clear guidance for what that means or where the lines are. It should/must be more than just psychoeducation counseling and, in my opinion, should be contextually framed around clients' communication or impact(s) experienced via their communication difference(s), disorder(s), or deficit(s), but again that line is not quite clear. For example, if you, the speech-language pathologist, aren't aware of what contributes to identify/role formation or change, or what's necessary for change, cognitive reframing, or to motivate change in desires, expectations (especially for the long-term therapy) might be more of a lost ferryboat guide in the bog vs. a skilled navigator with a map. In stuttering therapy, we are attempting to change behaviors, attitudes, beliefs, perspectives, and overall practices. With this comes impact on and transition with identity and perceived roles. Especially with the teenage client, a skilled speech-language pathologist has to know what to do when they encounter resistance and when to generally expect what types of reactions so they can plan ahead with how to address them. For example, as discussed early in the text, MI is a very important approach/skill/strategy to use with adolescents and other older clients. Instead of pushing back against their angst and resistance, go along with it and try to align yourself to their experiences while being that skilled guide, supporting clients' self-recognitions and changes. Help them shift from that extreme sense of loss of control in regard to their stuttering to agency and an internalized locus of control through increased self-efficacy and self-actualizations.

Summary

Beyond the messages carried by verbal communication, people evaluate, make judgments, and form opinions based on cognitive, emotional, behavioral, and social factors. Stuttering creates a context for negative reinforcements of anticipation, avoidance, and perceived and/or actual consequences. An acceptance-based approach identifies communication exchange and personhood as priorities over fluency. Of course, this process is complicated, because persons who stutter frequently encounter reinforcement of self-doubts, judgments, criticality, and overall sense of devalued self-worth. Some of this is external and some is internal to the individual. Open and nonjudgmental conversations with peers and personal sharing help decrease the sense of social isolation and prime them for more openness and cognitive flexibility. Exposure experiences, such as pseudostuttering or simply interacting in challenging contexts, is paired with resilience building. Pseudostuttering alters one's internal representation of locus of control as external to internal by taking control of when the stutters occur. Likewise, vicarious exposure via peers, podcasts, TEDx talks, and films can also provide opportunities for reframing what success is or can be. Positive experiences, including successful engagement in exposure activities, increase self-efficacy. When persons who stutter gain personalized experiences with success, it may be more meaningful. A sense of control over physiological states may also be a source of self-efficacy, as the PWS becomes desensitized to emotional valence, pre/peri/post reactions, elements of attribution, and physical representations of emotions. Detaching self from deeply embedded beliefs allows persons who stutter to explore those responses and how to manage them. This could include mindfulness, meditation, progressive relaxation, and tension reduction/relaxation techniques. The intent of such experiences includes awareness building, creation of objective experiential templates, expanding discussions regarding successes, and other influential factors. Techniques like motivational interviewing are a good fit for older clients.

References

Ambrose, N. G., Cox, N. J., & Yairi, E. (1997). The genetic basis of persistence and recovery in stuttering. *Journal of Speech, Language, and Hearing Research, 40*(3), 567-580.

Ardila, A., Bateman, J., Niño, C. R., Pulido, E., Rivera, D. B., & Vanegas, C. J. (1994). An epidemiologic study of stuttering. *Journal of communication disorders, 27*(1), 37-48.

Berquez, A., & Kelman, E. (2018). Methods in stuttering therapy for desensitizing parents of children who stutter. *American Journal of Speech-Language Pathology, 27*(3S), 1124-1138.

Briley, P. M., Gerlach, H., & Jacobs, M. M. (2021). Relationships between stuttering, depression, and suicidal ideation in young adults: Accounting for gender differences. *Journal of Fluency Disorders, 67*, 105820.

Coleman, C. (2018a). Community-centered assessment and treatment. In Amster, B. J. & Klein, E. R. (Eds.), *More than fluency: The social, emotional, and cognitive dimensions of stuttering* (1st ed., p. 215). Plural Publishing.

Coleman, C. E. (2018b). Comprehensive stuttering treatment for adolescents: A case study. *Language, speech, and hearing services in schools, 49*(1), 33-41.

de Oliveira, B. V. D., Domingues, C. E. F., Juste, F. S., Andrade, C. R. F. D., & Moretti-Ferreira, D. (2012). Familial persistent developmental stuttering: Genetic perspectives. *Revista da Sociedade Brasileira de Fonoaudiologia, 17*(4), 489-494.

de Oliveira, C. M. C., Cunha, D., & dos Santos, A. C. (2013). Risk factors for stuttering in disfluent children with familial recurrence. *Audiology-Communication Research, 18*(1), 43-49.

Flynn, T. W., & St. Louis, K. O. (2011). Changing adolescent attitudes toward stuttering. *Journal of Fluency Disorders, 36*(2), 110-121. https://doi.org/10.1016/j.jfludis.2011.04.002

Rezaeian, M., Akbari, M., Shirpoor, A. H., Moghadasi, Z., Nikdel, Z., & Hejri, M. (2020). Anxiety, social phobia, depression, and suicide among people who stutter; a review study. *Journal of Occupational Health and Epidemiology, 9*(2), 98-109.

Sheehan, J. G. (1970). *Stuttering: Research and therapy*. Harper and Row.

Tichenor, S. E., & Yaruss, J. S. (2019). Stuttering as defined by adults who stutter. *Journal of Speech, Language, and Hearing Research, 62*(12), 4356-4369.

Yaruss, J. S., & Quesal, R. W. (2004). Stuttering and the international classification of functioning, disability, and health (ICF): An update. *Journal of Communication Disorders, 37*(1), 35-52.

Yaruss, J. S., Quesal, R. W., Reeves, L., Molt, L. F., Kluetz, B., Caruso, A. J., . . . & Lewis, F. (2002). Speech treatment and support group experiences of people who participate in the National Stuttering Association. *Journal of Fluency Disorders, 27*(2), 115-134.

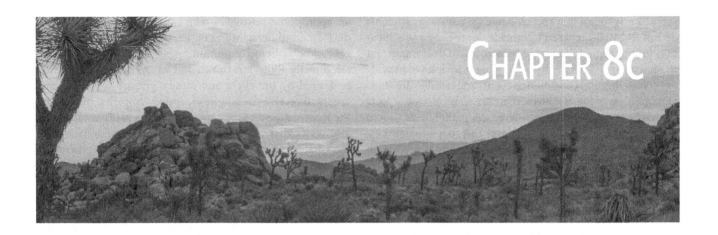

Special Topics and Disorders
Acquired Medical

Rebecca H. Affoo, PhD, CCC-SLP, SLP-Reg, SLP(c);
Miriam Carroll-Alfano, PhD, CCC-SLP; and Julia Fischer, PhD, CCC-SLP

Counseling Individuals With Dysphagia and Their Families

Rebecca H. Affoo, PhD, CCC-SLP, SLP-Reg, SLP(c)

Humans are innately capable of meeting nutritional needs via eating and swallowing; we are born ready to swallow, we develop swallowing skill over childhood, and it is one of the last functions lost in old age. Swallowing impairment, or ***dysphagia***, affects the preparation and transportation of saliva and ingested materials along the digestive tract and is commonly defined as reduced safety of the swallow, resulting in the misdirection of ingested material into the airway (aspiration) and/or reduced efficiency of the swallow, resulting in residual material left behind in the throat after the swallow has been completed (Logemann, 1998). A host of negative physical and mental health consequences are associated with dysphagia, including mortality (Altman et al.,

2010; Feng et al., 2019). Dysphagia may increase the risk of a person developing aspiration pneumonia, dehydration, and malnutrition (Crary et al., 2013; Namasivayam & Steele, 2015; Namasivayam-MacDonald et al., 2018; Takeuchi et al., 2014; van der Maarel-Wierink et al., 2011; Whelan, 2001). Furthermore, dysphagia is associated with negative psychosocial consequences that adversely impact a person's well-being and quality of life. Individuals with dysphagia frequently report having symptoms of depression and decreased quality of life, and they experience isolation from loss of the social aspects of eating food by mouth, anxiety or panic at mealtimes, and loss of self-esteem (Chen et al., 2009; Ekberg et al., 2002; Kim et al., 2019; Vesey, 2013).

It is well-established that dysphagia is a symptom of dysfunctions and disorders that affect the brain, nervous system, and/or the structure and function of the head and neck (Carrau et al., 2017; García-Peris et al., 2007; Takizawa et al., 2016). Because dysphagia is a symptom of a wide variety of different conditions affecting a heterogenous group of individuals across the age spectrum and because it causes serious adverse effects on physical and mental health, it can be very challenging to counsel individuals with dysphagia. In fact, a

Hoepner, J. K. (Ed.). *Counseling and Motivational Interviewing in Speech-Language Pathology* (pp. 175-186).

recent study found that speech-language pathology students do not feel well-prepared to provide counseling and education in dysphagia (Caesar & Merertu, 2020). It is important to remember that while the underlying principles of providing counseling and education to clients and families are similar regardless of the diagnosis, there are some unique aspects of dysphagia care that speech-language pathologists should consider. Some counseling situations that may be commonly experienced by the dysphagia clinician are described in the following to highlight the unique aspects of dysphagia-related care.

Breaking Bad News

Speech-language pathologists are often the first clinician to inform clients of a swallowing impairment and the potential consequences associated with that diagnosis. Patients experiencing dysphagia secondary to traumatic brain injury (TBI) or right hemisphere brain injury may demonstrate reduced insight and be unaware of any difficulties or distress associated with swallowing. Additionally, evidence suggests that as many as 30% of patients with dysphagia may experience silent aspiration (Garon et al., 2009), defined as aspiration without cough or other signs of distress. Impaired laryngeal and/or pharyngeal sensation can be one reason for experiencing silent aspiration and may also contribute to reduced awareness of any swallowing problems. For these individuals, receiving a diagnosis of dysphagia may be unexpected, resulting in a disruption of psychological well-being and high levels of anxiety and depression. For other patients, they may have received a diagnosis known to cause swallowing impairment but may or may not be aware that dysphagia is something they should expect as part of the disease trajectory. Other patients may suspect that something is wrong with their ability to swallow, or it may be one of the reasons they sought medical attention in the first place. In all these situations, the speech-language pathologist needs to be aware that their role may include breaking bad news and adjust their counselling strategies accordingly.

The Patient Self-Determination Act of 1991 means that patients should be allowed to participate fully in decisions regarding their health care (Koch, 1992). Speech-language pathologists are obligated to provide information about the swallowing diagnosis, the results of the evaluation that led to the diagnosis, the characteristics of the dysphagia, the underlying etiology that is causing the dysphagia, the prognosis, and any proposed treatment options. This also includes information about the anticipated outcomes of all options including the outcomes associated with not pursuing any of the proposed treatment options (i.e., doing nothing). However, *how* to do this has not been well studied. The SPIKES protocol (Kaplan, 2010) is a stepwise framework that clinicians can use to plan how they will engage in difficult discussions. SPIKES is an acronym for Setting, Perception, Invitation for information, Knowledge, Empathy, Summarize or strategize. Using the SPIKES framework, a clinician would find an appropriate setting in which to deliver the bad news, develop an understanding of what the client and family already knows before communicating any new information, ask directly about how much and what kind of information is desired by the client and family, prepare the client and family to receive the bad news, convey empathy, summarize the information in a way the patient can easily understand, and verify that the client and family have understood the information. Evidence from literature examining breaking bad news to individuals with cancer suggests that patients prefer someone with expertise to provide information about a diagnosis and treatment options as soon as it is available, but support during this stage was also rated as very important (Parker et al., 2001). Similarly, findings from a scoping review examining the health and social care needs of older adults with multiple chronic conditions and their caregivers revealed that people overwhelmingly want information that is clear and timely. They want to understand their health conditions (McGilton et al., 2018). Understanding leads to people being able to participate fully in decisions regarding their health care. Swallowing is a complex process that requires more than 25 pairs of muscles in the oral cavity, pharynx, larynx, and esophagus, and the control of swallowing represents a coordination among the brain stem and cortical central pathways (Doty, 1951; Doty & Bosma, 1956; Jean, 1984, 2001). Moreover, food and drink are an important part of many cultures, religions, and social interactions and are connected with a variety of emotions. As such, being able to educate clients and families about swallowing, the reason swallowing is impaired, and what that means in the context of the client's life, all while responding adequately to the reactions of the client and family, providing support, and facilitating the client to identify their own goals, direction, and plans is no easy feat. A dysphagia clinician's ability to counsel is very firmly interconnected with their knowledge and ability to share that knowledge in a way that is clear, culturally responsive, and accessible to clients and families but not simplified to the point of being inaccurate.

Swallowing Intervention

As per the American Speech-Language-Hearing Association (ASHA) clinical topic on Adult Dysphagia, the goals of swallowing intervention are as follows:

safely support adequate nutrition and hydration and return to safe and efficient oral intake (including incorporating the patient's dietary preferences and consulting with family members/caregivers to ensure that the patient's daily living activities are being considered); determine the optimum feeding methods/technique to maximize swallowing safety and feeding efficiency; minimize the risk of pulmonary complications; reduce patient and caregiver burden while maximizing the patient's quality of life; and develop treatment plans to improve safety and efficiency of the swallow.

Swallowing intervention is typically organized into three different approaches: compensatory, rehabilitative, or preventative types of interventions. Swallowing intervention should be person-centered and individualized to the client based on their goals. As mentioned previously, people need to understand their health condition in order to participate fully in decisions regarding their health care. The concept of "patient noncompliance" is a term that may be heard in reference to patients who are not following the swallowing-related recommendations of the speech-language pathologist; however, this term seems incongruent with the tenets of person-centered care. The evidence pertaining to adherence to dysphagia recommendations is limited. In fact, a systematic review completed by Krekeler et al. (2018) identified only 12 studies reporting patient adherence data. Some barriers to adherence to dysphagia recommendations that have been reported in the literature include dissatisfaction with food and/or fluid modification recommendations, issues with motivation, therapy buy-in, difficulty completing intervention tasks, or burden on caregivers (Colodny, 2005; Krekeler et al., 2018). Many of these barriers could be addressed by a dysphagia clinician who is able to provide education that is clear, culturally responsive, and accessible to clients and families. For example, if a client is noncompliant with food or fluid texture recommendations, the speech-language pathologist should consider the following questions: Did I collaborate with the client and family when we developed this management plan? Are these recommendations consistent with the client's goals of care? Did I provide adequate education about these recommendations? Clients and families should have an understanding of the rationale for dysphagia recommendations, and they should be supported in order to follow through with them. In addition, when effectively educating clients and families and practicing person-centered care, speech-language pathologists must be aware that swallowing interventions likely represent some kind of change in typical or baseline behavior for the client and therefore counseling in this scenario will rely heavily on the underlying principles of motivational interviewing (see Chapter 5).

Tube Feeding

Enteral tube feeding may be recommended for patients in the event they are unable to safely meet their nutritional needs by mouth. Tube feeding may represent a life-saving treatment option for individuals with a variety of different diagnoses, across the age spectrum. Individuals who have experienced an acute but severe decline in swallowing function that is expected to improve over time, such as those who have experienced a stroke or TBI, may require a temporary feeding tube as they recover (Ojo & Brooke, 2016). Returning to oral intake may be motivating for some patients and facilitate therapy buy-in. Moreover, swallowing therapy may include training with food or fluid boluses, which may be pleasurable

as well as motivating. Some individuals may require a long-term feeding tube secondary to structural oropharyngeal changes associated with radiotherapy for the treatment of head and neck cancer (Nugent et al., 2010). These individuals may be unable to take food by mouth due to the severity of their dysphagia and due to the distress and discomfort they experience when eating and drinking by mouth. Other individuals with neurodegenerative diseases like amyotrophic lateral sclerosis (ALS) may choose to receive enteral nutrition and hydration (Stavroulakis & McDermott, 2016) but enjoy some oral intake for pleasure early in the disease progression. Children may require a feeding tube to meet their nutritional requirements as they grow and develop but the decision-making process around enteral feeding may be quite distressing for parents (Hazel, 2006). The evidence suggests that for some individuals, enteral tube feeding improves quality of life (Ojo et al., 2019); however for others, the negative psychosocial impacts of this treatment may be quite serious (Martin et al., 2012). Tube feeding may result in the loss of pleasure and gustatory stimulation associated with mealtimes. Additionally, tube feeding may impact social engagement. A meal may no longer be associated with contact and managing problems related to tube function may interfere with social life. Moreover, enteral tube feeding transfers treatment responsibility and activity to patients and their caregivers to a large extent.

Certain patients may not be good candidates for enteral tube feeding. For example, the American Geriatrics Society published a position statement recommending that tube feeding be avoided in older adults with dementia and instead offer careful handfeeding (American Geriatrics Society Ethics Committee and Clinical Practice and Models of Care Committee, 2014). This does not mean that the speech-language pathologist abandons a person-centered approach when working with persons with dementia. For example, in the case of a person with dementia whose dysphagia severity does not match the degree of cognitive impairment (i.e., swallowing is severely impaired but cognitive status may only be moderately impaired) whose goals of care include prolonging life and promoting independence in activities of daily living, enteral feeding may be a reasonable option. Decisions about artificial nutrition and hydration for persons with advanced dementia are some of the most difficult and emotionally troubling decisions a family will make. "I don't want my loved one to starve to death" is a statement very commonly expressed by family members. As a speech-language pathologist, these are some of the hardest conversations to have with clients and families. There are numerous issues associated with feeding tube use for patients with dementia, including highly complex ethical, moral, and cultural considerations. Please see Gillick (2000) for an excellent review of these considerations. Ultimately, it is the responsibility of the speech-language pathologist to stay up to date on the evidence around tube feeding, and they must be able to communicate with clients and family members about the trajectory of disease and associated dysphagia and elicit goals of care.

Caregiver Burden

It is well-known that persons with dysphagia experience negative psychosocial consequences that adversely impact their well-being and quality of life, including isolation, anxiety, and depression (Ekberg et al., 2002; Vesey, 2013). Evidence suggests that dysphagia also negatively impacts familial or informal caregivers. Recent work has identified that caregivers of aging spouses with dysphagia report increased emotional burden as compared with caregivers of aging spouses without dysphagia (Shune & Namasivayam-MacDonald, 2020a). Caregivers of aging parents with dysphagia report increased physical and emotional burden (Shune & Namasivayam-MacDonald, 2020a). It is important for speech-language pathologists to be knowledgeable about how dysphagia impacts patients as well as families and modify their practice accordingly to support clients as well as caregivers. See Shune and Namasivayam-MacDonald (2020b) for a comprehensive review on caregiver burden.

Palliative Care

Palliative care is defined by the World Health Organization (2002) as "an approach that improves the quality of life of individuals and their families facing the problems associated with life threatening illness, through prevention and relief of suffering by means of early identification and impeccable assessment and treatment of pain and other problems, physical, psychosocial and spiritual" (p. 84). Many life-limiting illnesses are known to cause swallowing impairments and it is generally accepted that speech-language pathologists play an important role in the care of people receiving palliative care. That role includes assessing and managing dysphagia, assisting patients in fulfilling their wishes or advanced directives throughout the illness trajectory, advocating for patients to live with dignity and comfort, educating and counselling the patient and family about swallowing impairments, educating the interprofessional team about swallowing impairments, and participating in overall patient care as a member of the interprofessional team (O'Reilly & Walshe, 2015). Speech-language pathologists may also play a critical role in introducing a patient with a life-limiting illness to the concept of palliative care and counselling patients and families about transitioning dysphagia treatments to maximize quality of life (Puntil-Sheltman, 2013).

Key Takeaways

- Dysphagia results in serious adverse physical and mental health consequences and is a symptom of a wide variety of different conditions affecting a heterogenous group of individuals across the age spectrum. The prognoses and treatment options for dysphagia are highly dependent on the underlying etiology causing the dysphagia as well the client's personal factors and environmental context.

- Speech-language pathologists may be required to communicate bad news about a swallowing impairment to clients and families. Using a communication framework and providing clear and timely information is advised.

- Educational counseling is a critical component of person-centered dysphagia care. Clients and families cannot participate fully in health care decisions unless they understand the health condition.

- The nature of the swallowing impairment, the prognoses, and the goals of care all influence the selection of the most appropriate treatment options. Person-centered care and education that is clear, culturally responsive, and accessible to clients and families is vital to facilitate adherence to dysphagia recommendations.

- Enteral tube feeding may be recommended for clients who cannot safely meet their nutritional needs by mouth, but this decision may be accompanied by significant emotional distress for clients and family members. Speech-language pathologists should be very knowledgeable about the efficacy of tube feeding and the associated ethical, moral, and religious factors that may influence client and family decision-making. A person-centered approach is advised.

- Speech-language pathologists must be knowledgeable about the burden of dysphagia on family caregivers and modify their practice to support clients as well as caregivers.

- Speech-language pathologists support patients receiving palliative care by introducing a patient with a life-limiting illness to the concept of palliative care, assessing and managing dysphagia in a way that is consistent with goals of care, and educating the patient, family, and the interprofessional team about swallowing impairments.

References

Altman, K. W., Yu, G. -P., & Schaefer, S. D. (2010). Consequence of dysphagia in the hospitalized patient: Impact on prognosis and hospital resources. *Archives of Otolaryngology-Head & Neck Surgery, 136*(8), 784. https://doi.org/10.1001/archoto.2010.129

American Geriatrics Society Ethics Committee and Clinical Practice and Models of Care Committee. (2014). American Geriatrics Society feeding tubes in advanced dementia position statement. *Journal of the American Geriatrics Society, 62*(8), 1590-1593. https://doi.org/10.1111/jgs.12924

American Speech-Language-Hearing Association. (n.d.). *Adult dysphagia*. (Practice Portal). https://www.asha.org/practice-portal/clinical-topics/adult-dysphagia/

Caesar, L., & Merertu, K. (2020). Speech-language pathologists' perceptions of their preparation and confidence for providing dysphagia services. *Perspectives of the ASHA Special Interest Groups, 5*(6), 1666-1682. https://doi.org/10.1044/2020_PERSP-20-00115

Carrau, R. L., Murry, T., & Howell, R. J. (Eds.). (2017). *Comprehensive management of swallowing disorders* (2nd ed.). Plural Publishing.

Chen, P. -H., Golub, J. S., Hapner, E. R., & Johns, M. M. (2009). Prevalence of perceived dysphagia and quality-of-life impairment in a geriatric population. *Dysphagia*, *24*(1), 1-6. https://doi.org/10.1007/s00455 -008-9156-1

Colodny, N. (2005). Dysphagic independent feeders' justifications for noncompliance with recommendations by a speech-language pathologist. *American Journal of Speech-Language Pathology*, *14*(1), 61-70. https://doi.org/10.1044/1058-0360(2005/008)

Crary, M. A., Humphrey, J. L., Carnaby-Mann, G., Sambandam, R., Miller, L., & Silliman, S. (2013). Dysphagia, nutrition, and hydration in ischemic stroke patients at admission and discharge from acute care. *Dysphagia*, *28*(1), 69-76. https://doi.org/10.1007/s00455-012-9414-0

Doty, R. W. (1951). Influence of stimulus pattern on reflex deglutition. *The American Journal of Physiology*, *166*(1), 142-158. https://doi.org /10.1152/ajplegacy.1951.166.1.142

Doty, R. W., & Bosma, J. F. (1956). An electromyographic analysis of reflex deglutition. *Journal of Neurophysiology*, *19*(1), 44-60. https://doi.org /10.1152/jn.1956.19.1.44

Ekberg, O., Hamdy, S., Woisard, V., Wuttge-Hannig, A., & Ortega, P. (2002). Social and psychological burden of dysphagia: Its impact on diagnosis and treatment. *Dysphagia*, *17*(2), 139-146. https://doi.org /10.1007/s00455-001-0113-5

Feng, M.-C., Lin, Y.-C., Chang, Y.-H., Chen, C.-H., Chiang, H.-C., Huang, L.-C., Yang, Y.-H., & Hung, C.-H. (2019). The mortality and the risk of aspiration pneumonia related with dysphagia in stroke patients. *Journal of Stroke & Cerebrovascular Diseases*, *28*(5), 1381-1387. https://doi.org/10.1016/j.jstrokecerebrovasdis.2019.02.011

García-Peris, P., Parón, L., Velasco, C., de la Cuerda, C., Camblor, M., Bretón, I., Herencia, H., Verdaguer, J., Navarro, C., & Clave, P. (2007). Long-term prevalence of oropharyngeal dysphagia in head and neck cancer patients: Impact on quality of life. *Clinical Nutrition (Edinburgh, Scotland)*, *26*(6), 710-717. https://doi.org/10.1016/j.clnu .2007.08.006

Garon, B. R., Sierzant, T., & Ormiston, C. (2009). Silent aspiration: Results of 2,000 video fluoroscopic evaluations. *The Journal of Neuroscience Nursing: Journal of the American Association of Neuroscience Nurses*, *41*(4), 178-187.

Gillick, M. R. (2000). Rethinking the role of tube feeding in patients with advanced dementia. *The New England Journal of Medicine*, *342*(3), 206-210. https://doi.org/10.1056/NEJM200001203420312

Hazel, R. (2006). The psychosocial impact on parents of tube feeding their child. *Paediatric Nursing*, *18*(4), 19-22.

Jean, A. (1984). Brainstem organization of the swallowing network. *Brain, Behavior and Evolution*, *25*(2-3), 109-116. https://doi.org/10.1159 /000118856

Jean, A. (2001). Brain stem control of swallowing: Neuronal network and cellular mechanisms. *Physiological Reviews*, *81*(2), 929-969. https:// doi.org/10.1152/physrev.2001.81.2.929

Kaplan, M. (2010). SPIKES: A framework for breaking bad news to patients with cancer. *Clinical Journal of Oncology Nursing*, *14*(4), 514-516.

Kim, J., Lee, Y. W., Kim, H., & Lee, E. (2019). The mediating and moderating effects of meaning in life on the relationship between depression and quality of life in patients with dysphagia. *Journal of Clinical Nursing*, *28*(15/16), 2782-2789. https://doi.org/10.1111/jocn.14907

Koch, K. A. (1992). Patient self-determination act. *The Journal of the Florida Medical Association*, *79*(4), 240-243.

Krekeler, B. N., Broadfoot, C. K., Johnson, S., Connor, N. P., & Rogus-Pulia, N. (2018). Patient adherence to dysphagia recommendations: A systematic review. *Dysphagia*, *33*(2), 173-184. https://doi.org/10.1007 /s00455-017-9852-9

Logemann, J. A. (1998). The evaluation and treatment of swallowing disorders. *Current Opinion in Otolaryngology & Head & Neck Surgery*, *6*(6), 395-400.

Martin, L., Blomberg, J., & Lagergren, P. (2012). Patients' perspectives of living with a percutaneous endoscopic gastrostomy (PEG). *BMC Gastroenterology*, *12*, 126. https://doi.org/10.1186/1471-230X-12-126

McGilton, K. S., Vellani, S., Yeung, L., Chishtie, J., Commisso, E., Ploeg, J., Andrew, M. K., Ayala, A. P., Gray, M., Morgan, D., Chow, A. F., Parrott, E., Stephens, D., Hale, L., Keatings, M., Walker, J., Wodchis, W. P., Dubé, V., McElhaney, J., & Puts, M. (2018). Identifying and understanding the health and social care needs of older adults with multiple chronic conditions and their caregivers: A scoping review. *BMC Geriatrics*, *18*(1), 231. https://doi.org/10.1186/s12877-018-0925-x

Namasivayam, A. M., & Steele, C. M. (2015). Malnutrition and Dysphagia in long-term care: A systematic review. *Journal of Nutrition in Gerontology and Geriatrics*, *34*(1), 1-21. https://doi.org/10.1080/21551 197.2014.1002656

Namasivayam-MacDonald, A. M., Slaughter, S. E., Morrison, J., Steele, C. M., Carrier, N., Lengyel, C., & Keller, H. H. (2018). Inadequate fluid intake in long term care residents: Prevalence and determinants. *Geriatric Nursing*, *39*(3), 330-335. https://doi.org/10.1016/j.gerinurse .2017.11.004

Nugent, B., Lewis, S., & O'Sullivan, J. M. (2010). Enteral feeding methods for nutritional management in patients with head and neck cancers being treated with radiotherapy and/or chemotherapy. *The Cochrane Database of Systematic Reviews*, *3*, CD007904. https://doi.org/10.1002 /14651858.CD007904.pub2

Ojo, O., & Brooke, J. (2016). The Use of Enteral Nutrition in the Management of Stroke. *Nutrients*, *8*(12), 827. https://doi.org/10.3390 /nu8120827

Ojo, O., Keaveney, E., Wang, X.-H., & Feng, P. (2019). The effect of enteral tube feeding on patients' health-related quality of life: A systematic review. *Nutrients*, *11*(5), 1046. https://doi.org/10.3390/nu11051046

O'Reilly, A. C., & Walshe, M. (2015). Perspectives on the role of the speech and language therapist in palliative care: An international survey. *Palliative Medicine*, *29*(8), 756-761. https://doi.org/10.1177 /0269216315575678

Parker, P. A., Baile, W. F., de Moor, C., Lenzi, R., Kudelka, A. P., & Cohen, L. (2001). Breaking bad news about cancer: Patients' preferences for communication. *Journal of Clinical Oncology: Official Journal of the American Society of Clinical Oncology*, *19*(7), 2049-2056. https://doi .org/10.1200/JCO.2001.19.7.2049

Puntil-Sheltman, J. (2013). Clinical decisions regarding patients with Dysphagia and palliative care. *Perspectives on Swallowing and Swallowing Disorders (Dysphagia)*, *22*(3), 118-123. https://doi.org/10 .1044/sasd22.3.118

Shune, S. E., & Namasivayam-MacDonald, A. M. (2020a). Swallowing impairments increase emotional burden in spousal caregivers of older adults. *Journal of Applied Gerontology*, *39*(2), 172-180. https://doi.org /10.1177/0733464818821787

Shune, S. E., & Namasivayam-MacDonald, A. (2020b). Dysphagia-related caregiver burden: Moving beyond the physiological impairment. *Perspectives of the ASHA Special Interest Groups*, *5*(5), 1282-1289. https://doi.org/10.1044/2020_PERSP-20-00067

Stavroulakis, T., & McDermott, C. J. (2016). Enteral feeding in neurological disorders. *Practical Neurology*, *16*(5), 352-361. https://doi.org/10 .1136/practneurol-2016-001408

Takeuchi, K., Aida, J., Ito, K., Furuta, M., Yamashita, Y., & Osaka, K. (2014). Nutritional status and dysphagia risk among community-dwelling frail older adults. *The Journal of Nutrition, Health & Aging*, *18*(4), 352-357. https://doi.org/10.1007/s12603-014-0025-3

Takizawa, C., Gemmell, E., Kenworthy, J., & Speyer, R. (2016). A systematic review of the prevalence of oropharyngeal Dysphagia in stroke, Parkinson's disease, Alzheimer's disease, head injury, and Pneumonia. *Dysphagia*, *31*(3), 434-441. https://doi.org/10.1007/s00455-016-96 95-9

van der Maarel-Wierink, C. D., Vanobbergen, J. N. O., Bronkhorst, E. M., Schols, J. M. G. A., & de Baat, C. (2011). Meta-analysis of dysphagia and aspiration pneumonia in frail elders. *Journal of Dental Research*, *90*(12), 1398-1404. https://doi.org/10.1177/0022034511422909

Vesey, S. (2013). Dysphagia and quality of life. *British Journal of Community Nursing*, *Suppl 5*, S14-S19. https://doi.org/10.12968/bjcn .2013.18.sup5.s14

Whelan, K. (2001). Inadequate fluid intakes in dysphagic acute stroke. *Clinical Nutrition, 20*(5), 423–428. https://doi.org/10.1054/clnu.2001 .0467

World Health Organization (WHO). (2002). *National cancer control programmes: Policies and managerial guidelines* (2nd ed.). WHO.

Counseling Individuals With Laryngectomies

Miriam Carroll-Alfano, PhD, CCC-SLP

Total laryngectomy is the complete surgical removal of the larynx, resulting in loss of voice due to complete and permanent separation of the upper and lower airway (Ceachir et al., 2014). This procedure is primarily performed due to cancer in the larynx or surrounding structures. Other causes can include trauma to the neck or damage due to radiation treatment. According to the American Cancer Society (2021), more than 12,000 cases of laryngeal cancer will be diagnosed annually, with more than 75% of these cases being diagnosed in men. Most people diagnosed with laryngeal cancer are over age 55 years, and Black men are more likely to be diagnosed and die from laryngeal cancer than White men (American Cancer Society, 2021). Alcohol and tobacco use are the greatest risk factors for laryngeal cancers (National Cancer Institute, 2021). Laryngeal cancers account for less than 1% of all cancers, and incidence and mortality rates have been falling due in part to fewer people smoking and newer and advanced treatments when cancer is diagnosed (National Cancer Institute, 2021). While incidence and prevalence are low, these individuals have significant and unique needs that require the knowledge and skills of a speech-language pathologist.

Undergoing a laryngectomy is a life-altering event. Not only has the person been given a serious medical diagnosis that leads to the surgery, but they will experience physical changes to respiration, communication, and swallowing, along with changes to their social, vocational, and physical activities (American Cancer Society, 2021; Brook, 2018; Jenson, 2013). Due to the removal of the laryngeal cartilages and vocal folds, an alternative means of communication is necessary. A patient's wants, needs, and postsurgical anatomy and functioning must be considered. Structural and physiological changes following surgery result in changes to the oral, pharyngeal, and esophageal phases of swallowing.

Because undergoing a laryngectomy is such a profound experience, it is essential that a person undergoing laryngectomy receive education and counseling by a speech-language pathologist both before and after their laryngectomy (i.e., pre- and postsurgical counseling). It can be challenging to prepare someone for such a life-changing event, and some might say you can never be adequately prepared.

Studies have consistently demonstrated that up to half of laryngectomy recipients report not receiving adequate education and counseling both before and after surgery (Carroll-Alfano, 2019; Salva & Kallail, 1989; Zeine & Larson, 1999). Women are significantly less likely to report receiving adequate education and counseling before surgery relative to men (Carroll-Alfano, 2019; Salva & Kallail, 1989) and have been found to experience strong feelings of fear and anxiety after a laryngectomy at twice the rate of men (Salva & Kallail, 1989). Persons with a tracheoesophageal prosthesis (TEP) are more likely to report adequate education and counseling before and after surgery than persons using other alaryngeal speech methods (Carroll-Alfano, 2019). This difference may be a result of the increased interactions that persons with TEP have with speech-language pathologists relative to persons using other communication methods (Culton & Gerwin, 1998). Prior to surgery, doctors were the highest rated source of education and counseling, followed by speech-language pathologists, the internet, and support groups. After surgery, all four groups were rated statistically equal (Carroll-Alfano, 2019).

Presurgical Counseling

Presurgical counseling is vital to prepare persons undergoing laryngectomy for the changes and challenges they will face. Presurgical counseling can be difficult to deliver depending upon the path taken to the laryngectomy. In some cases, the time between learning that surgery is required to having the surgery can be compressed to a period of 1 week or less, due to the location and staging of their cancer or trauma. In other cases, one can live with head and neck cancer for many years, but eventually require the surgery due to stenosis, side effects of radiation, or recurrence of cancer. The availability and quality of presurgical counseling can depend upon the location at which the procedure is being performed. Laryngectomies are typically performed in large urban and suburban medical centers. Consolidation of these low-volume procedures to large medical centers improves outcomes (Gourin et al., 2019). These larger facilities often have established patient care protocols that include presurgical and postsurgical education and counseling.

During presurgical education and counseling, it is essential that at a minimum, the speech-language pathologist makes it clear that the patient will not be able to speak following surgery due to loss of voice, as studies have found that approximately 20% of laryngectomy recipients report not being aware of this critical fact (Salva & Kallail, 1989; Zeine & Larson, 1999). Additionally, the speech-language pathologist will provide information about the available communication options, including TEP, electrolarynx, esophageal speech, writing, picture communication boards, and augmentative devices (text to speech app or designated communication device). Initial communication method following surgery will be different from long-term communication method due to the need for recovery from the surgery and possible radiation treatment (i.e., swelling and tenderness precludes use of an electrolarynx or TEP). The speech-language pathologist should also discuss possible swallowing disorders, and the potential need for an altered diet or alternative, nonoral nutrition. Informing the patient and family about these changes to communication and swallowing can help them better anticipate the adjustments ahead, and provide encouragement going into the surgery knowing that there is a plan in place for recovery of communication and swallowing. Although presurgical consultation with the speech-language pathologist is ideal, there are cases when this does not occur.

Postsurgical Counseling

Postsurgical education and counseling should begin immediately after surgery. The speech-language pathologist will make sure a short-term communication method is in place and work with the patient through the course of their recovery to find a long-term communication method that works for the patient. As the patient recovers from surgery, the speech-language pathologist will trial different communication methods. Although there are many different options for alaryngeal speech, these methods will be different from laryngeal speech. It will take time for a person with a laryngectomy to accept and adapt to their new method of communication. They will experience a range of emotions and challenges learning to communicate with their new voice and may require counseling at various times during this process. The TEP has become the most common method of postlaryngectomy communication and the prosthesis can be placed during the laryngectomy surgery or at a later time; however, everyone is not a candidate for a TEP and this will be determined by the surgeon. One benefit of the rise in popularity of TEP is that this communication method will require the person with a laryngectomy to see a speech-language pathologist regularly for prothesis changes, providing an opportunity for education and counseling over an extended period of time.

Education about postsurgical swallowing will also occur, with treatment of dysphagia initiated when appropriate. The surgeon will place a feeding tube for nutrition, either via temporary placement of a nasogastric tube or long-term surgical placement of a gastrostomy tube (i.e., G-tube). As the patient recovers, oral feeding will be introduced. The speech-language pathologist will work with the person with laryngectomy to provide education, strategies, and treatment as needed for a return to the safest and least restrictive diet.

Persons with laryngectomy have long-term counseling needs and thus postsurgical education and counseling should continue for some time. Many persons with laryngectomies will say that they have never met another person with a laryngectomy. This is unfortunate, since they can be a great resource and support for each other. All persons with laryngectomy should be encouraged to participate in support groups; however, support group participation can vary based on a variety of factors, and speech-language

pathologists should tailor their support group recommendations accordingly. Persons in rural areas are less likely to participate in in-person support groups compared to those from suburban or urban areas, likely due to lack of in-person groups in their area (Carroll-Alfano, 2019). These persons should be provided information about virtual or social media support groups that would be appropriate for them. Men should be especially encouraged to participate in support groups, as they are less likely to participate in support groups of any kind compared to women (Carroll-Alfano, 2019). Finally, persons using esophageal speech or text-to-speech are much less likely to participate in in-person support groups relative to those who use a TEP (Carroll-Alfano, 2019). This may be due to lower intelligibility of these alternative methods relative to TEP (Singer et al., 2013), lack of confidence in using these methods in public, and persons using these methods having less interaction with speech-language pathologists leading to fewer referrals to in-person support groups.

Support groups, whether in-person, virtual, and or social media groups are a great way for persons with laryngectomy to communicate with each other. Support group members can share experiences and questions about daily care, challenges and frustrations, identity and role changes, return to activities of daily living such as work and travel, and many other topics. Support group members have the lived experience of having a laryngectomy, and in conjunction with the professional expertise provided by the speech-language pathologist, make a great team of support for the person with a laryngectomy.

Boxes 8c-1 and 8c-2 provide case illustrations for individuals who had laryngectomees.

References

American Cancer Society (2021a). *Cancer Facts and Figures 2021.* https://www.cancer.org/research/cancer-facts-statistics/all-cancer-facts-figures/cancer-facts-figures-2021.html

American Cancer Society (2021b). *Surgery for laryngeal and hypopharyngeal cancers.* https://www.cancer.org/cancer/laryngeal-and-hypopharyngeal-cancer/treating/surgery.html

Brook, I. (2018). *The laryngectomee guide expanded edition.* Self-published.

Carroll-Alfano, M. (2019). Education, counseling, support groups, and provider knowledge of total laryngectomy: The patient's perspective, *Journal of Communication Disorders, 82,* 105938. https://doi.org/10.1016/j.jcomdis.2019.105938

Ceachir, O., Hainarosie, R., & Zainea, V. (2014). Total laryngectomy—Past, present, future. *Maedica (Buchar), 9*(2), 210-216.

Culton, G. L., & Gerwin, J. M. (1998). Current trends in laryngectomy rehabilitation: A survey of speech-language pathologists. *Otolaryngology-Head and Neck Surgery, 118*(4), 458-463. https://doi.org/10.1177/0194599898118004

Gourin, C., Stewart, C., Frick, K., Fakhry, C., Pitman, K., Eisele, D., & Austin, M. (2019). Association of hospital volume with laryngectomy outcomes in patients with larynx cancer. *JAMA Otolaryngology—Head Neck Surgery, 145*(1), 62-70.

Jenson, K. (2013). *The modern laryngectomee.* Practical SLP Info.

Box 8c-1
Peter

Peter is a 55-year-old man who experienced a hoarse voice for about 6 months. He was referred to an ENT after multiple doses of antibiotics were unsuccessful at treating his symptoms and was diagnosed with laryngeal cancer. He was treated with radiation, and the treatment was initially successful. About 1 year later at a follow-up appointment with his ENT, it was discovered that his cancer had returned. He was told he needed a laryngectomy, and surgery was scheduled for 1 week later. Although he knew that his larynx was going to be removed, he did not fully understand how this would affect his ability to talk. He did not meet with a speech-language pathologist presurgically.

Peter's recovery was complicated due to a fistula between the tracheoesophageal wall. He was nothing by mouth and without a verbal communication method for 3 months while the fistula healed, using writing for communication during this time. He received a referral for outpatient speech therapy.

Peter was not a candidate for a TEP due to his fistula. The speech-language pathologist educated Peter and his wife about his communication options, and worked with them to identify the electrolarynx as his method of alaryngeal speech.

Box 8c-2
Bill

Bill is a 58-year-old man diagnosed with squamous cell carcinoma of the trachea. Due to the tumor's proximity to the larynx, and the fast rate of growth of these tumors, a laryngectomy was recommended and scheduled to be performed in 14 days.

Bill met with the hospital speech-language pathologist, and she referred him to a laryngectomy support group that met in the area. Bill, his wife, and his daughter were able to attend a meeting of the support group before his surgery. They met with the speech-language pathologist who hosted the group and group members with laryngectomy, asked questions of the group members, and were educated about the changes to his communication and swallowing that he would experience following the surgery. Bill was able to see different communication methods in action including TEP, electrolarynx, and esophageal speech, and learned that although having a laryngectomy is life changing, it is not life ending.

Bill underwent his surgery, followed by 30 sessions of radiation treatment. He had a TEP placed during his surgery, and met with the speech-language pathologist to learn how to use it and make adjustments as his body healed. He returned to the support group 2 months later, this time by himself. He continued to learn from the group members and speech-language pathologist. A year later, his speech-language pathologist asked him to become a mentor for other patients who were scheduled for a laryngectomy, and he continues to do this regularly.

National Cancer Institute. (2021). *Cancer stat facts: Laryngeal cancer—cancer stat facts.* https://seer.cancer.gov/statfacts/html/laryn.html

Salva, C., & Kallail, K. (1989). An investigation of the counseling needs of male and female laryngectomees. *Journal of Communication Disorders, 22,* 291-304.

Singer, S., Wollbruck, D., Dietz, A., Schock, J., Pabst, F., Vogel, H.-J., . . . & Meuret, S. (2013). Speech rehabilitation during the first year after total laryngectomy. *Head & Neck, 35*(11), 1583-1590.

Zeine, L., & Larson, M. (1999). Pre- and post-operative counseling for laryngectomees and their spouses: An update. *Journal of Communication Disorders, 32,* 51-71.

Counseling in the Context of AAC Intervention for Adults With Amyotrophic Lateral Sclerosis

Julia M. Fischer, PhD, CCC-SLP

Counseling is an integral part of augmentative and alternative communication (AAC) intervention. AAC is an area of clinical practice that focuses on maximizing the efficiency and effectiveness of communication for individuals who are unable to communicate via traditional means alone (ASHA, n.d., a). AAC intervention is dynamic and ongoing as decisions are made and training is implemented with clients and their communication partners. People who may benefit from AAC intervention are faced with learning new or different ways to communicate while dealing with differing emotions, feelings, and thoughts related to their condition, diagnosis, and prognosis. The use of both informational and personal adjustment counseling (ASHA, n.d., b) is an essential component of effective AAC intervention. Clinicians who use appropriate counseling techniques increase the opportunity for optimal outcomes (Holland, 2007).

Three Phases of AAC for Amyotrophic Lateral Sclerosis

Early Phase

Ball et al. (2007) described a three-phase intervention model for providing AAC services to people with ALS. The timing and type of counseling will vary for each person depending on the degree of dysarthria and how the person is coping with their diagnosis. According to Chiò et al. (2009), the median survival rate is approximately 30 months from the time of onset. However, 10% to 20% of people diagnosed with ALS live 5 years post diagnosis. Factors such as age at time of onset, bulbar versus spinal symptoms at onset, and rate of disease progression were found to contribute to the variable timeline (Chiò et al., 2009). Informational counseling during the early phase is best described as proactive. The clinician will monitor speech changes, provide information about voice and messaging banking, and educate the person with ALS and their communication partners about possible changes to speech performance over time that will impact future needs for communication supports. Some people with ALS are accepting and prepared to learn about various AAC strategies and techniques as communication options in the early phase of intervention. However, there are also people with ALS who are at different stages of acceptance and may

not be ready to hear information about the deterioration of speech and potential communication challenges. In that situation, the clinician will integrate personal adjustment counseling skills, such as active listening and empathy, into the intervention (Beck & Kulzer, 2018). According to Luterman (2020), personal adjustment counseling helps clients deal with the grief of losing the life they thought they may have or had hoped to have. The time that adults with ALS need to accept that their speech will deteriorate to the point they may need AAC varies (Brownlee & Palovcak, 2007). "When diagnosed with ALS, people commonly experience emotional upheaval and grief. They may go through different phases of grief in the process of accepting the diagnosis and relentless disease progression" (Ball et al., 2007, p. 293). The clinician's knowledge and use of good counseling skills, such as listening without judging and viewing each person with compassion (Goldberg, 2007), can help determine what and how much information the person is ready to learn. In this and subsequent phases, acknowledging the emotional and psychosocial aspects of ALS will be an important part of counseling (Yorkston et al., 2013). The clinician must establish a follow-up mechanism to monitor when acceptance occurs and prepare for additional intervention.

Middle Phase

Informational counseling plays a central role during the middle phase of AAC intervention. However, the clinician must be sensitive to all aspects of the person's care as the disease progresses. People with ALS and their families may be making difficult decisions about the use of ventilators and feeding tubes to prolong life at this time. It may be difficult for people to process and make decisions related to communication if they are overwhelmed with medical concerns. Similar to the early phase of intervention, clinicians need to actively listen to the person with ALS and their communication partners to ensure preferences, wishes, and desires are reflected in the recommendations for AAC intervention. During this phase, the focus shifts toward completing a formal AAC assessment with recommendations for communication supports and a training intervention on how to use the supports to augment and/or provide an alternative mode of communication (Ball et al., 2007). Information is shared about the range of AAC supports that are available and those that are a good match based on the assessment results.

Late Phase

The final phase of intervention includes adaptations to AAC strategies, techniques, devices, and supports to address changes in capabilities and communication needs as well as accommodate any changes in the person's living situation (Ball et al., 2007). These adaptations and accommodations ensure each person with ALS has an effective and efficient means of communicating until the end of life (Bardach, 2015). Yorkston et al. (2013) stated that effective communication preserves a sense of control for people with ALS that can facilitate improved management of both personal and medical decisions. Skillful counseling is needed to determine which adaptations and accommodations may be needed to best support the person with ALS and their communication partners. The need for comprehensive counseling as part of AAC intervention is highlighted here. Box 8c-3 provides a case illustration of Rose, a woman who was diagnosed with ALS.

Key Takeaways

- Counseling is an integral component of AAC intervention.
- Both informational and personal adjustment counseling are needed during all phases of intervention.
- Consider each person's stage of grief and level of acceptance of their diagnosis during intervention.

References

American Speech-Language-Hearing Association (n.d., a). *Augmentative and alternative communication* (Practice Portal). www.asha.org/Practice-Portal/Professional-Issues/Augmentative-and-Alternative-Communication/

American Speech-Language-Hearing Association (n.d., b). *Counseling for professional service delivery* (Practice Portal). www.asha.org/Practice-Portal/Professional-Issues/Counseling-For-Professional-Service-Delivery/

Ball, L. J., Beukelman, D. R., & Bardach, L. (2007). Amyotrophic lateral sclerosis. In D. R. Beukelman, K. L. Garrett, & K. M. Yorkston (Eds.), *Augmentative communication strategies for adults with acute or chronic medical conditions* (pp. 287-316). Brookes Publishing.

Bardach, L. G. (2015). Enhancing communication in hospice settings. In S. W. Blackstone, D. R. Beukelman, & K. M. Yorkston (Eds.), *Patient-provider communication: Roles for speech-language pathologists and other health care professionals* (pp. 271-301). Plural Publishing.

Beck, K., & Kulzer, J. (2018). Teaching counseling microskills to audiology students: Recommendations from professional counseling educators. *Seminars in Hearing, 39*(1), 91-106. https://doi.org/10.1055/s-0037-1613709

Beukelman, D. R. & Light, J. C. (2020). *Augmentative and alternative communication: Supporting children and adults with complex communication needs* (5th ed.). Brookes Publishing.

Brownlee, A., & Palovcak, M. (2007). The role of augmentative communication devices in the medical management of ALS. *NeuroRehabilitation, 22*(6), 445-450.

Chiò, A., Logroscino, G., Hardiman, O., Swingler, R., Mitchell, D., Beghi, E., Traynor, B. G., & Eurals Consortium. (2009). Prognostic factors in ALS: A critical review. *Amyotrophic lateral sclerosis: official publication of the World Federation of Neurology Research Group on Motor Neuron Diseases, 10*(5-6), 310-323. https://doi.org/10.3109/17482960802566824

Costello, J. M. (2011, 2016). *Message banking, voice banking, and legacy messages.* Boston Children's Hospital. https://www.childrenshospital.org/centers-and-services/programs/a-_-e/als-augmentative-communication-program/protocol-of-assessment-considerations/voice-preservation/message-banking/examples-of-message-banking

Goldberg, S. (2007). There's an elephant in the room: Issues in death and dying. In A. L. Holland (Ed.), *Counseling in communication disorders: A wellness perspective* (pp. 261-279). Plural Publishing.

Hanson, E., Yorkston, K., & Britton, D. (2011). Dysarthria in amyotrophic lateral sclerosis: A systematic review of characteristics, speech treatment, and augmentative and alternative communication options. *Journal of Medical Speech-Language Pathology, 19*(3), 12-30.

Holland, A. L. (2007). *Counseling in communication disorders: A wellness perspective.* Plural Publishing.

Luterman, D. (2020). On teaching counseling: Getting beyond informational counseling. *American Journal of Speech-Language Pathology, 29*(2), 903-908. https://doi.org/10.1044/2019_AJSLP-19-00013

Nordness, A., Ball, L., Fager, S., Beukelman, D., & Pattee, G. (2010). Late AAC assessment for individuals with amyotrophic lateral sclerosis. *Journal of Medical Speech-Language Pathology, 18*(1), 48-54.

Yorkston, K. M., Miller, R. M., Strand, E. A., & Britton D. (2013). *Management of speech and swallowing disorders in degenerative diseases* (3rd ed.). PRO-ED.

Box 8c-3
Rose

Rose, a 58-year-old woman, was diagnosed with ALS after experiencing increasing difficulty with her speech and swallowing over a period of 6 months. She retired early from her job as an elementary school librarian after she received the formal medical diagnosis. Rose lived at home with her husband of 35 years.

Approximately 12 months after Rose reported noticing her initial symptoms, I received a referral from her neurologist to see Rose for an AAC assessment. Timely referrals for an AAC assessment are crucial so people with ALS can be proficient in the use of AAC strategies before they need to rely on them for everyday communication (Nordness et al., 2010). The first phase of AAC intervention for Rose included an assessment of her speech, discussion of voice and message banking, and a conversation about her understanding of ALS and concerns she had about communication. I began each session by asking, "How can I help you today?" I utilized several counseling skills during that initial meeting. I actively listened to her as we discussed her medical diagnosis, so I could determine her level of understanding of how her speech may change over time as well as her interest in exploring AAC options that are available should she need them in the future. I directly ask each person, "What is your understanding of your diagnosis?" I focused on listening to what she was saying as well as her nonverbal communication. I have found that many people with ALS and their communication partners become emotional during these discussions about the degeneration of function and eventual death. It is important to honor our clients by providing facial tissues and allowing moments of silence or making an empathic statement such as, "I see this is very difficult," during those conversations. Beck and Kulzer (2018) discuss the importance of conveying empathy, that is the clinician communicates their understanding of the person's point of view accurately and with an unconditional positive regard. I paraphrased a summary of what I heard her share in our conversation about her speech changes and potential need for communication support. I then asked for feedback to verify that I captured their statements correctly by stating, "I heard you say . . ." and asking, "Did I understand you correctly?" Informational counseling played a role in the early phase when I explained voice banking and message banking (see Costello 2011, 2016 for more information) and demonstrated several types of AAC supports to Rose and her husband. I scheduled a follow-up appointment with them for 3 months in the future and gave them all my contact information in case they had any questions prior to that meeting.

Rose had moved into the middle phase of intervention at the time of our next meeting. I began the session by asking, "How can I help you today?" and determined her current communication needs by asking, "Are you having any difficulties communicating with particular people, in certain environments, and about certain topics?" For example, Rose stated that people did not understand her on the telephone, so she could no longer call her medical providers to ask questions. I acknowledged this new communication need and assured her we would address it during this session. Rose's speech rate had slowed to 50 words per minute and her speech intelligibility was 60% at the sentence level with unfamiliar communication partners. Hanson et al. (2011) recommended that AAC should be considered when a person's speech rate falls below 50% of their normal rate. Therefore, the goal for that session was to complete a comprehensive AAC assessment and make recommendations (see Beukelman & Light, 2020, for information about the comprehensive AAC assessments for people with ALS). Rose still had use of her fingers, hands, and arms, which allowed her to access the touchscreen on a computer with her right index finger. Counseling during this phase included education about the assessment process, funding options for an AAC device, and intervention options. I have found that some people with ALS and their communication partners are overwhelmed during the AAC assessment process due to the amount of information that is gathered and decisions that must be made. It is important to pay attention to the body language and facial expressions of individuals to ensure they are understanding the information and to answer any questions that arise. The person with ALS and their communication partners are important team members involved in making recommendations. Take care to listen carefully to their preferences and choices and not rush them during the decision-making process. Rose and her husband asked several questions during the assessment and stated their preferences. I completed the funding paperwork and Rose received her speech-generating device (SGD). We scheduled intervention sessions to train Rose how to operate the system and use the

(continued)

Box 8c-3 (continued)

Rose

different features for efficient and effective communication as well as support her adjustment to using an alternative mode of communication.

My next meeting with Rose and her husband was 8 months later. She was anarthric and had lost most of her ability to use her upper limbs, hands, or fingers to access her SGD. I reassessed her options for access and recommended an eye tracking camera. After the camera was purchased and added to her SGD, she attended additional sessions for training. Counseling continued to play an important role in the late phase of intervention as it extended beyond the in-person sessions. It was important that Rose and her husband knew they could contact me with questions or concerns about her SGD and communication needs. I was a resource for them when they had questions and listened when they expressed sadness and frustration as her physical condition continued to decline. Adapting access to Rose's SGD with the eye tracking camera allowed her to effectively communicate for another 4 months before she died.

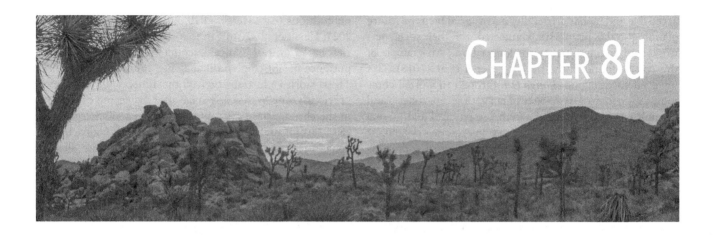

CHAPTER 8d

Special Topics and Disorders
Aphasia and Acquired Cognitive-Communication

Deborah Hersh, PhD, FSPA;
Natalie Douglas, PhD, CCC-SLP; and Jerry K. Hoepner, PhD, CCC-SLP

Counseling in the Context of Aphasia

Deborah Hersh, PhD, FSPA

How best to offer counseling for a person with aphasia after stroke, and for their family members, is a complex area and one that is challenging for speech-language pathologists (Brumfitt, 2009; Northcott et al., 2018; Sekhon et al., 2015; 2019) and for stroke health professionals more generally (Baker et al., 2021). It can be difficult to know how to answer emotional questions from clients like, "Why me? Why is this happening?" (Simmons-Mackie & Damico, 2011) or common questions like, "Will I get better?" (Cheng et al., 2020). Audrey Holland (2007) noted: "In counseling post-stroke clients, the crystal ball is always cloudy" (p. 163) so, even though there is an expectation toward recovery after stroke, clinicians need to know how and when to manage people's fears, uncertainty, and psychological distress. This is particularly so because of the very high rates of depression after stroke (Baker et al., 2018) and the impact of emotional distress and low mood in the longer term on quality of life (Baker et al., 2021; Cruice et al., 2011). Cruice et al. (2011) called for more formal assessment to identify people with aphasia with poor psychological well-being. Hilari et al. (2010) found that people with more severe strokes were likely to experience distress in the early period, but that concerns continued with loneliness and decreasing social networks highlighted at 3 and 6 months poststroke. The need to support psychological well-being extends to family members as well as people with aphasia themselves (Grawburg et al., 2013), but best practice approaches, such as routine screening and treatment of depression, stepped psychological care, and a biopsychosocial approach, are not always employed (Baker et al., 2021).

While recognizing role boundaries (Flasher & Fogle, 2012; Holland, 2007), this context highlights the need for speech-language pathologists to feel able to address emotional well-being when working with clients with aphasia and their families. They need to be able to recognize "counseling moments" (Flasher & Fogle, 2012; Holland & Nelson, 2014) and embed counseling skills into aphasia therapy sessions. Specific counseling skills are discussed throughout this book but in this context require active listening, collaborative problem-solving, patience, optimism, flexibility, the ability to make conversations and counseling techniques

Hoepner, J. K. (Ed.). *Counseling and Motivational Interviewing in Speech-Language Pathology* (pp. 187-204).

accessible and "aphasia-friendly," and a social focus on future planning so that people stay connected with their social networks and communities in the longer term. An example of this can be found in the study by Hersh et al. (2018). This involved encouraging **change talk** through supported communication for a 61-year-old woman with severe aphasia and hemiplegia poststroke, and a complex physical and mental health history. She was being seen by an exercise physiologist who was trying to find ways to manage her patient's resistance to engaging in any programs that would increase her levels of physical activity. The exercise physiologist was unsure how to offer motivational interviewing considering the severity of her patient's language impairment. I introduced the concept of supported communication, which we then used to adapt the strategies of motivational interviewing to be aphasia friendly. We used visual ratings, values card sorting, personalized photos, and visualized goals and timelines. We involved the patient's family, found ways to link going to the gym with the social opportunities that she was more interested in, and celebrated small successes so that she was proud of her achievements. This approach helped her resolve her ambivalence, transitioning from reluctance to regular rehabilitation exercise attendance. As well as showing that even severe aphasia should not be a barrier to **change talk**, this case demonstrated the value of interprofessional collaboration, where the adapted counseling approach not only aided inclusion of a patient who might not otherwise have received this intervention but also increased the confidence of a colleague to be a communication partner for her patient with severe aphasia.

Hallowell (2017) notes that there are key times when psychological distress may be particularly overwhelming:

- At onset of an acquired brain injury
- When people receive assessment and prognostic information
- When they return home after a stay in hospital
- If they perceive their recovery starting to plateau
- At discharge from therapy

Counseling moments may arise often and at any time as people realize what is lost and what the changes might mean for their lives. For people with aphasia, the ability to talk through problems with family, to make plans, and to share thoughts on how to cope are all potentially impeded by the language difficulties, so speech-language pathologists have a special role supporting communication and in conversation partner training (Baker et al., 2021). People may need support to come to terms with physical, social, and financial changes and to manage transitions as services are withdrawn (Hersh, 2009). A person-centered and family-centered approach should underpin practice, along with an awareness of stages of grief, and people's need for information, trusting relationships, support, and hope (Bright et al., 2013).

One of the ways to share ideas or suggestions about clinical practice is through stories (Strong et al., 2018), an approach that I have used in teaching as well as in research

publications (e.g., Hersh, 2010, 2015; Hersh & Armstrong, 2021; Hersh et al., 2018). In this chapter, I will use two stories, based on real clinical encounters, to illustrate the importance of noticing and managing "counseling moments." These stories illustrate two of the timepoints mentioned previously, one in the early stage after stroke and the second in the chronic stage after an unsatisfactory discharge. They raise several useful points when considering counseling in aphasia practice. See Boxes 8d-1 and 8d-2 for case illustrations of individuals with aphasia.

References

Baker, C., Worrall, L., Rose, M., Hudson, K., Ryan, B., & O'Byrne, L. (2018). A systematic review of rehabilitation interventions to prevent and treat depression in post-stroke aphasia. *Disability and Rehabilitation*, 40(16), 1870-1892. https://doi.org/10.1080/09638288.2017.1315181

Baker, C., Worrall, L., Rose, M., & Ryan, B. (2021). Stroke health professionals' management of depression after post-stroke aphasia: A qualitative study. *Disability and Rehabilitation*, 43(2), 217-228. https://doi.org/10.1080/09638288.2019.1621394

Bright, F., Kayes, N. M., McCann, C. M., & McPherson, K. M. (2013). Hope in people with aphasia. *Aphasiology*, 27(1), 41-58. https://doi.org/10.1080/02687038.2012.718069

Brumfitt, S. (2009). *Psychological wellbeing and acquired communication impairment*. Wiley-Blackwell.

Cheng, B., Worrall, L. E., Copland, D. A., & Wallace, S. J. (2020). Prognostication in post-stroke aphasia: How do speech pathologists formulate and deliver information about recovery? *International Journal of Language & Communication Disorders*, 55(4), 520-536. https://doi.org/10.1111/1460-6984.12534

Cruice, M., Worrall, L., & Hickson, L. (2011). Reporting on psychological well-being of older adults with chronic aphasia in the context of unaffected peers. *Disability and Rehabilitation*, 33(3), 219-228. https://doi.org/10.3109/09638288.2010.503835

Flasher, L. V., & Fogle, P. T. (2012). *Counseling skills for speech-language pathologists and audiologists* (2nd ed). Delmar Cengage.

Grawburg, M., Howe, T., Worrall, L., & Scarinci, N. (2013). A qualitative investigation into third-party functioning and third-party disability in aphasia: Positive and negative experiences of family members of people with aphasia. *Aphasiology*, 27(7), 828-848. https://doi.org/10.1080/02687038.2013.768330

Hallowell, B. (2017). *Aphasia and other acquired neurogenic language disorders: A guide for clinical excellence*. Plural Publishing.

Hersh, D. (2009). How do people with aphasia view their discharge from therapy? *Aphasiology*, 23(3), 331-350. https://doi.org/10.1080/02687030701764220

Hersh, D. (2010). Aphasia therapists' stories of ending the therapeutic relationship. *Topics in Stroke Rehabilitation*, 17(1), 30-38.

Hersh, D. (2015). "Hopeless, sorry, hopeless": Co-constructing narratives of care with people who have aphasia post-stroke. *Topics in Language Disorders*, 35(3), 219-236. https://doi.org/10.1097/TLD.0000000000000060

Hersh, D. (2016). Therapy in transit: Managing aphasia in the early period post stroke. *Aphasiology*, 30(5), 509-516. https://doi.org/10.1080/02687038.2015.1137555

Hersh, D. & Armstrong, E. (2021). Information, communication, advocacy, and complaint: How the spouse of a man with aphasia managed his discharge from hospital. *Aphasiology*, 35(8), 1067-1083. https://doi.org/10.1080/02687038.2020.1765304

Box 8d-1

Brian and Edith

I was working in a publicly funded hospital where I was one of a team carrying inpatient and outpatient caseloads. One early afternoon, I received a phone call from Edith. She sounded distraught. Her husband, Brian, had been discharged and sent home 2 days earlier from the hospital following a left hemisphere stroke after only a short admission. The medical team had judged his deficits as mild; another speech-language pathology colleague had assessed him as able to swallow, eat, and drink without modifications. He had good upper and lower limb mobility and his communication abilities had not been viewed as a reason to remain in hospital. Edith had been told Brian would be referred for an outpatient speech-language pathology appointment and be seen in about 2 weeks. Her tone on the phone confirmed she could not wait. I invited them to the hospital to see me immediately, and they arrived by taxi within the hour looking highly anxious. They were both in their mid-70s and retired. They had two adult children and two grandchildren, none living locally. Edith was at a loss as to why Brian could not manage a normal conversation with her, why his speech was full of errors, why he was not himself. Brian looked shell-shocked and upset that Edith was so panicked. It was increasingly clear that neither of them really understood what was going on. They might have been told that the referral to outpatient speech-language pathology was for aphasia, but they did not absorb the word itself or what it meant. Edith confided that she thought Brian's changed communication meant that he was going mad, and she was scared it might get worse.

I explained aphasia and tried to relate it to Brian's language profile, demonstrating through some basic initial assessment that he could understand conversational language well, and at what point he was having difficulty. We talked specifically about his conduction aphasia, using analogies to explain his phonemic paraphasias and conduit d'approche behaviors, particularly evident on confrontation naming, sentence-level repetition, and reading aloud. *Conduit d'approche* is a term used to describe patients with conduction aphasia who are trying to reach the correct sounds for a target word. They make multiple phonemic errors but gradually improve as their errors approximate the target word. We discussed the fact that this was not a disorder of personality, intelligence, or judgment. The couple looked relieved. Edith then explained that, as a younger woman, she had cared for her father who had an early dementia, and she was fearful that Brian's odd communication was an indicator of a similar trajectory. She cried and said she felt guilty about getting it all wrong and thinking that her husband might be dementing. Brian was surprised by this story, as Edith had not shared her fears with him. With the information they now had, the couple were able to look at their situation more clearly. We talked a little more, including about their children and grandchildren, and they seemed to relax. We put tentative plans in place for further speech-language pathology sessions including some at home. We talked about Brian's strengths and abilities, the likelihood of further improvement, what he might like to work on in therapy, and made plans for the couple to link with a local community aphasia group when they felt ready to go.

This situation of high stress for the couple sits in the context of the sudden and dramatic change experienced after stroke, even one without major physical deficits, like hemiparesis. Perhaps the first key point from this case is that counseling needs to be timely. Edith needed someone to talk to immediately, and Brian's ability to focus on his adjustment to being at home was being derailed by his concerns for his wife. Waiting could have perpetuated their anxiety and have negatively impacted their relationship. Second, the couple needed accessible and tailored information about stroke and aphasia, about what supports were available, and what aphasia might mean for them (Rose et al., 2019). Stroke ward environments are very busy (Hersh, 2016), and the couple did not seem to have had the time to talk about the stroke sufficiently to prepare mentally or emotionally for going home. Third, this case illustrated the importance of not making assumptions about the implications of changed communication for patients and families (Hersh & Armstrong, 2021). Even when a diagnosis is explained and apparently understood, the repercussions of that information for particular individuals may be more complex than initially realized. The fact that Brian was physically able to return home quickly, and was deemed mildly impaired, did not necessarily mean that Edith was prepared for the communication changes he was experiencing. His expressive language errors not only caused Brian frustration but triggered a range of emotions in Edith that neither were expecting. The session the couple attended that afternoon combined counseling, information, and support that together allowed Edith to reflect on her own fears, gave a chance for Brian to share that understanding, and defused their anxiety sufficiently for them to start planning ahead.

Box 8d-2

Ken

Ken was a single man who lived alone in a small apartment. He had recently had his 50th birthday. Three years earlier, he had had a stroke that left him initially with a nonfluent aphasia and a dense right-sided hemiplegia. He used a wheelchair when he was out but managed with a tripod walking stick at home. Prior to his stroke, Ken had been a heavy smoker and drinker and had worked as a laborer. He now received a disability pension. I was asked to see Ken for a short burst of aphasia therapy after he contacted his local doctor requesting a referral to speech-language pathology.

Ken's first session was spent in discussion. He had clearly made significant improvement since his early phase of rehabilitation, and his aphasia was now mainly characterized by residual word-finding difficulties and slowness when reading and typing on his home computer. He found the word-finding problems embarrassing. We talked about what had prompted Ken to request more therapy; it was, he said, because he had just turned 50 and wanted to work out where he was going in life. He needed to talk through things that continued to make him angry. In particular, he recalled a conversation with a speech-language pathologist whom he had seen over a 3-month period after leaving rehabilitation soon after his stroke. Ken's memory was that they had worked together each session on pictures and talking about pictures. She then told him, "This is as good as it gets," and he was discharged.

I asked Ken if he thought he had improved since that time, and he laughed and said his improvement showed how wrong she was. But he reported that her comment had made him feel very depressed and that after discharge from therapy, he hardly left his apartment for over a year, watched TV, and cut himself off from previous contacts. He was angry that this happened to him when he was young, that he was left with little money, was physically and socially restricted, and couldn't drive or travel easily. It took him a long time to ask his doctor for a referral, but now he said he wanted to turn things around, particularly as he had received a few comments from neighbors that he was talking better.

I asked him what he might like to change, what was important to change, and how confident he felt to make those changes. We jotted these down on a piece of paper and visualized informal rating scales to get a sense of where he felt he was along the rating regarding his goals. He said he didn't want to feel angry all the time, was bored, and wanted to catch up with his old friends more. I asked him what might help him make that happen, and we brainstormed key ideas: getting out of the wheelchair outside without fear that he would fall, feeling confident with public transport, being able to manage people who were not patient or who irritated him. We developed an initial plan together: a block of aphasia therapy to help him re-establish contact with old friends (focus on text messages, confidence on the phone, strategies to manage word-finding difficulties); a referral to physiotherapy for a program to increase use of the walking stick outside; an offer to go with him to a local community aphasia group, as he did not want to go alone; and a session with the community occupational therapist to explain about the Men's Shed program (https://mensshedswa.org.au/) and other options for increasing participation.

Ken continued therapy with me for 6 more weeks. He saw the community physiotherapist and focused on his ability to walk outside and manage steps and uneven surfaces. I introduced him to the local community aphasia group. Three months later, I heard he was volunteering with the aphasia group as someone to talk to group members who had a more severe aphasia than he did.

This case was interesting because Ken had actually achieved much of his adjustment prior to seeing me. He had initiated the visit to his local doctor and requested referral. He recognized his own feelings of anger and his desire to turn things around. The session that I ran included use of a motivational interviewing technique where the ideas of what needed to change came from him. Our session gave him an opportunity to talk without being judged, a time to reflect, and a structure for further work. Our focus on aphasia was only a part of what he wanted to change. He also sought confidence to access his community physically, to get back to meeting people, and to reconnect with friends. In addition, by volunteering and helping others, Ken was able to gain a sense of satisfaction that he was contributing and was able to start building a positive sense of self and of life's potential. Ken's story highlights the issues that can arise in the chronic phase. It shows how speech-language pathologists can quietly integrate counseling into therapy,

(continued)

Box 8d-2 (continued)

Ken

consider referral to other members of the multidisciplinary team, and work in a way that builds people's autonomy and ability to problem-solve. It is also a reminder that community aphasia groups and aphasia organizations offer crucial, ongoing support for people in the longer term, and that our counseling is more effective when accompanied by practical options to help people manage life with chronic aphasia.

Hersh, D., Newitt, R., & Barnett, F. (2018). Change talk when talk has changed: Theoretical and practical insights into motivational interviewing in aphasia. *Aphasiology, 32*(Suppl. 1), 85-87. https://doi.org/10.1080/02687038.2018.1487003

Hilari, K., Northcott, S., Roy, P., Marshall, J., Wiggins, R. D., Chataway, J., & Ames, D. (2010). Psychological distress after stroke and aphasia: the first six months. *Clinical Rehabilitation, 24*(2), 181-190. https://doi.org/10.1177/0269215509346090

Holland, A. L. (2007). *Counseling in communication disorders: A wellness perspective*. Plural Publishing.

Holland, A. L., & Nelson, R. L. (2014). *Counseling in communication disorders: A wellness perspective* (2nd ed.). Plural Publishing.

Northcott, S., Simpson, A., Moss, B., Ahmed, N., & Hilari, K. (2018). Supporting people with aphasia to 'settle into a new way to be': Speech and language therapists' views on providing psychosocial support. *International Journal of Language & Communication Disorders, 53*(1), 16-29. https://doi.org/10.1111/1460-6984.12323

Rose, T., Wallace, S., & Leow, S. (2019). Family members' experiences and preferences for receiving aphasia information during early phases in the continuum of care. *International Journal of Speech-Language Pathology, 21*(5), 470-482. https://doi.org/10.1080/17549507.2019.1651396

Sekhon, J. K., Douglas, J., & Rose, M. L. (2015). Current Australian speech-language pathology practice in addressing psychological well-being in people with aphasia after stroke. *International Journal of Speech-Language Pathology, 17*(3), 252-262. https://doi.org/10.3109/17549507.2015.1024170

Sekhon, J. K., Oates, J., Kneebone, I., & Rose, M. (2019). Counselling training for speech-language therapists working with people affected by post-stroke aphasia: a systematic review. *International Journal of Language & Communication Disorders, 54*(3), 321-346. https://doi.org/10.1111/1460-6984.12455

Strong, K. A., Lagerwey, M. D., & Shadden, B. B. (2018). More than a story: My life came back to life. *American Journal of Speech-Language Pathology, 27*(1S), 464-476. https://doi.org/10.1044/2017_AJSLP-16-0167

Counseling Individuals With Dementia and Their Families

Natalie Douglas, PhD, CCC-SLP

The diagnosis of dementia is quite overwhelming to individuals and their loved ones (Kovaleva et al., 2021). There are many etiologies of dementia such as Alzheimer's disease, Parkinson's disease, dementia with Lewy bodies, frontotemporal lobar degeneration, Huntington's disease, and vascular disease (Bayles et al., 2020), and this information can be taxing and confusing to receive (Teel & Carson, 2003). The events leading up to the diagnosis of dementia are often frightening, and the progressive loss of memory, communication, executive functions, and independence in activities of daily living leave individuals and families feeling frustrated and worried about the future (Teel & Carson, 2003).

For individuals who are in earlier stages of the disease process or perhaps diagnosed with mild cognitive impairment, fear of the future and how to prevent further deterioration are often paramount concerns (Kessler et al., 2012). Individuals and families may lack knowledge of dementia and its progression, or they may even have misinformation about the topic from well-intended family and friends. As the dementia syndrome progresses, individuals with dementia and their families grapple with options for the optimal living situation. People living with dementia may live at home and with personal companion visitors, home health aides, and/or participation in specialized day programs (Brush & Mills, 2014). Over time, the person living with dementia may transition to independent senior living, assisted living, memory care, nursing homes, and eventually palliative or hospice care (Alzheimer's Association, n.d.). They may also need rehabilitation services for other medical conditions that arise while living with dementia. The transition to another living space for a person living with dementia is quite challenging and should be handled with care.

Legal and financial concerns arise for individuals and families living with dementia as well. Upon diagnosis of dementia, it is important for families to ensure that advanced directives are up to date and that items such as estate planning, emergency preparedness, and long-term care insurance are considered (National Institutes of Health, n.d.). Many families are often unprepared for the onslaught of these issues, and direction to resources is needed.

Speech-language pathologists working with individuals with dementia and their families commonly encounter these significant challenges requiring counseling. As the other special topics in this chapter, dementia requires person-centered, culturally responsive care that supports the individual living with dementia and their family as much as possible (Hickey & Douglas, 2021; Hyter & Salas-Provance, 2019). Speech-language pathologists may also support communication at the end of life or provide education about nonoral feeding options to inform family decision making

(Chang & Bourgeois, 2020). Indeed, decisions about oral intake, autonomy, safety, and quality of life take center stage and may cause significant burden on individuals and families that speech-language pathologists may ease.

Person-centered care means that we are centering the person with dementia above the progression of the dementia syndrome, focusing on the abilities of the person living with dementia, and designing strengths-based programming (Chenoweth et al., 2019; Fazio et al., 2018; Kim & Park, 2017). The diagnosis of dementia may exacerbate a current mental health diagnosis both in the person living with dementia and their care partner (Etters et al., 2008). For example, if a person has a diagnosis of anxiety or depression at baseline, this could worsen due to stressors that accompany dementia.

Strengths-based programming for individuals living with dementia may involve the implementation of external memory aids (Bourgeois et al., 2001), spaced retrieval training (Benigas et al., 2016), augmentative or alternative communication (Bourgeois et al., 2001), and the leveraging of technology such as tablets or home control devices (Lorenz et al., 2019) to facilitate conversation with loved ones and to participate as much as possible in desired activities. Other individuals and families living with dementia may also have dysphagia (Espinosa-Val et al., 2020) and require either direct therapeutic exercises such as expiratory muscle strength training or other dietary modifications or compensatory strategies (Rogus-Pulia & Plowman, 2020). Discussions around oral and mouth care also often ensue (Lauritano et al., 2019).

Most families living with individuals with dementia require care partner training to support meaningful interaction and engagement (O'Rourke et al., 2018). Care partner training may include modifying language, environmental modifications to support communication, and enhancing sensory input such as vision and hearing (Bourgeois, 2014). Care partners of people living with dementia, both family and in health care settings, are at risk for caregiver burden (Brush & Mills, 2014). They may experience a wide range of feelings including guilt, anger, grief, along with the exacerbation of whatever relationship dynamics were present prior to the diagnosis of dementia. It is important to encourage self-care, overcoming guilt, making time for oneself and resources about where to look for help such as respite or support programs.

All individuals and families living with dementia benefit from interprofessional practice as speech-language pathologists are charged with educating both family and other caregivers in optimizing both swallowing and cognitive-communication skills. An orientation toward counseling can ground our services to better serve individuals with dementia and their families (Holland & Nelson, 2020). In the following cases, I will highlight some personal experiences in counseling individuals with dementia and their families while bringing attention to some key concepts. Box 8d-3 provides a case illustration for Mrs. Smith and Box 8d-4 provides a case illustration for Mr. Jones. Both cases are followed by descriptions of how each case was approached.

Box 8d-3
Mrs. Smith

Mrs. Smith returned to your skilled nursing facility after completing a videofluoroscopy swallow study at the hospital. The speech-language pathologist completing the study recommended strict nothing by mouth due to aspiration of multiple consistencies. Prior to the study, Mrs. Smith was on a pureed diet with thin liquids. Her oral intake has decreased in the past several weeks. Mrs. Smith's daughter is coming for a care planning meeting today, and she wants support in deciding what to do next.

Box 8d-4
Mr. Jones

Mr. Jones worked as a groundskeeper in a local park, and he has been struggling with the transition to an assisted living environment with memory care. In addition to a diagnosis of dementia of the Alzheimer's type, Mr. Jones also experienced a stroke a few weeks back that caused weakness on his right side requiring the use of a walker for stability. Mr. Jones has been receiving speech therapy for cognitive-communication needs. He found a meaningful role of sweeping the fenced-in patio area; however, nursing reports that there is not enough staff to supervise him outside. Mr. Jones wants to go outside by himself, but he often forgets his walker, and it was deemed unsafe to go outside without it. Nursing has reported that he has been found wandering the halls, refusing other therapies, and experiencing general restlessness and malaise. The care team is looking for input.

Decisions About Nonoral Feeding

Approach to the Case

Before the care plan meeting, it was important to gather technical information from the interprofessional team (Holland & Nelson, 2020). This included information about Mrs. Smith's overall medical prognosis and medical status. Also, a summary of the evidence concerning feeding tubes in people with dementia was needed. As Mrs. Smith is living with moderate dementia, it was critical to have a summary of evidence for Mrs. Smith's daughter in a way that is accessible, as well as communication and conversational supports for

Mrs. Smith to participate in the conversation. This might include writing key words and/or picture supports (Bourgeois, 2014).

I also had to prepare myself personally for this meeting. In this case, I reflected on my own biases about this topic (Boysen & Vogel, 2008). Explicitly becoming aware of my own biases helped me to arrive at a place of nonjudgment for when the meeting began (Holland & Nelson, 2020). My goal was to approach the conference from a place of meeting both Mrs. Smith and her daughter where they were, without anticipating their responses, to set up the conversation for mutual respect.

Several opportunities for counseling arose during the care plan meeting. Mrs. Smith's daughter appeared sad, tearful, frustrated, and confused. I realized that although I had gathered technical information, the most important aspect right then was holding space and active listening (Holland & Nelson, 2020). Ensuring that I took an intentional pause prior to offering any technical information was key. It allowed me to validate Mrs. Smith's daughter's emotions without judgment. I used phrases such as, "I can see how you would feel this way," "You seem to love your mother so very much," and "We are here for you" to facilitate this process.

After moments of silence, I used a strategy to transition into technical information by asking, "Would you like to hear information about feeding tubes in people with dementia?" or "Is it an OK time to move forward with some information about how your mom is doing medically?" Once Mrs. Smith's daughter agreed to hear the further information, the physician on the team offered information about Mrs. Smith's overall medical diagnosis, noting that Mrs. Smith appears to be approaching the active dying process and that palliative care services may be of benefit (Riedl et al., 2020).

Upon hearing this, Mrs. Smith's daughter became quite tearful and requested to leave the room. It became evident that perhaps Mrs. Smith's daughter was not aware of palliative care services as she noted, "I see you're giving up on her." I took this opportunity to gather resources I had made about the differences between palliative and curative care. I ensured that communication supports were also available for Mrs. Smith (Bourgeois, 2014).

Mrs. Smith's daughter eventually came back to the room and apologized. I continued to encourage holding space, validation of feelings, and allowing room for the grief that Mrs. Smith's daughter was experiencing (Luterman, 2017). I did my best to remain fully present even though part of me was concerned that now I had two items of technical information to provide (palliative care and feeding tubes), and the clock was ticking. Mrs. Smith's daughter appeared ready to receive information about palliative care. I provided the information slowly, pausing to allow for questions, and I was grateful to note some relief that was appearing to wash over Mrs. Smith's daughter.

Next, I provided an external memory aid/communication support to Mrs. Smith (Chang & Bourgeois, 2019). A black-and-white line drawing of a feeding tube was presented along with a template stating "yes," "no," or "maybe." Immediately upon seeing the feeding tube line drawing, Mrs. Smith cried and pushed the drawing away from her. Mrs. Smith then looked to her daughter who was still quite teary, so I continued to allow room for silence and grieving.

After this emotional meeting, I took a moment to engage in an intentional mindfulness activity on my drive home from work. Instead of listening to a podcast, I took some time for silence to reflect upon today's events, cultivating gratitude for the role that I played in this family's life.

Decisions About Autonomy and Safety

Approach to the Case

Prior to meeting with Mr. Jones, I gathered information as to what these behaviors could mean (Holland & Nelson, 2020). I called Mr. Jones's family and reviewed his medical records again. I found that Mr. Jones was extremely hesitant to move into assisted living, according to his son. Mr. Jones's son reported that moving to assisted living was abrupt as Mr. Jones's spouse suddenly passed away. I also discovered that Mr. Jones was only recently diagnosed with dementia due to Alzheimer's disease. It seems that Mr. Jones had significant cognitive-communication deficits that his wife often compensated for prior to her passing.

With this brief but critical preparation time, I began to recognize that this situation about the walker and the freedom to be outside was the tip of the iceberg. I started to consider the various levels of loss that Mr. Jones could be experiencing at this time—the loss of his wife, the loss of his home, the loss of his identity, the loss of his independence (Luterman, 2017). I also started to consider the timing of Mr. Jones's diagnosis of Alzheimer's disease and wondered about his level of knowledge about the disease itself. I collected accessible information about Alzheimer's disease and dementia, connected with the facility social worker about potential grief resources, and gathered detailed information about staffing patterns with an eye on Mr. Jones's desire to spend more time outside.

After checking with other staff to assess which time of day might be best for Mr. Jones to talk, I met Mr. Jones outside in the courtyard. I explained that today's session would be a bit different as I learned new information and wanted to support him being outside more frequently. I started with an open-ended question, "Mr. Jones, tell me about moving here to Pine Grove." Mr. Jones went on to state that none of his children care about him and threw him into this place after he lost his Patty [spouse]. Instead of saying anything else, I was fully present, I paused, my body was facing Mr. Jones, and with silence, I created a place of safety. After a period of silence, I validated Mr. Jones's feelings by stating, "That must have been so very difficult." Mr. Jones started to cry, and stated, "I don't even know what's wrong with me. Just a few months ago, Patty was bringing me my pills, we were going out to eat, and everything was fine."

After continued silence and validating of Mr. Jones's feelings, I stated, "It sounds like you have a had a lot of loss in the past months—your wife, your independence, the home that you knew." Mr. Jones went on to say that everyone was so worried about his stroke that no one seemed to care that he lost his wife and has been kicked out of his home. "Who cares about my walker?" he said. "What's the point?"

After the session, I started to feel full of guilt and shame because I conducted several sessions without the knowledge of Mr. Jones's recent losses. I was focused on his recent stroke, memory strategies, and functional communication, but I missed important opportunities to provide holistic care (Cohen-Mansfield, 2021). After work, I took some time to attempt to cultivate self-compassion, acknowledging my mistakes, telling myself that mistakes are part of what it means to be human, and allowing myself to be mindful of this situation as an opportunity for future growth (Bluth & Neff, 2018).

This counseling opportunity shifted my approach in cognitive-communication treatment as well. For instance, I provided extensive education about Alzheimer's disease. With visual supports, I explained the typical progression of the disease along with several examples of people living successfully with dementia. I connected Mr. Jones to the social worker who was facilitating a support group for people who have lost their spouses, and I worked to facilitate Mr. Jones's independence throughout the assisted living community. I provided strategies to the social worker for Mr. Jones to optimally engage including external memory aids and communication supports, removing distractions, speaking in shorter sentences, slowing rate of speech, and ensuring Mr. Jones's attention prior to speaking (O'Rourke et al., 2018). Finally, I solicited facility volunteers to support Mr. Jones's sweeping outside more frequently. Mr. Jones's participation steadily improved as he was allowed room for grief and the explicit acknowledgment of his many losses.

Key Takeaways

- The diagnosis of dementia is overwhelming for individuals and their families due to multiple etiologies of the disease, the frightening nature of symptoms, and the significant impact it has on almost all areas of life.
- Individuals living with dementia and their families are often not prepared for the many financial and legal matters that may arise with a diagnosis of dementia.
- Speech-language pathologists can support individuals and families living with dementia through supporting decisions about quality of life and autonomy while providing optimal cognitive-communication and swallowing interventions.
- Care partners of individuals living with dementia often require communication partner training in addition to resources for coping and self-care.

- An orientation toward person-centered, culturally responsive, and interprofessional practice will facilitate working with individuals with dementia and their families through strengths-based programming.

References

Alzheimer's Association (n.d.). Long-term care. https://www.alz.org/help-support/caregiving/care-options/long-term-care

Bayles, K., McCullough, K., Tomoeda, C. (2020). *Cognitive-communication disorders of MCI and dementia: Definition, assessment, and clinical management* (3rd ed.). Plural Publishing.

Benigas, J. E., Brush, J. A., & Elliot, G. M. (2016). *Spaced retrieval step by step*. Health Professions Press.

Bluth, K., & Neff, K. D. (2018). New frontiers in understanding the benefits of self-compassion. *Self and Identity, 17*(6), 605-608. https://doi.org/10.1080/15298868.2018.1508494

Bourgeois, M. (2014). *Memory and communication aids for people with dementia*. Health Professions Press.

Bourgeois, M., Dijkstra, K., Burgio, L., & Allen-Burge, R. (2001). Memory aids as an augmentative and alternative communication strategy for nursing home residents with dementia. *Augmentative and Alternative Communication, 17*(3), 196-210. https://doi.org/10.1080/aac.17.3.196.210

Boysen, G. A., & Vogel, D. L. (2008). The relationship between level of training, implicit bias, and multicultural competency among counselor trainees. *Training and Education in Professional Psychology, 2*(2), 103-110. https://psycnet.apa.org/doi/10.1037/1931-3918.2.2.103

Brush, J., & Mills, K. (2014). *I care: A handbook for care partners of people with dementia*. Balboa Press.

Chang, W. Z. D., & Bourgeois, M. S. (2020). Effects of visual aids for end-of-life care on decisional capacity of people with dementia. *American Journal of Speech-Language Pathology, 29*(1), 185-200. https://doi.org/10.1044/2019_AJSLP-19-0028

Chenoweth, L., Stein-Parbury, J., Lapkin, S., Wang, A., Liu, Z., & Williams, A. (2019). Effects of person-centered care at the organisational-level for people with dementia. A systematic review. *PloS One, 14*(2), e0212686. https://doi.org/10.1371/journal.pone.0212686

Cohen-Mansfield, J. (2021). The rights of persons with dementia and their meanings. *Journal of the American Medical Directors Association, 22*(7), 1381-1385. https://doi.org/10.1016/j.jamda.2021.03.007

Espinosa-Val, C., Martín-Martínez, A., Graupera, M., Arias, O., Elvira, A., Cabré, M., Palomera, E., Bolivar-Prados, M., Clave, P., & Ortega, O. (2020). Prevalence, risk factors, and complications of oropharyngeal dysphagia in older patients with dementia. *Nutrients, 12*(3), 863. https://doi.org/10.3390/nu12030863

Etters, L., Goodall, D., & Harrison, B. E. (2008). Caregiver burden among dementia patient caregivers: A review of the literature. *Journal of the American Academy of Nurse Practitioners, 20*(8), 423-428. https://doi.org/10.1111/j.1745-7599.2008.00342.x

Fazio, S., Pace, D., Flinner, J., & Kallmyer, B. (2018). The fundamentals of person-centered care for individuals with dementia. *The Gerontologist, 58*(suppl 1), S10-S19. https://doi.org/10.1093/geront/gnx122

Hickey, E., & Douglas, N. F. (2021). *Person-centered memory and communication interventions for dementia*. Plural Publishing.

Holland, A. L., & Nelson, R. L. (2020). *Counseling in communication disorders: A wellness perspective*. Plural Publishing.

Hyter, Y. D., & Salas-Provance, M. B. (2019). *Culturally responsive practices in speech, language, and hearing sciences*. Plural Publishing.

Kessler, E. -M., Bowen, C. E., Baer, M., Froelich, L., Wahl, H. W. (2012). Dementia worry: A psychological examination of an unexplored phenomenon. *European Journal of Ageing, 9*(4), 275-285. https://dx.doi.org/10.1007%2Fs10433-012-0242-8

Kim, S. K., & Park, M. (2017). Effectiveness of person-centered care on people with dementia: A systematic review and meta-analysis. *Clinical Interventions in Aging, 12,* 381. https://dx.doi.org/10.2147%2FCIA.S117637

Kovaleva, M., Spangler, S., Clevenger, C., & Hepburn, K. (2018). Chronic stress, social isolation, and perceived loneliness in dementia caregivers. *Journal of Psychosocial Nursing and Mental Health Services, 56*(10), 36-43. https://doi.org/10.3928/02793695-20180329-04

Lauritano, D., Moreo, G., Della Vella, F., Di Stasio, D., Carinci, F., Lucchese, A., & Petruzzi, M. (2019). Oral health status and need for oral care in an aging population: A systematic review. *International Journal of Environmental Research and Public Health, 16*(22), 4558. https://doi.org/10.3390/ijerph16224558

Lorenz, K., Freddolino, P. P., Comas-Herrera, A., Knapp, M., & Damant, J. (2019). Technology-based tools and services for people with dementia and carers: Mapping technology onto the dementia care pathway. *Dementia, 18*(2), 725-741. https://doi.org/10.1177%2F1471301217691617

Luterman, D. M. (2017). *Counseling persons with communication disorders and their families* (6th ed.). Pro-Ed.

National Institutes of Health. (n.d.). *Legal and financial planning for people with dementia.* National Institute on Aging. https://www.nia.nih.gov/health/legal-and-financial-planning-people-alzheimers

O'Rourke, A., Power, E., O'Halloran, R., & Rietdijk, R. (2018). Common and distinct components of communication partner training programmes in stroke, traumatic brain injury and dementia. *International Journal of Language & Communication Disorders, 53*(6), 1150-1168. https://doi.org/10.1111/1460-6984.12428

Riedl, L., Bertok, M., Hartmann, J., Fischer, J., Rossmeier, C., Dinkel, A., Ortner, M., & Diehl-Schmid, J. (2020). Development and testing of an informative guide about palliative care for family caregivers of people with advanced dementia. *BMC Palliative Care, 19*(1), 1-8. https://doi.org/10.1186/s12904-020-0533-3

Rogus-Pulia, N. M., & Plowman, E. K. (2020). Shifting tides toward a proactive patient-centered approach in dysphagia management of neurodegenerative disease. *American Journal of Speech-Language Pathology, 29*(2S), 1094-1109. https://doi.org/10.1044/2020_AJSLP-19-00136

Teel, C. S., & Carson, P. (2003). Family experiences in the journey through dementia diagnosis and care. *Journal of Family Nursing, 9*(1), 38-58. https://doi.org/10.1177/1074840702239490

Counseling Individuals With Traumatic Brain Injuries and Their Families

Jerry K. Hoepner, PhD, CCC-SLP

Traumatic brain injuries (TBI) disrupt lives in a way that is hard to fully understand unless you have experienced it. Truly listening to our clients, seeing them as experts, and learning from their lived experience is an important starting point. A challenge for counseling individuals with TBI is the heterogeneity of this population but this is just a good reminder to follow an individualized, person-centered approach.

Common Issues for Adults With Traumatic Brain Injuries

The *first few days* after a brain injury are often a time of total shock and a completely overwhelming state for both individuals with TBI and their partners, across the severity continuum. We must be mindful of their emotional and cognitive state and readiness for the deluge of information shared with them at this point. Individuals with TBI and their partners highly value compassion, a sense that they're being listened to and collaborating in care, and a balance of reality and hope.

Visitors and Bouncers

Following a serious injury like TBI, individuals with TBI and their families are often inundated with well-intended visitors. Too many visitors, left unregulated, talking over and around the individual with TBI, can cause overstimulation and potentially agitation for the individual with TBI. Families are often uncomfortable or too overwhelmed to even begin to regulate this. Also, they may not recognize the implications of overstimulation on their loved one's recovery. Our role is to explain to the family (outside of these moments) the potential for overstimulation and the need to broker how many people visit at one time and support the way they interact. Volunteer to take on the role of bouncer and educate visitors briefly with compassion.

Acute Confusional States

For individuals with moderate to severe brain injuries, they may encounter a period of recovery that includes an acute confusional state. During this time, they are disoriented to person, place, time, and situation. This disoriented state, often coupled by prefrontal damage that further reduces inhibition, can result in many inappropriate behaviors that are uncharacteristic for the individual. For family and visitors, this is a painful shock that they are likely not prepared to deal with without some advance warning and education. Two things to consider: (1) the family needs to know that this is a typical part of recovery and in most cases it means that the person is getting better; and (2) they need to know that nothing the individual with TBI does or says is directed at them personally. Box 8d-5 provides an illustration of acute confusional states.

Mild Traumatic Brain Injuries and Concussion

Ever heard of a catch-22? We're told that people with mild TBI/concussion are more likely to have persistent symptoms if we talk too much about symptoms or feed into their reports of symptoms. We're told that it's better to tell them that there are symptoms early on but they pass quickly. That's

Box 8d-5

Acute Confusional State

Dawson was a 43-year-old man who sustained a moderate to severe TBI in a snowmobile accident. He was intoxicated at the time and was flighted to a regional trauma center. Upon admission, he was comatose for 1 day. Within a day of regaining consciousness, he was alert, disoriented, and agitated. He was married, although they had been separated and contemplating divorce prior to the accident due to his ongoing problems with alcohol use. He has an adult son, who lives 3 hours away, and another 15-year-old son in high school. As a result of his confused, agitated state, he spoke in a string of profanities and often removed his hospital gown and pants because the feeling of cloth on his skin further irritated him. That combination made visits, particularly for his 15-year-old son, very difficult to predict and manage. Part of the speech-language pathologist's role was to explain his recovery and current behaviors to Dawson's wife and sons. Visits remained important, so timing best opportunities for a good visit had to be strategic. Scaffolding to reduce the likelihood of inappropriate words or behaviors was implemented, along with a plan to just leave the interaction if signs of agitation began to arise. (Dawson's wife and sons were educated regarding those signs and a staff member was present to safeguard and look for signs as well.) Dawson's wife was very supportive and conveyed her intentions to help him out, until he reached a point where he could either care for himself or be placed in a setting where care would be provided.

A few weeks later, Dawson was released to home, under his wife's care and with her full support. He received outpatient day programming (5 days a week, 3 hours per day across occupational therapy, physical therapy, and speech-language pathology therapy) until he reached a point where sessions dwindled down to one or two speech-language pathology therapy sessions per week. Once able to care for himself safely, he began a transition back to his factory assembly line position, and his wife began to finalize their divorce. She remained an important support and checked in on Dawson regularly, even after their separation and eventual divorce.

---

all fine and dandy for those individuals who have symptoms that pass, but it is insulting and disenfranchising for those who have persistent issues. And we know that some people do have persistent issues and that there is evidence for underlying organic pathology (not always recognized in early neuroimaging scans). Even *if* the persistent symptoms some report were not "organic" or imageable with our current technologies, we cannot simply dismiss them, as the impact can be devastating for these individuals. We must find a middle ground and treat these individuals with compassion.

Learning Readiness

Learning readiness is a big factor in provision and acceptance of services for persons with TBI. Impaired self-awareness is ubiquitous to TBI, and this alters their ability to recognize the need for supports, particularly chronic, community-based supports. Community-based groups and support networks exist that provide crucial ongoing supports to individuals with TBI in the chronic phase of recovery but these lifelines are often rejected early on. This is not surprising, as recognition of impairments is impaired, even more so early on. Therefore, it is important to provide information to individuals with TBI and their families early on but also establish pathways for continued connection with those individuals. This may include connecting with their providers to emphasize the chronicity of TBI and provide referrals to support groups and networks, particularly at points when the client and their family may be more receptive to such supports.

Impaired Self-Awareness and Self-Regulation

For individuals with TBI, impairments in self-awareness and self-regulation compromise interpersonal relationships at home, with friends, at school/work, and a host of other social settings. While self-regulation is contingent upon multiple factors—including contextual demands, environment, partner support/demands, and self-awareness—improving self-awareness is often a first step in improving self-regulation. A number of cognitive rehabilitation and counseling approaches have been applied to address this challenging issue. In this case, the cognitive and counseling approaches are typically integrated.

Mark Ylvisaker and Tim Feeney have written extensively about coaching and self-regulation techniques for children, adolescents, and adults with TBI. They suggest the use of multiple approaches used in conjunction with one another. Ylvisaker and Feeney (2009) advocated for an apprenticeship model to scaffold development of self-regulation. This includes think-aloud techniques, delivered by the clinician, to model one's thinking approach to addressing a challenging task. This includes emotional reactions in the moment and how those challenges are overcome. For instance, if I'm working on a homework task, I might say, "Argh, this is really frustrating. The teacher didn't even tell me what I'm supposed to do for this assignment. It makes me mad, because I feel like I have to teach myself. But, maybe she did that on purpose. Maybe that's part of the assignment, to figure it out. Maybe there isn't just one right way to do it. I can get this. I'll show her that I can get this. Okay, so there are a few ways I could do this . . ." In this manner, executive functions are learned vicariously through context-sensitive interventions, fostering self-regulation and self-determination (Ylvisaker & Feeney, 2002, 2009). Paired with the reflective framework of obstacle-goal-plan-do-review, this creates a rich context for planning and self-evaluating performance (Ylvisaker & Feeney, 1998, 2009). Obstacle-goal-plan-do-review helps clients to (1) identify tangible obstacles to effective performance, (2) predict performance, (3) identify goals for successful task completion, (4) design an actionable plan or script for actually carrying out the task, and (5) implement that plan and review the performance. Hmm . . . sounds like a motivational interviewing framework. The great thing about this approach is it is malleable to use with physical tasks (e.g., cooking a meal, cleaning the house) and social interactions within context. Clients are encouraged to identify metaphors that are meaningful and "package several pieces of information into one thought unit" (Ylvisaker & Feeney, 2000, p. 414), thus guiding thinking. Leanne Togher and colleagues are developing an online training program based on these tenets (presented at the 2021 Cognitive Communication Symposium in Manchester, UK). Simple but eloquent examples of metaphors for conversation include, "When speaking, your role is to 'pass the ball,'" "When listening, your role is to 'catch the ball.'" Likewise, clients are encouraged to identify meaningful life narratives, particularly those where the client has overcome a challenge. Emulation is another metaphoric tool, as clients are encouraged to identify someone to emulate as they approach certain tasks. For instance, if a client wants to be better at conversation, they may emulate a friend or family member or even an actor to serve as their model. All of these techniques are pulled together in Ylvisaker's (2006) self-coaching model. This approach draws upon environmental cues to trigger self-regulatory thoughts and behaviors. Scripts are developed to address communication and other behaviors in contexts known to be challenging. While the focus is on self-determination, providing contextualized models of behavior can help provide a roadmap to successful interactions.

Video self-modeling (VSM) can be used to address self-awareness and self-regulation in the context of dyadic conversations between individuals with TBI and their communication partners (Douglas et al., 2014, 2019; Hoepner et al., 2021; Hoepner & Olson, 2018). Joint VSM draws heavily upon the self-coaching approach (Ylvisaker, 2006) and principles of joint communication partner training (Togher et al., 2013). Self-coaching encourages identification of one's own successes and challenges as a way to move toward more effective communication behaviors. Video is often used

to provide a tangible and reviewable context for identifying these successes and challenges, reducing demands on memory and scaffolding self-assessment. Joint communication partner training is more effective than solo training in producing meaningful conversational change in TBI (Togher et al., 2013). Motivational interviewing OARS microskills (i.e., open-ended questions, affirmations, reflections, and summarization) are used to structure all interactions. Open-ended questions are used to elicit self-assessments, accurate self-assessments are affirmed, and reflections/summaries are used in metacognitive debriefing about interactions. Joint VSM begins by identifying social communication challenges through direct video review of a conversation between the individual with TBI and their partner, using the La Trobe Communication Questionnaire (Douglas et al., 2000). A *self-* and *other*-form of the La Trobe Communication Questionnaire allow each individual to rate frequency of challenging behaviors within that conversation, increasing accuracy for both the individual with TBI and their partner, while improving consensus on communication challenges (Hoepner & Turkstra, 2013). This supports the dyad in identifying potential communication goals, drawing upon communication challenges such as interrupting, perseveration, or speaking too softly for which they had good consensus (i.e., items that they agreed were a challenge/potential problem for their interactions). Once goals are identified by the dyad, goal attainment scales are collaboratively developed as a mechanism to measure progress toward goals. Weekly homework includes recording conversational interactions at home and throughout the community to serve as a context for supported video review within sessions. Clinicians play back clips of the conversations within sessions, pausing the video at opportune moments (i.e., just after a successful or challenging communication moment occurred in the video), prompting the individual with TBI and their partner to assess their *own* behavior in that clip, avoiding assessment of each other as much as possible. Clinicians typically view the video for the first time, in the moment of reviewing the clip with the dyad—this eliminates the need for time consuming video review outside of the session and allows them to be flexible in the moment regarding their prompting. While clinicians prompt identification of both successes and challenges, the focus is on accurate self-assessment on the part of the individual with TBI and their partner. This process is intended to be errorless, as the clinician can replay the video clip and scaffold identification of behaviors; beginning with open-ended questions or providing goal-related cues (e.g., "You've been working on not raising your voice when you're upset. In this clip, how do you think you did?" Regardless of whether the individual responds, "I raised my voice" or "I kept my cool, didn't raise my voice," our response is positive—"You did raise your voice but it's good you recognized it," or "Yes, you completely kept your cool"). If the individual doesn't respond to goal-related cues, the clinician can replay the clip and simply ask, "Did you raise your voice?" Because a consequence of improved self-awareness is increased self-criticism and rumination (Hoepner & Olson, 2018; Hoepner et al., 2021), controlling the selection of video clips to review is an important element of flexibility on the part of clinicians. For instance, when the individual with a TBI begins to increase self-critical comments (e.g., "I really suck at conversation, I'm a burden to my partner"), the clinician can intentionally shift her prompts to clips that include a successful interaction, skipping over problem spots they noticed but don't want to use to elicit self-identification of a challenge. Outcomes suggest that individuals with TBI improve their ability to accurately self-identify both successes and challenges, increase positive communication behaviors and decrease challenging behaviors, and begin to self-regulate in the moment. Likewise, partners decrease behaviors that serve as a barrier to the individual with a TBI and increase supports (Douglas et al., 2014; Douglas et al., 2019; Hoepner et al., 2021; Hoepner & Olson, 2018).

Return to Work

Returning to work is often a priority and pressing goal for individuals with TBI. Unfortunately, expectations about returning to work do not always align with the reality of their current context. Individuals with TBI may be inclined to return to work before they are ready, ignoring advice of rehabilitation staff. Others may have impairments that preclude them from returning to work, at least in the near term. Speech-language pathologists should also be careful not to write off the possibility and do their best to follow the client's needs, helping them to explore realities instead of telling them what they cannot do. Effective transitions back to work come with a plan. When we oppose or forbid return to work, it can result in pushback in the form of returning on their own. This sets the individual up for failure and is not a fair indication of their potential. Box 8d-6 illustrates the challenges of returning to work following a TBI.

Some things to consider for effective transitions:

- Don't deny the possibility of returning to work.
- Let the client explore their own abilities and self-confront through role plays and hands-on trials (recreating workplace scenarios).
- Plan, plan, plan—collaborate with the client to identify potential barriers and a plan to address them.
- Script and practice key conversations such as phone calls, interviews, "big asks" such as accommodations, and disclosing about the brain injury.
- It helps to have a speech-language pathologist by your side for some disclosure conversations, as it is easier for the speech-language pathologist to say, "She's very capable and intelligent, she just needs breaks and a plan for . . ." than it is for the client to say that about themselves.
- Disclose information about the brain injury and deficits on a need-to-know basis. Telling everyone can sometimes cause problems. Something is wrong, oh—that must have been the person with a TBI who did that.

Box 8d-6
Only on My Terms . . .

Early in my clinical career, I was working with a woman with a moderate TBI who wanted to return to her position as an executive in a branch of an international business. While I did not deny her the possibility of returning to work, I was cautious and suggested a timeline that didn't match hers. She pushed back and returned to work before she was ready. The result was a disaster, as her interpersonal interactions with those she supervised were harsh and inflexible. I'm not sure whether a well-coordinated and collaborative transition plan would have made a difference. Being the top executive at that company may not have been in the cards. Either way, it was not a good indicator of her potential. A couple of years later, she decided she wanted to return to the workforce and apply for a position as a waitress, a position she held often in college. Wiser about transitions at that point (thanks in part to her), I said this seemed like a good next step. In my mind, I was thinking—"Oh, great! Good idea, pick a stressful job at a busy restaurant that requires outstanding executive functions and interpersonal skills. Yep, let's start with that job." So, that's what we did. Responding to her with a positive affirmation actually allowed us to collaborate on steps needed to return to work successfully. We worked through the process of applying—easy for her—check! We role played interviewing—easy for her—check! We scripted and practiced the big ask—"Can I start out with a few hours a week, see how it goes and gradually add hours if it goes well?" The answer was a resounding yes. She was hired, conquered two 4-hour shifts per week, conquered four 4-hour shifts, conquered five 4-hour shifts, and said—that's good, I don't want to work more than that; it is enough but not too much. Within a few weeks, she was their best waitress—meticulous with her service, outstanding with the customers, fully dependent on her notepad but who cares.

Often, clients will come to their own realizations about what is reasonable, if you are patient enough to let them walk through the process, rather than imposing your will and expertise by telling them what is and is not possible.

Communication measures, such as social inference and speed of verbal reasoning skills, are predictive of stable employment within skilled jobs after TBI (Meulenbroek & Turkstra, 2016). Deficits in interpersonal skills are the

Box 8d-7

Return to College

Check out this episode of the Full Prefrontal podcast episode #73 with Dr. Mary Kennedy as she discusses her work on returning to college following brain injuries.

https://rb.gy/v9bn1

primary reason for workplace separation following TBI (Meulenbroek et al., 2016; Meulenbroek & Turkstra, 2016). Politeness markers (e.g., "If it's not too much trouble . . .", "I was wondering . . .", "If you don't mind . . .") are crucial in workplace communication (Meulenbroek & Cherney, 2019). Therefore, a big focus of your return to work should be on social communication skills and self-regulation.

Return to College

A dynamic, individualized coaching approach can be used to address returning to college after a TBI (Hoepner et al., 2019; Kennedy & Krause, 2011; Kennedy et al., 2012; O'Brien et al., 2018). The program begins by identifying academic challenges through the College Survey for Students with Brain Injury (Kennedy & Krause, 2010). A follow-up, semistructured interview is used to elicit students' own solutions to addressing those challenges and supports them in setting their own goals. The approach relies heavily on motivational interviewing as a tool to foster self-assessment, goal identification, and identification of the student's own solutions and strategies. The OARS framework is used to keep the focus on self-regulation, avoiding the pitfall of advice or solution giving. Thus, rather than simply tutoring or re-teaching students, the approach focuses on developing self-regulation and strategic behaviors through this counseling process. Outcomes include increases in metacognitive statements, improved self-regulation, increased use of strategies, and improved grades (Hoepner et al., 2019; Kennedy & Krause, 2011; Kennedy et al., 2012; O'Brien et al., 2018). The approach is highly contextualized, using the students' actual homework, rather than contriving cognitive exercises that are not likely to generalize. For further details on the dynamic coaching program, readers are encouraged to read Mary Kennedy's (2017) textbook *Coaching College Students with Executive Function Problems* (see Box 8d-7 to hear Mary Kennedy discuss the program in the Full Prefrontal podcast).

Sexuality and Intimacy

Sexuality and intimacy are normal human needs that can be affected by TBI. We need to be prepared to have these important conversations. Individuals with TBI may be hypersexual, disinhibited, and/or have problems maintaining arousal. Early on, memory and awareness can be impaired, so intimacy should be discouraged when the person is in a disoriented state or memory problems preclude appropriate decision making (refer back to Box 3-1 for a case example). If the individual acting in a disinhibited manner is confused and disoriented, we need to redirect them to a more positive activity. This is not a counseling moment. On the other hand, if they are gaining awareness and are oriented, we should facilitate self-reflection and self-regulation (e.g., "How do you think that might make the people around you feel?" or "Tell me a bit about that statement."). In either case, it is not appropriate to tell them to stop (aside from an immediate threat of assault), as this is unlikely to change behavior. Prompting a conversation about it, while it may be uncomfortable for us, is usually a better way to handle disinhibited behaviors or comments. Dating is a common goal after brain injury, particularly for young persons. Letting the individual know that we are open to having conversations about dating and related intimacy topics is a good start. Sexuality and intimacy are discussed further in the segment by Emma Power et al., later in this chapter.

Friends Are Often Fickle

Unfortunately, loss of preinjury friends is a common phenomenon after TBI. Changes to the individual's social discourse, self-regulation, social-vocational roles, and several other factors contribute to loss of friendships. Individuals with severe TBI identified an average of 3.35 friends, which drops to 1.52 when paid carers and family are excluded (Douglas, 2020). Post-TBI friendships were broadly characterized as "going downhill," which included four phases: losing contact, being misunderstood, wanting to share, and hanging on (Douglas, 2020). There is evidence that while the number of friends decreases, the quality of friendships for remaining friends is high (Flynn et al., 2018). Salas et al. (2018) examined social isolation and friendships in the chronic phase, identifying four main themes: the impact of long-term cognitive and behavioral problems on relationships, loss of old friends (old referring to friends prior to TBI), difficulties making new friends, and relating to other survivors in order to fight social isolation. Thus, it is important to recognize the importance of family and paid carers as part of the social networks for persons with TBI, nurture the remaining strong relationships, and connect individuals with TBI with peers.

Support Groups

Support groups are an important resource for individuals with TBI in the subacute to chronic phase of recovery. TBI is a lifelong issue for many and the challenges they experience do not go away. If anything, new challenges arise as people enter new phases of life. Do your best to create pathways that connect your current clients to groups now but potentially in the future, when they are more receptive and recognize the need for themselves. Peer support programs have been shown to improve knowledge of TBI, quality of life, and overall outlook, while reducing anxiety and depression (Anson & Ponsford, 2006; Appleton et al., 2011; Bedard et al., 2003; Keegan et al., 2019). Group interventions also improve self-regulation and psychosocial functioning (Harrison-Felix et al., 2018; Ownsworth et al., 2000).

Peer support and mentorship programs, provided to individuals with TBI and their family members, are another useful form of group programming. In this model, peers with TBI mentor newer individuals with TBI and partners mentor new family members. It results in improved ability to cope with anger, anxiety, depression, and sadness, thus improving overall quality of life for individuals with TBI (Hibbard et al., 2002). Family members identified improved communication with professionals as a key outcome. Similarly, Hoepner (2021) trained peers to deliver basic motivational interviewing techniques to peers in a community-based brain injury group in an eight-session program. Over time, some peers recognized the purpose and value of evoking rather than directly prescribing solutions. Those peers became powerful models within role plays and during debriefings. All eight regular attendees reached emerging proficiency in OARS techniques and a mindset shift from egocentric advice givers toward collaborators who inhibit their own experience and solutions in order to evoke a peer's own potential solutions.

Group cognitive behavioral approaches (CBT) also result in positive outcomes. Walker et al. (2010) found that a group CBT approach significantly reduced participants' anger and improved their ability to control feelings of anger. Similarly, Backhaus et al. (2010) observed positive outcomes for individuals with TBI and their caregivers, following a CBT approach. Perceived self-efficacy, an important factor for long-term adjustment, improved significantly and was maintained over time. A follow-up study by Backhaus et al. (2016) compared a coping skills/peer support group to a CBT group, noting improvements in self-efficacy and emotional stability for both groups.

Depression and Suicide

Given the heterogeneity of experiences following TBI, it is difficult to make definitive statements about incidence and prevalence of depression or suicide. Further, while there is overlap between depression and suicide, we certainly cannot equate the two.

Depression in Traumatic Brain Injuries

The SHEFBIT study is a large cohort study (N = 827) that was carried out at Sheffield Teaching Hospital in the United Kingdom (Singh et al., 2018). Fifty-six percent of participants had depression at 10 weeks (Hospital Anxiety and Depression Scale–Depression subscale score of less than 8). Those with depression had more postconcussive symptoms and worse psychosocial and global outcome ratings. Prevalence dropped to 41% at 1-year post onset (Singh et al., 2019). Scholten et al. (2016) noted that 25% to 50% of individuals with TBI will experience major depression in the first year of recovery. More than 60% experience depression within 7 years of onset (Fann et al., 2009). Major depressive episodes are associated with social isolation, hostility, and cognitive impairments (Mauri et al., 2014).

Suicide in Traumatic Brain Injuries

A large longitudinal study of the prevalence of depression and suicidal behavior after TBI was conducted through follow-up data from TBI Model Systems (Fisher et al., 2016). This study examined 20 years of follow-up data, finding a rate of depression ranging from 25% to 28%, suicidal ideation ranging from 7% to 10%, and suicide attempts over the past year ranging from 0.8% to 1.7%. Importantly, those who experienced depression and/or suicidal behaviors at 1-year post onset demonstrated persistently elevated rates of depression and suicidal behaviors 5 years post. Box 8d-8 includes two case illustrations of suicidal thoughts by individuals with TBI.

Potential Issues for Partners

Preinjury Relationships

Certainly, TBIs can affect all types of people. That being said, individuals who make less than ideal choices put themselves at greater risk for brain injuries. This sometimes means that their preinjury relationships are already strained or problematic. Supporting a partner who was on the cusp of a divorce or separation prior to the injury holds some unique challenges. It's important to drop any assumptions and begin by listening more than talking. Time invested in listening can be very helpful when you move toward discharge planning, particularly what their role will be in that transition. Strained preinjury relationships may be a part of the history between parents with TBI and their children or vice versa. Again, listening more than talking initially is a good rule of thumb in order to create a safe place for partners to share their perspectives. For family who may be a key element of care provision and support upon return home, understanding these relationships is crucial.

Learning Readiness

Yes, this doesn't just apply to individuals with TBI. Adjusting to the trauma of nearly losing their partner, less than ideal sleep, the stress of role changes and taking on their partner's duties (e.g., paying bills, household duties), and information overload can make it hard for partners to take

Box 8d-8

Suicidal Thoughts, Two Cases

Shani was a 25-year-old paramedic at the time of her brain injury. She sustained a mild to moderate brain injury in a motor vehicle crash. Following her injury, she had chronic, persistent headaches, tinnitus, light sensitivity, sound sensitivity, fatigue, and irritability. She was described by her partner as a bubbly, energetic person who was dedicated to helping others. After her injury, she struggled with returning to her previous life. Just about everything about ambulance runs exacerbated her symptoms. The motion made her feel nauseated, the sounds of the siren irritated her and amplified her headaches, which ultimately disrupted her ability to do her job, a job she loved. She had also enrolled in a nursing degree program shortly before her injury, but decided to delay that program given her symptoms. Nevertheless, she was proactive, seeking resources to address her symptoms and attending our community brain injury group. (I should mention, she wasn't my client and that I only knew her from group.) We always begin sessions with a check-in, noting that we have a plan for the evening but are happy to drop that plan if necessary. That's when Shani dropped a bomb on the group. She said that things were heading in a downward spiral at work, at home, and life in general. She was thinking about ending it all. Almost reflexively, I asked, "Do you have a plan for doing this?", a question I have unfortunately had to ask a few times in my clinical career. To my dismay, she said, "Yes, I do," which set the next steps into motion. I said, "Can we take a walk?" and she agreed. Since we were in a medical center, we walked directly to the emergency department, and I sat with her until she was admitted. Meanwhile, I had left the group alone, so when I returned, we debriefed. The challenge was to keep the focus of the conversation on their reaction to the situation, as I could not discuss her situation further. A few days later, she was released from the hospital. I called to check on her. She said that things were much better, and I was relieved. A day later, I received word that she had ended her life. My head began to spin.

Dawson had a lot to deal with after his brain injury. He had already been processing the imminent separation and divorce, what that would mean for his children, a challenging return to work, and a shift to living alone. As he transitioned back to work, thanks to a great employer, he started gradually, with a plan to eventually get back to a bit less than full time. That allowed us to continue outpatient sessions and focus on real issues related to work, managing things at home, and continued cognitive rehabilitation. One day he said, "I can't do it anymore," which prompted me to ask, "What do you mean?" He explained that he was through with fighting it, being a burden on everyone, he was going to end it. I responded with, "Do you have a plan?" and he explained what it was. My office was right beside the physical therapy gym, so I asked one of the physical therapists if they could join me on a walk with Dawson. Yes, the physical therapist had other things to do, and no, I didn't give any further explanation. On the neurotrauma floor, the way you say something and the look on your face is all it takes. We walked together to our behavioral health unit, and I sat with Dawson through the intake process. After he was admitted, I connected with the behavioral health team, the neuropsychologist, and Dawson's new mental health counselor. They shared their plan and I asked how I could help. After just a couple of days, Dawson was released. Not everything was perfect but when he returned to outpatient therapy, he was focused on a plan—a plan to return to work, for staying connected with his ex-wife and their family. We asked her to join us in a session, which she gladly agreed to do. She offered to help with things he had been overwhelmed by, such as bills, his checkbook, and health insurance.

in new information as well. Keeping your verbal messages concise and to the point, supported by written resources and information, and establishing clear lifelines of where to get any of the information they missed is critical.

Visitors and Well-Intentioned Friends

Early on, shortly after an individual is hospitalized, it is typical for lots of family and friends to visit, extending their support to family members. This is when they offer, "Let me know if there is anything you need." Of course partners, at that point, are so overwhelmed, they don't know what they need. Down the road, when they recognize what they need, it's pretty tricky to make a cold call and say, "Remember when you said, you'd help out with anything I need?" Preparing partners for this likely type of proposal can be helpful. A simple script like, "I don't even know now, but I'm sure I will. Is it OK if I reach out to you later?" is like getting permission to ask later.

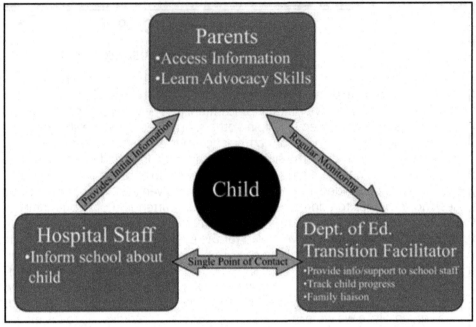

Figure 8d-1. STEP model (Reproduced with permission from Glang, A., Todis, B., Ettel, D., Wade, S. L., & Yeates, K. O. (2018). Results from a randomized trial evaluating a hospital-school transition support model for students hospitalized with traumatic brain injury. *Brain Injury, 32(5)*, 608-616.).

Common Issues for Children With Traumatic Brain Injuries

Latent Onset of Challenges

Be aware of the potential for challenges that will emerge later in the child's life. Having a good transition plan and contingencies is crucial. This includes a system for flagging issues that may not currently be on anyone's radar. Because younger children are not fully developed, we do not expect them to demonstrate fully refined executive functions. For many, demands do not increase until the middle school years and then they ramp up in high school. If a child is in elementary school or earlier at the time of their injury, you will not be able to detect executive dysfunction until those demands change. If years pass between injury and these upticks in demands, educators may not correlate the challenges with the TBI and may instead attribute them to something else. Multiple safeguards and pathways are necessary to deal with this concern.

Return to School Transitioning

A plan of care for return to school is crucial to their success. This means establishing communication between medical speech-language pathologists, school-based speech-language pathologists, teachers, school counselors, coaches, parents, and the student with a TBI. Students with disabilities related to the TBI are entitled to formal supports under federal law through Section 504 (Rehabilitation Act of 1973, 29 USC § 794) and the Individuals with Disabilities Education Act (IDEA). 504 Plans can provide accommodations for course schedules, physical access adaptations, and instructional accommodations. Glang et al. (2018) found

that about 60% of students received no academic services upon returning to school. Lundine et al. (2021) report that 45% of students with TBI had an Individualized Education Plan (IEP) for 1 year after returning to school. Unfortunately, only 35% received services through the IEP, 9.5% received services under both IEP and 504 Plans, 8.5% through a 504 plan, and 47% received only informal or no services. Boys with severe TBIs and those with parents who advocated for services were most likely to receive ongoing special education services 1 year later. Girls with TBI and those students with less severe impairments were unlikely to receive services. This all suggests that counseling parents about potential services and accommodations is crucial, along with establishing a transition plan collaboration between medical and school speech-language pathologists, along with other educators and professionals. Lundine et al. (2021) provided a nice list of potential accommodations to consider, including test accommodations such as extra time for tests and assignments, placement in a resource room or learning center, extra help from teachers during and outside of class, speech-language pathology services, a modified course schedule, use of notes during tests, physical and mobility accommodations, in-school counseling, vision/hearing supports, small group instruction in regular education classrooms, peer assistance, relocation of desk, a one-to-one teaching assistant in select classes, note taker, visual aids, reduced stimuli, and audio recordings. These accommodations were drawn from a survey of TBI research experts, special educators, and parents (Glang et al., 2018). Glang et al. (2018) developed the School Transition and Re-entry Program (STEP) to address the need for an efficient model to address counseling and communication with parents, educators, and transition facilitators (Figure 8d-1).

Letting Go

When children and adolescents sustain moderate to severe brain injuries, parents confront issues of death and loss or uncertainty regarding the vision of what their child would become. Parents see their child on life support, unconscious, and have the images and emotions of the fateful day deeply etched into their psyche. Meanwhile, the child awakens and moves forward with no recollection of that time period. They begin the process of moving forward, but it is often difficult for parents to do the same. This can result in justifiable feelings of cautiousness and a need to shelter that child. Parents can become torn between feelings of wanting to support the best outcome for their child while setting a conservative agenda, which can be difficult to navigate.

References

Anson, K., & Ponsford, J. (2006). Who benefits? Outcome following a coping skills group intervention for traumatically brain injured individuals. *Brain Injury, 20*(1), 1-13.

Appleton, S., Browne, A., Ciccone, N., Fong, K., Hankey, G., Lund, M., Miles, A., Wainstein, C., Zach, J., & Yee, Y. (2011). A multidisciplinary social communication and coping skills group intervention for adults with acquired brain injury (ABI): A pilot feasibility study in an inpatient setting. *Brain Impairment, 12*(3), 210-222.

Bedard, M., Felteau, M., Mazmanian, D., Fedyk, K., Klein, R., Richardson, J., Parkinson, W., & Minthorn-Biggs, M. B. (2003). Pilot evaluation of a mindfulness-based intervention to improve quality of life among individuals who sustained traumatic brain injuries. *Disability and Rehabilitation, 25*(13), 722-731.

Douglas, J. (2020). Loss of friendship following traumatic brain injury: A model grounded in the experience of adults with severe injury. *Neuropsychological Rehabilitation, 30*(7), 1277-1302. https://doi.org/10.1080/09602011.2019.1574589

Douglas, J. M., Knox, L., De Maio, C., & Bridge, H. (2014). Improving communication-specific coping after traumatic brain injury: Evaluation of a new treatment using single-case experimental design. *Brain Impairment, 15*(3), 190-201.

Douglas, J. M., Knox, L., De Maio, C., Bridge, H., Drummond, M., & Whiteoak, J. (2019). Effectiveness of communication-specific coping intervention for adults with traumatic brain injury: Preliminary results. *Neuropsychological Rehabilitation, 29*(1), 73-91.

Douglas, J. M., O'Flaherty, C. A., & Snow, P. C. (2000). Measuring perception of communicative ability: The development and evaluation of the La Trobe Communication Questionnaire. *Aphasiology, 14*(3), 251-268.

Fann, J. R., Hart, T., & Schomer, K. G. (2009). Treatment for depression after traumatic brain injury: A systematic review. *Journal of Neurotrauma, 26*(12), 2383-2402. https://doi.org/10.1089/neu.2009.1091

Fisher, L. B., Pedrelli, P., Iverson, G. L., Bergquist, T. F., Bombardier, C. H., Hammond, F. M., Hart, T. Ketchum, J. M., Giacino, J., & Zafonte, R. (2016). Prevalence of suicidal behaviour following traumatic brain injury: Longitudinal follow-up data from the NIDRR Traumatic Brain Injury Model Systems. *Brain Injury, 30*(11), 1311-1318. https://doi.org/10.1080/02699052.2016.1195517

Flynn, M. A., Mutlu, B., Duff, M. C., & Turkstra, L. S. (2018). Friendship quality, friendship quantity, and social participation in adults with traumatic brain injury. *Seminars in Speech and Language, 39*(5), 416-426.

Glang, A., Todis, B., Ettel, D., Wade, S. L., & Yeates, K. O. (2018). Results from a randomized trial evaluating a hospital-school transition support model for students hospitalized with traumatic brain injury. *Brain Injury, 32*(5), 608-616.

Harrison-Felix, C., Newman, J. K., Hawley, L., Morey, C., Ketchum, J. M., Walker, W. C., Bell, K. R., Millis, S. R., Braden, C., Malec, J., Hammond, F. M., Eagye, C. B., & Howe, L. (2018). Social competence treatment after traumatic brain injury: A multicenter, randomized controlled trial of interactive group treatment versus noninteractive treatment. *Archives of Physical Medicine and Rehabilitation, 99*(11), 2131-2142.

Hibbard, M. R., Cantor, J., Charatz, H., Rosenthal, R., Ashman, T., Gundersen, N., Ireland-Knight, L., Gordon, W., Avner, J., & Gartner, A. (2002). Peer support in the community: Initial findings of a mentoring program for individuals with traumatic brain injury and their families. *Journal of Head Trauma Rehabilitation, 17*(2), 112-131.

Hoepner, J. K., & Olson, S. E. (2018). Joint video self-modeling as a conversational intervention for an individual with a traumatic brain injury and his everyday partner: A pilot investigation. *Clinical Archives of Communication Disorders, 3*(1), 22-41. http://dx.doi.org/10.21849/cacd.2018.00262

Hoepner, J. K., Salo, M., & Weich, H. (2019). Replication of a dynamic coaching program for college students with acquired brain injuries. *Clinical Archives of Communication Disorders, 4*(2), 98-112.

Hoepner, J. K., Sievert, A., & Guenther, K. (2021). Joint video self-modeling for persons with traumatic brain injury and their partners: A case series. *American Journal of Speech-Language Pathology, 30*(2S), 863-882.

Keegan, L. C, Murdock, M., Suger, C., & Togher, L. (2019). Improving natural social interaction: Group rehabilitation after traumatic brain injury. *Neuropsychological Rehabilitation, 24*, 1-26.

Kennedy, M. R. (2017). *Coaching college students with executive function problems.* The Guilford Press.

Kennedy, M. R. T., & Krause, M. O. (2010). Academic experiences of adults with and without traumatic brain injury using the College Survey for Students with Brain Injury (CSS-BI). *Brain Injury, 24*, 325.

Kennedy, M. R., & Krause, M. O. (2011). Self-regulated learning in a dynamic coaching model for supporting college students with traumatic brain injury: Two case reports. *Journal of Head Trauma Rehabilitation, 26*(3), 212-223.

Kennedy, M. R., O'Brien, K. H., & Krause, M. O. (2012). Bridging person-centered outcomes and therapeutic processes for college students with traumatic brain injury. *Perspectives on Neurophysiology and Neurogenic Speech and Language Disorders, 22*(4), 143-151.

Lavoie, S., Sechrist, S., Quach, N., Ehsanian, R., Duong, T., Gotlib, I. H., & Isaac, L. (2017). Depression in men and women one year following traumatic brain injury (TBI): A TBI model systems study. *Frontiers in Psychology, 8*, 634.

Lundine, J. P., Todis, B., Gau, J. M., McCart, M., Wade, S. L., Yeates, K. O., & Glang, A. (2021). Return to school following TBI: Educational services received 1 year after injury. *Journal of Head Trauma Rehabilitation, 36*(2), E89-E96.

Mauri, M. C., Paletta, S., Colasanti, A., Miserocchi, G., and Altamura, A. C. (2014). Clinical and neuropsychological correlates of major depression following post-traumatic brain injury, a prospective study. *Asian Journal of Psychiatry, 12*, 118-124. https://doi.org/10.1016/j.ajp.2014.07.003

Meulenbroek, P., & Cherney, L. R. (2019). The voicemail elicitation task: Functional workplace language assessment for persons with traumatic brain injury. *Journal of Speech, Language, and Hearing Research, 62*(9), 3367-3380.

Meulenbroek, P., & Turkstra, L. (2016). Job stability in skilled work and communication ability after moderate-severe traumatic brain injury. *Disability and Rehabilitation, 38*(5), 452-461.

O'Brien, K. H., Schellinger, S. K., & Kennedy, M. R. (2018). Self-regulation strategies used by students with brain injury while transitioning to college. *NeuroRehabilitation, 42*(3), 365-375.

Ownsworth, T. L., McFarland, K., & Mc Young, R. (2000). Self-awareness and psychosocial functioning following acquired brain injury: An evaluation of a group support programme. *Neuropsychological Rehabilitation, 10*(5), 465-484.

Salas, C. E., Casassus, M., Rowlands, L., Pimm, S., & Flanagan, D. A. (2018). "Relating through sameness": A qualitative study of friendship and social isolation in chronic traumatic brain injury. *Neuropsychological Rehabilitation, 28*(7), 1161-1178.

Scholten, A. C., Haagsma, J. A., Cnossen, M. C., Olff, M., van Beeck, E. F., & Polinder, S. (2016). Prevalence of and risk factors for anxiety and depressive disorders after traumatic brain injury: A systematic review. *Journal of Neurotrauma, 33*(22), 1969-1994. https://doi.org/10.1089/neu.2015.4252

Singh, R., Mason, S., Lecky, F., & Dawson, J. (2018). Prevalence of depression after TBI in a prospective cohort: The SHEFBIT study. *Brain Injury, 32*(1), 84-90.

Singh, R., Mason, S., Lecky, F., & Dawson, J. (2019). Comparison of early and late depression after TBI; (the SHEFBIT study). *Brain Injury, 33*(5), 584-591.

Togher, L., McDonald, S., Tate, R., Power, E., & Rietdijk, R. (2013). Training communication partners of people with severe traumatic brain injury improves everyday conversations: A multicenter single blind clinical trial. *Journal of Rehabilitation Medicine, 45,* 637-645.

Ylvisaker, M. (2006). Self-coaching: A context-sensitive, person-centered approach to social communication after traumatic brain injury. *Brain Impairment, 7*(3), 246-258.

Ylvisaker, M., & Feeney, T. J. (1998). *Collaborative brain injury intervention: Positive everyday routines.* Singular Publishing Group.

Ylvisaker, M., & Feeney, T. (2000). Reflections on Dobermans, poodles, and social rehabilitation for difficult-to-serve individuals with traumatic brain injury. *Aphasiology, 14*(4), 407-431.

Ylvisaker, M., & Feeney, T. (2002). Executive functions, self-regulation, and learned optimism in paediatric rehabilitation: A review and implications for intervention. *Pediatric Rehabilitation, 5*(2), 51-70.

Ylvisaker, M., & Feeney, T. (2009). Apprenticeship in self-regulation: Supports and interventions for individuals with self-regulatory impairments. *Developmental Neurorehabilitation, 12*(5), 370-379.

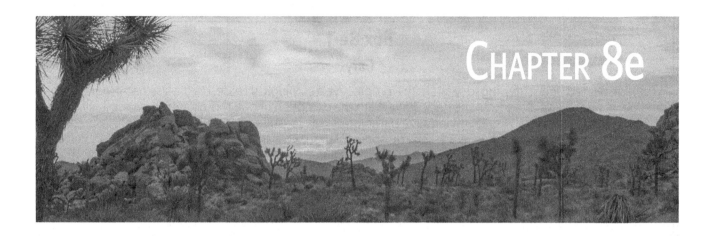

CHAPTER 8e

Special Topics and Disorders
Important Conversations

*Robin Pollens, MS, CCC-SLP; Nancy Petersen, MSW;
Emma Power, PhD, BAppSc, CPSP MSPAA; Margaret McGrath, PhD, MSc, BSc;
and Sandra Lever, MN, BHM, RN, CNC, NSLHD*

Counseling in Palliative Care Contexts

Robin Pollens, MS, CCC-SLP

Palliative care is a treatment approach that supports individuals who are living with serious chronic health conditions or declining health as they approach end of life. It is based upon the following goals: providing relief from pain and other distressing symptoms, offering a support system to help patients live as actively as possible until death, integrating the psychological and spiritual aspects of care, and offering a support system to help the family cope during the patient's illness (World Health Organization, 2019). It is a multiprofessional and systemic view of care in which patients, family, and practitioners are integrated in an interactive system (Gramm et al., 2020; Pollens, 2012).

As a speech-language pathologist engaging with patients in a palliative or end-of-life care context, the focus of care shifts away from treatment goals, which primarily address improvement of impairment-level communication, cognitive, or swallowing skills of the patient. Rather, the overall goals are to ease distress, support the patient and family's quality of life, help them to maintain social connectivity, and communicate with the care team (Pollens, 2004). Box 8e-1 illustrates this focus of care.

Interprofessional Collaborations

Speech-language pathologists in palliative care settings often provide care in unison with a multidisciplinary team. In this context, speech-language pathologists and social workers may collaborate to support the individual in areas such as self-determination, adjustment to illness, and access to resources for patients in palliative care (Pollens & Lynn, 2011). The speech-language pathologist may incorporate different approaches to facilitate this type of collaboration, including:

Hoepner, J. K. (Ed.). *Counseling and Motivational Interviewing
in Speech-Language Pathology* (pp. 205-216).
© 2024 Taylor& Francis Group.

Box 8e-1

Gary

Gary, age 58, had been surviving for years with a progressive neurologic disease. His disease had progressed, and he was unable to move from the neck down, with the exception of one thumb, which he used skillfully to navigate the computer. A speech-language pathologist was consulted to provide suggestions related to dysphagia. After a few sessions, Gary asked the speech-language pathologist to help him with his voice. While his articulation was clear, he did have reduced volume, breath support, and quality of voice. The speech-language pathologist observed Gary communicating with his daily care attendant. She had no difficulty understanding his speech. The speech-language pathologist discussed this with Gary after the care attendant left the room.

Gary became quiet and somewhat teary. The speech-language pathologist remained quiet also. Many people need time in order to articulate their thoughts. He had difficulty initiating the muscle movements for voicing due to the disease, and the additional overlay of heightened emotion increased his challenge in expressing his thoughts. When he was ready, he explained.

He had four buddies, long-time friends who came together and visited him. He thrived on hearing their banter. But he wished that he could enter the conversation. If he did talk, they often couldn't hear him. His body needed to be positioned reclined in a specialized chair, and this created a distance barrier. The speech-language pathologist identified, confirmed, and acknowledged his feelings. Gary appreciated that his friends were continuing to visit him, but he still felt lonely and isolated during the visit.

From this counseling moment, therapy tasks emerged. First, Gary and his speech-language pathologist collaborated on creating a short "handout" with tips on how to communicate with him (e.g., "Give me time to answer, it takes time for my muscles to move"). Next, the speech-language pathologist provided a voice amplifier with a long cord so the speaker rested at the end of Gary's recliner chair. With these adaptations, his visiting friends could hear him, and he began the process of contributing to the conversations.

It was important that this speech-language pathologist valued taking time to listen for and observe Gary's emotional state. Gary felt supported enough to express his emotional pain. And steps could then be addressed to support Gary's quality of life. In this way, counseling can be an integral part of the speech-language pathologist's interaction with individuals receiving palliative care.

- Using supportive conversation strategies (Kagan et al., 2001) to clarify the patient's ideas or concerns and convey these ideas to the social worker or other members of the interprofessional team.
- Educating the social worker on communication facilitation techniques that are effective for engaging with this patient for supportive counseling.
- Referring to the palliative care team social worker for more in-depth counseling. Social workers are trained to manage family dynamics, treat anxiety, and facilitate advance care planning conversations (Leff, 2021).

Counseling Family Members

Additionally, the speech-language pathologist often has a key role in counseling the family members of the patient who is receiving palliative care. The American Speech-Language-Hearing Association (ASHA; 2021) outlines two types of counseling: informational counseling and personal adjustment counseling. Box 8e-2 incorporates both of these types of counseling services when the speech-language

pathologist provides counseling with a family member in palliative care. It also illustrates the model of referring to a medical social worker for additional services on behalf of the family member.

Listening Carefully

According to the World Health Organization's definition of palliative care (World Health Organization, 2019), palliative care (1) integrates the psychological and spiritual aspects of patient care; and (2) offers a support system to help the family cope during the patient's illness and in their own bereavement. The services provided by the speech-language pathologist in this case scenario served these functions, with a special focus on supporting the psychological needs of the family member.

This case scenario also highlights the importance of listening carefully to the concerns of the patient or family. Speech-language pathology intervention in palliative care is often brief. By listening to and understanding the specific concerns of the patient or family, intervention goals and

---

Box 8e-2

Eleanor and Greg

A speech-language pathologist received a referral for a woman, Eleanor, with a prior diagnosis of dementia and a new diagnosis of stroke. When the speech-language pathologist arrived at her home, she was reclined in a hospital bed in the small living room. Although dementia had resulted in a gradual declining trajectory of ability, a recent sudden and marked reduction in Eleanor's ability to ambulate and communicate was very distressing to the husband. He had no close family in the community. He continued tearfully that one doctor had told him that she may soon benefit from hospice services.

The speech-language pathologist spoke directly with Eleanor, and she provided brief responses but did not initiate any verbal communication. She could read large-print single words on a whiteboard but was variable in pointing to it conversationally.

In the next visit, Eleanor was sleeping and aroused only briefly to voice and touch. Her husband, Greg, said she had not slept during the night, and she was very tired. The speech-language pathologist told the husband they could use the time to talk together, and the speech-language pathologist asked him, "How are *you* doing?" Greg spoke for the next half hour, describing many concerns. The speech-language pathologist adopted a listening approach and provided empathic engagement, which enabled this husband to express his distress.

Greg felt very alone in the care of his wife. At times, she became distressed if he was not near, but he still had to do all of the household duties. He was concerned that if he even went outside to get the mail or take out the trash, his wife would call for him, and he would not hear her. He also described his wife's agitation due to her reduced memory. If he needed to get her ready to take her to an appointment or if a therapist was coming, she became very distressed by what to her was an unexpected intrusion.

Greg became especially tearful when talking about the future. He had questions related to finances, as well as a lack of familiarity with the care that hospice could provide or what it would mean to accept this approach.

The speech-language pathologist responded by acknowledging these challenges and offering that the following visits could focus on these concerns. She also recommended a referral for the medical social worker to assist with the financial concerns and to understand the hospice process. He agreed to these recommendations.

In the follow-up visits, interventions were initiated, which directly responded to the husband's concerns. An alert button connected to a beeper was demonstrated. His wife could push the button if she wanted her husband to tend to her and he was not in the room. Repeated modeling was required, but the patient expressed satisfaction with this button, and the husband felt relieved that he was honoring her need for constant connection. Additionally, use of a whiteboard was initiated. Each morning the husband wrote the key events of the day and reviewed it with his wife. As each event occurred, he showed her the whiteboard. This reduced the agitation and frequency of anger directed at the husband when a transition event occurred.

---

resource provision can specifically relate to what is needed at that time to ease distress or to improve the quality of the person's life as they approach death (Goldberg, 2014; Pollens, 2020; Wallace, 2013). One approach to strengthen the practitioner's ability to discern a patient's or family's need is using a mindfulness approach. Bernstein (2019) defined mindfulness as follows:

> The ability to pay attention to what is happening "right now," in this room with this patient, and not be distracted by other demands and concerns, creates space to use your wisdom and knowledge effectively and with care for the dignity of each patient. (p. 16)

Counseling Amid Other Interventions

It may not always be easy to differentiate **counseling** from other **treatment** approaches when working with families whose loved ones are in palliative care. For example, a daughter is tearful because her mom with end-stage renal disease "won't eat" and the speech-language pathologist gently explains that her mom's swallowing ability has declined significantly, and that people often have minimal appetite as they approach the end of their life. The speech-language pathologist further acknowledges that this is very hard because we want to try to feed our loved ones—and that nurturing her mom in other ways may be helpful. Is this dysphagia treatment or a counseling moment? Likely, these elements are inseparable and interdependent.

An individual who survived surgery and radiation for oral cancer may now be able to resume many life activities but is no longer able to eat beyond taking small sips. The loss of the pleasure of eating compounded by the loss of the social connection of eating at meals with others is profound. For a speech-language pathologist to not acknowledge this reality and only focus on "tongue-based exercises" would diminish the value of the clinical relationship and be a missed opportunity for the individual to express their emotions.

Listening for important cultural, familial, or ethnic views of illness and healing may also support the emotional needs of care partners who provide palliative care for a loved one. For example, educating a Hmong daughter how to carefully provide rice water by spoon or teaching a rural farmer how to provide his wife with small tastes of their homegrown peach juice sprang from an openness to understanding what is valued by the care provider during this time of great distress.

Developing the presence of a "listening mind" and a compassionate presence is important in all areas of work for a speech-language pathologist. "Each time we quiet our mind, our listening becomes sharp and clear, deep and perceptive. . . . and can reach out and hear, as if from inside, the heart of someone's pain" (Dass & Gorman, 1985, p. 223).

As a speech-language pathologist working in a palliative care framework, a counseling relationship can result in the provision of meaningful and authentic goals. The family can feel supported in your understanding of their concerns. Most importantly, your skills as a speech-language pathologist may be a key factor that enables a person to communicate what is essential to them during palliative or end-of-life care.

References

American Speech-Language Hearing Association. (2021). Counseling for professional service delivery. https://www.asha.org/PracticePortal/Professional-Issues/Counseling-For-Professional-Service-Delivery/

Bernstein, S. (2019). Mindfulness and nursing practice. *Nursing, 49*(6), 14-17. http://doi.org/10.1097/01.NURSE.0000558105.96903.af

Dass, R., & Gorman, P. (1985). *How can I help: Stories and reflections on service.* Alfred a Knopf.

Goldberg, S. (2014). There's an elephant in the room: Issues in death and dying. In A. Holland, & R. Nelson, (Eds.), *Counseling in communication disorders: A wellness perspective* (2nd ed.). Plural Publishing.

Gramm, J., Trachsel, M., & Berthold, D. (2020). Psychotherapeutisches arbeiten in palliative care. *Verhaltenstherapie, 30*(4), 323-333.

Kagan, A., Black, S. E., Duchan, J. F., Simmons-Mackie, N., & Square, P. (2001). Training volunteers as conversation partners using "Supported Conversation for Adults With Aphasia" (SCA). *Journal of Speech, Language, and Hearing Research, 44*(3), 624-638. http://doi.org/10.1044/1092-4388(2001/051)

Leff, V. (March 22, 2021). *On the value of social work in palliative care.* PallMed: A Hospice and Palliative Medicine Blog. https://www.pallimed.org/2021/03/on-value-of-social-work-in-palliative.html

Pollens, R. (2004). Role of the speech-language pathologist in palliative hospice care. *Journal of Palliative Medicine, 7*(5), 694-702. http://doi.org/10.1089/jpm.2004.7.694

Pollens, R. (2012). Integrating speech-language pathology services in palliative end-of-life care. *Topics in Language Disorders, 32*(2), 137-148. http://doi.org/10.1097/TLD.0b013e3182543533

Pollens, R. (2020). Facilitating client communication in palliative end-of-life care: Impact of speech-language pathologists. *Topics in Language Disorders, 40*(3), 264-277. http://doi.org/10.1097/TLD.0000000000000220

Pollens, R. & Lynn, M. (2011). Social work and speech pathology: Collaborating for communication in palliative care. In T. Altilio, & S. Otis-Green (Eds.), *Oxford textbook of palliative social work.* Oxford University Press.

Wallace, G. (2013). Speech-language pathology: Enhancing quality of life for individuals approaching death. *ASHA SIG 15 Perspectives on Gerontology, 18*(3), 112-120. https://doi.org/10.1044/gero18.3.112

World Health Organization. (2019). Definition of palliative care. http://www.who.int/cancer/palliative/definition/en/

Counseling in Death, Dying, and Bereavement Contexts

Nancy Petersen

Look closely and you will see almost everyone carrying bags of cement on their shoulders. That's why it takes courage to get out of bed in the morning and climb into the day.

~ Edward Hirsch, Gabriel: A Poem *(2014)*

Death, dying, and grieving loss is a universal human experience. Despite the ability of science to extend life far longer than ever imagined, there is currently no way to extend life infinitely. At least not yet. That discovery will inevitably lead to innumerable issues we can only imagine now, and will change the landscape of death, but the underlying human issue will remain. Loss will continue. And loss comes in all shapes and sizes, and the effect of loss varies in every instance, yet it is often ignored, despite its constant presence in our lives and the lives of those we serve. There is also joy, happiness, optimism, and those are celebrated and expected.

As I hope you are aware by now, the decision to work with humans every day, especially in a clinical setting as a speech-language pathologist, means you will soon find yourself sitting in a room with someone suffering a loss. It means a real potential to encounter any or all human thoughts and feelings, including grief resulting from their personal loss or grief from various losses, and the possibility of their own death. To be clear, this should be something we as humans are prepared for at any time. We should be able to support those around us when they experience a death, or offer emotional strength when someone close is facing constant small losses due to chronic illness or even natural aging. And some of us seem far more prepared than others. Some have learned by experiencing loss themselves, some are naturally empathic. But there are those who are truly petrified, who may believe death is a word to avoid or even a word with innate power. Given that you will be in a particularly intimate situation with patients and families, and may find yourself face to face with your client's emotions, including grief, it might be to your advantage to seriously consider where you fit in this continuum of comfort.

Serving the Whole Patient

Considering the American educational system's bent toward separating instead of integrating, students in a multitude of medical or human service fields are taught for hours about their specific study area of choice. All you need to know about the anatomy of the ear or lobes of the brain is taught and tested—drugs and dosages, resources, and statistics—until you can impress many in conversation, but often the human you will be treating is far more than those parts. Many important conversations are left untouched with the hope that each student came to school with fully fledged skills in "being human." Often graduates are sent into the world without the basic tools needed to serve their whole patient. In our death-denying culture, we often move from a home and community where we are protected from death to an "educational silo" that fails to expand the human understanding further than required by the degree. We choose a career path and are then released into the world to serve an entire, complex human, only to feel unprepared if an interaction takes an unexpected turn.

Denying and Avoiding Conversations About Death

As history proves, American death denial wasn't accidental. Someone or something went to great lengths to remove all upsetting language, experiences, and even emotions from death. These "someones" have told us for many years that they are "protecting" us from the "difficulty" of death, and that we need not be "bothered" by the details of our loss so, here we are. The use of words like *lost*, *gone*, *passed*, *moved on*, and *crossed over* do not help us avoid the truth of death, and if they are intended to soften the blow, many can tell you, they do not. The real, gut-wrenching loss and grief remain. And after all the so-called protection we've paid for, many are unprepared when it hits, hard.

Americans have a unique inability to see death for what it is and a fairly new desire to avoid getting our hands dirty. How quickly the body is taken away. How impersonal the salons we rent to stare at a person often referred to as unrecognizable. No more spending time preparing, grieving, loving our person, as we did not two or three generations ago. So, few are aware that a living room is called such because it is where the living gathered while supporting family and friends after a death. Now we allow strangers to take them away and prepare them, sanitize them. And this change in death care can be traced directly to the funeral industry, who financially benefit from our fears—fears that have arisen from seeds the burgeoning industry planted when they realized the money that could be made if death became taboo. Starting during the Civil War, the funeral industry has become a billion dollar per year industry, claiming to help us at a most difficult time when, in fact, many would argue it often serves to make it worse.

In short, death in America has become a commodity. Our customs and traditions are dictated by industry, rather than spirituality or values. Our fear of getting old and dying prevents us from talking about it, so we perpetuate the same customs—customs designed specifically for profit.

~Nicole Archer, CNET

Our culture's determination to avoid death, as if it is a choice we make, has taken all kinds of strange turns since the Civil War. Millions, or most likely billions, are spent on youth preserving products, advertised as though maintaining youth is paramount. Vitamins in our water, collagen in our lip balm, hair regrowing from our heads, poison being injected to reduce wrinkles, and the list goes on. Death is even described often using references to sports and war in an effort to incorrectly reframe one of life's only unavoidable truths:

You've written that in America, we tend to think of dying as losing and being alive as winning, which I agree with. When we look at the language around death—"he lost his battle to cancer"—it's sports terms.... terms that we use about competition that we're applying to life and to death when really, of course, death is not losing and being alive is not winning.

~ Megan O'Rourke and Hanya Yanagihara, 2017

So where does that leave you? My hope is this will open your eyes to things you've not noticed before. Death is something that should be considered and discussed far more than it is in public spaces with thoughtful audiences. What place does death and grief have in our society? How do other cultures embrace death and grief and all its meanings? Does our current pushback of all things death benefit us in any way? Do our aging loved ones suffer because of our own fears and rejection of the inevitable? Are we prepared to make important decisions when a loved one gets ill or injured? Does our health care system sway under the financial burden of our denial? Should costs of caring for our loved ones post death be dictated by political lobbyists? Can we afford death the American way, financially or mentally? These questions need to be asked and thoughtfully answered.

Now with all that knowledge swirling about in your brain, what can we do to better serve our patients? Are there thoughts and perhaps insights on how these societal issues may show up in your day-to-day professional life? Most importantly, how you can react in a way that benefits those you serve, without feeling you've gotten in over your head or crossed out of your professional lane? Let's discuss practical ideas you can use in many aspects of your whole life.

Expressions of Grief

Human emotion and need cannot be constrained to any particular hour of the day or place on a map. Humans, in this particular situation, American humans, have often been taught to be strong in and around death or to keep grief hidden, as if showing emotion is an embarrassment or weakness. So, where this grief may show itself has no real boundaries and may come to the surface at what seems to you like a mundane or completely unrelated time, like during a session when you are discussing what the patient plans to make for dinner that evening. You may have no idea that Barney's recently deceased mother, Lorraine, always made spaghetti on Tuesday nights when he was growing up, and today is his first Tuesday since returning from the funeral. And Barney begins to cry. The most important thing to know as a speech-language pathologist and a human is how to listen and be patient, even if it means stopping the speech-language pathology part of your session and caring for Barney while he grieves. And yes, you can do this and should feel comfortable sitting in the grief with Barney so he isn't alone. Sitting in silence with someone in emotional pain, especially grief, is one of the greatest gifts you can offer another human being, and it can also be one of the hardest things you'll do as a clinician or person. There is no right or wrong answer, sometimes there aren't even questions, so do not worry, you can't fix it, but you can be with him while he experiences it. We want to help and fix, but real grief has to be felt and leaned into in order to move through it.

Grief and loss happen to everyone. We've all felt misunderstood during times of great pain. We've also stood by, helpless, in the face of other people's pain. We've all fumbled for words, knowing no words can ever make things right.

~Megan Devine, It's OK that you're Not OK: Meeting Grief and Loss in a Culture that Doesn't Understand

The palliative care section of ASHA (2021) outlines two types of counseling: informational counseling and personal adjustment counseling. Sitting with a patient as they manage through grief clearly falls under the second, and allows you to switch to a service just as vital as the more concrete care plan goals you've written.

Remember, grief can be loud, quiet, messy, confusing. All are acceptable expressions of deep intense feelings. A few examples of real patient interactions can hopefully frame the previous discussion and show a few of many possible

---

Box 8e-3
Dr. Barbara

Barbara, a single, 78-year-old stroke patient and retired physician, was very upset and crying when I found her in a small room, missing therapy. She was very angry at another staff member whom she believed was treating her like a child. She admitted she had told the staff member to "shut up" a number of times and wasn't interested in ever seeing her again. After sitting with her a while, I asked if she wanted to share what had upset her so much. She explained that her 15-year-old cat, Merlin, was dying. She told Merlin the morning she had the stroke that she'd be home soon, but had been in one institution or another for 18 months since the stroke and never returned home to tell him she loved him. There is no happy ending for Barbara or Merlin, but listening and caring about her grief was helpful. We discussed all the other losses she has endured since the stroke, and she seemed to better understand the sadness, anger, and grief she felt was proportionate to the situation. She returned to therapy and has returned every day since.

---

practical applications. Boxes 8e-3, 8e-4, and 8e-5 provide case illustrations of individuals experiencing grief and loss.

Your gifts will take you far and choosing a profession to better the lives of others puts you in elite company. Truly caring for others is the first and most important tool you can possess as you embark on your own journey. With a willingness to try, you have the power to offer what they need at that moment. Not every time, but enough times.

When we honestly ask ourselves which person in our lives mean the most to us, we often find that it is those who, instead of giving advice, solutions, or cures, have chosen rather to share our pain and touch our wounds with a warm and tender hand. The friend who can be silent with us in a moment of despair or confusion, who can stay with us in an hour of grief and bereavement, who can tolerate not knowing, not curing, not healing and face with us the reality of our powerlessness, that is a friend who cares.

—Henri Nouwen, Out of Solitude: Three Meditations on the Christian Life (2004)

Box 8e-4
Molly

She looked just like her! The patient looked just like one of my best friends, and I was paralyzed for a moment. I had to go into her room for our session, but I needed a moment to take a deep breath and gather myself. Molly was a 31-year-old young lady with long, wavy golden red hair and the spitting image of a friend I'd had for 10 years. Except Molly was dying. I was working on the cancer ward at a large hospital, and Molly was waiting for me. The direct grief wasn't mine to experience, as family and friends would, but the intimacy brought on by a likeness meant it took a moment to gather my wits. We chatted a while and discussed the weather and the latest *Friends* episode. I invited her to the next unit support group gathering, and she hesitated. I did my best not to cajole or encourage her in an attempt to lessen my uncomfortable feelings, but instead let the silence hang in the air out of a simple fear of saying the wrong thing. She said we could discuss it later, and maybe she'd change her mind, but for now she wanted to call her mom. She discharged a few days later. There was much bustling about in her room that day, and I never got to talk to her much more, but I hope still that my presence brought only kind support and that I added nothing to her burden.

Box 8e-5
Dwight

Dwight was a giant of a man, worshipped by many who had experienced his mentoring and coaching over the years and fiercely protected by his amazing children and dedicated wife. But the stroke was massive. Dwight felt defeated but couldn't help smile at the cheerleaders at his bedside. He had only a few words and fewer movements available to him. The rehab program was discussed and the intensive therapies available thrilled the family, who just knew it was the answer to Dwight's deficits. He started with a daughter by his side, but while she was out of the treatment room, Dwight looked intently at the speech-language pathologist and asked in barely a whisper, "Why?" It was clear to her that the effort Dwight was giving was not for himself, but for the family who so adored him. He looked and felt exhausted and managed to communicate this was not how he wanted to spend what was left of his life. He seemed to know he would not be getting better. He hated to let his family down. And how could he give up when he'd spent his life encouraging and pushing those who didn't think they could? The therapist spoke to the daughter and used all her skills to explain what she and Dwight discussed. Not a week later it was decided he would stay home, and not a month later we all learned he died. At home with his family. The therapist was not a part of his care for a long time, but clearly was there at the right time.

Key Takeaways

- Listening is key. You need no special training, special knowledge, or magical answers to listen.
- Meet your patient where they are. Try to keep your personal thoughts out of the interactions and listen to where they are and how they are coping in their unique situation.
- Death and loss are real. Each one of these are human experiences, often made worse by ignoring or denying their existence.
- There isn't *one* person assigned to assist someone with these feelings. You may happen to be the one present when they surface, and that makes you the person at that moment.
- Your own comfort with your own feelings of death, grief, and loss can be a great help as you enter this intimate human practice of speech-language pathology. The service you provide may be much broader than you once thought.
- Finally, death and grief aren't the only taboo subjects in our society. Human sexuality has also been made "dirty" or "inappropriate" in almost all situations, yet it remains one of the quintessential human experiences that many face with far less knowledge or comfort than is deserved. This topic will be discussed further in this section and it will be important in your professional career and human experience to give it notice and thought.

Suggested Readings

Robert Neimeyer has written extensively about using the narrative approach to help people process grief and renegotiate identity following loss. If you're interested in further readings, check out these works by Neimeyer and colleagues.

Neimeyer, R. A. (2001). *Meaning reconstruction & the experience of loss.* American Psychological Association.

Neimeyer, R. A. (2001). Reauthoring life narratives: Grief therapy as meaning reconstruction. *The Israel Journal of Psychiatry and Related Sciences, 38*(3/4), 171.

Neimeyer, R. A. (2001). The language of loss: Grief therapy as a process of meaning reconstruction. In R. A. Neimeyer (Ed.), *Meaning reconstruction & the experience of loss* (pp. 261-292). American Psychological Association. https://doi.org/10.1037/10397-014

Neimeyer, R. A., Klass, D., & Dennis, M. R. (2014). A social constructionist account of grief: Loss and the narration of meaning. *Death Studies, 38*(8), 485-498.

Neimeyer, R. A., Prigerson, H. G., & Davies, B. (2002). Mourning and meaning. *American Behavioral Scientist, 46*(2), 235-251.

Stewart, A. E., & Neimeyer, R. A. (2001). Emplotting the traumatic self: Narrative revision and the construction of coherence. *The Humanistic Psychologist, 29*(1-3), 8-39.

References

Archer, N. (2020). Funerals are expensive, broken and exploitative. They have to change. CNET. https://www.cnet.com/features/funerals-are-expensive-broken-exploitative-they-have-to-change/

Devine, M. (2017). *It's ok that you're not ok: Meeting grief and loss in a culture that doesn't understand.* Sounds True, Inc.

Hirsch, E. (2014). *Gabriel: A poem.* Knopf.

Nouwen, H. (2004). *Out of solitude: Three meditations on the Christian life.* Ave Maria Press.

O'Rourke, M., & Yanagihara, H. (2017). *The exchange: Why Americans can't cope with trauma: Writers Meghan O'Rourke and Hanya Yanagihara explore death and grief in the Facebook age.* https://foreignpolicy.com/2017/01/11/the-exchange-why-americans-cant-cope-with-trauma-meghan-orourke-hanya-yanagihara-the-long-goodbye-a-little-life/

Sexuality and Intimacy

Emma Power, PhD, BAppSc, CPSP MSPAA;
Margaret McGrath, PhD, MSc, BSc;
and Sandra Lever, MN, BHM, RN, CNC, NSLHD

The World Health Organization defines sexuality as "a central aspect of being human throughout life that encompasses sex, gender identities and roles, sexual orientation, eroticism, pleasure, intimacy, and reproduction. It is experienced and expressed in thoughts, fantasies, desires, beliefs, attitudes, values, behavior, practices, roles, and relationships. It is also influenced by the interaction of biological, psychological, social, economic, political, cultural, ethical, historical, religious and spiritual factors" (World Health Organization, 2006, 2010). For many speech-language pathologists (and health professionals more generally), this topic may not be a priority among the complex rehabilitation needs associated with stroke recovery, especially if this taboo topic is not raised by clients. However, we are at a fork in the road in our profession of how to approach sexuality and intimacy education and counseling with our clients. This fork in the road can be illustrated by two differing possible journeys for our client Liam and his wife Beth (See Box 8e-6).

Box 8e-6
Liam and Beth

Liam is a 38-year-old man who had a middle cerebral artery infarct 4 months earlier. He has a degree in engineering and, prior to his stroke, worked full-time for a construction company. He lives with his wife of 4 years, Beth, who is 33 years old. Liam speaks English and some Italian. He is popular with friends and family and enjoys keeping fit including going to the gym, playing soccer, and surfing.

Liam has moderate to severe aphasia characterized by nonfluent speech with simple phrases, word-finding difficulty, and phonological paraphasias. He has a reliable yes/no response but difficulty following two-step instructions. His reading and writing abilities follow a similar pattern. He uses gesture to express himself and responds well to supported conversation with written (key words and phrases) and pictorial supports. He has right-sided hemiparesis and can walk short distances but spends most days in a self-propelled wheelchair. He requires moderate assistance with activities of daily living including continence.

The speech-language pathologist sees him as an outpatient at the multidisciplinary outpatient center twice every week after a referral from the hospital inpatient team. The outpatient speech-language pathologist has conducted some assessment and talked about initial goal-setting with Liam and Beth, which has focused on linguistic recovery and exploring his social network goals using the social network tool.

Journey A—Current Practice to Date

The speech-language pathologist continues to develop communication goals with Liam that focus on (1) reducing his language impairment, (2) maximizing his participation in sports-related activities with his friends, (3) brief communication partner training for Beth, and (4) expressing his daily basic needs and wants at home. Beyond simple communication partner training, the speech-language pathologist does not raise the relationship in terms of intimacy and sexuality with either Liam or Beth. Liam receives 3 months of communication treatment before his discharge. Later, the couple go on to have a family with two children. However, when asked what help they got, Beth replies, "None. We had to work it out all by ourselves without help. It was really stressful and we just bumbled through alone . . . we nearly divorced."

A Commentary on Journey A

We know there are many barriers for clinicians and clients to initiate discussion about sexuality and intimacy (McGrath et al., 2021). Several of these barriers relate to our own values, attitudes, self-efficacy, and skills. In Journey A, the speech-language pathologist may have assumed that addressing sexuality and intimacy was not part of their role, or would be addressed by other team members (McGrath et al., 2021). It could be that the clinician consciously or subconsciously views people with stroke as representative mostly of an older stroke population who they believe are asexual and not interested in sex or intimacy (McGrath et al., 2019). Even when working with a younger stroke survivor like Liam, the speech-language pathologist might mistakenly believe that planning for having children, fertility, and sexual health are not relevant issues/goals after stroke (Cruz-Herranz et al., 2015; Mellor et al., 2013; Soriano et al., 2002). In addition to assumptions about ageism and ableism, the speech-language pathologist may associate sexuality and intimacy so specifically with the sexual act (Lever & Pryor, 2017), limiting broader views around intimacy and the role of communication impairment as a critical additional challenge for people with aphasia in their intimate lives. There is a possibility that when Liam and Beth do *not* raise the issue themselves, clinicians take this absence as confirmation of these values/attitudes (McGrath et al., 2021). Even if the speech-language pathologist did agree that sexuality and intimacy were part of their role, they still may believe that it is not a priority among other goals in a possibly constrained service delivery setting (McGrath et al., 2021). Alternatively, the speech-language pathologist might want to raise the topic with Liam and Beth, but does not believe they have the skills, resources, and referral pathways to do so, or that their institutions would be supportive (Lepage et al., 2020; McGrath et al., 2021). The speech-language pathologist may be uncomfortable with the topic personally, echoing the societal taboo, and possess little or narrow experience with it. Subsequently, they may prefer to avoid it, understandably not wanting to risk a negative reaction from the client or their family (McGrath et al., 2021). In Journey A, the speech-language pathologist and rehabilitation team are simply not aware that raising sexuality and intimacy poststroke is recommended practice; if they were, they might not be monitoring their own services to ensure information and support are provided according to guidelines (Royal College of Physicians Intercollegiate Stroke Working Party, 2016; Stroke Foundation, 2017; Winstein et al., 2016). As a result, sexuality is silenced (McGrath et al., 2019) and communication impairments then result in silence within the silence (Lemieux et al., 2001; McGrath et al., 2019).

Onward to Journey B—What Helps to Take a Different Journey With Our Clients?

The informative and adjustment counseling role requires ultimately for us to reflect on these issues and question what might stop us from raising this topic and seeing it as part of our role. Thus, a first step is to understand our own values, attitudes, lack of knowledge, and potential unconscious or conscious biases so we can seek assistance, give ourselves permission to not be experts, and ultimately reduce negative impacts on others. The second step is to apply frameworks (e.g., PLISSIT model; Annon, 1976) in a team approach over the continuum of care, to support the provision of sexuality education and counseling utilizing the principles of Stepped Care (Kneebone, 2016). The third step is to realize that while there are limitations on our knowledge and scope of role, speech-language pathologists have unique and specialized skills in supported communication (Simmons-Mackie et al., 2010), accessible communication formats (Rose et al., 2012), and a critical role in life's communication-related activities (Chapey et al., 2000). Embedding these principles into our practice allows us to create a different journey for Liam and Beth.

Journey B—Toward Better Practice

In relation to the speech-language pathologist's own reflection on values and knowledge, the speech-language pathologist considers sexuality and intimacy an integral part of life and rehabilitation poststroke. They understand sexuality and intimacy is more than sex, and that it extends to broader and deeper components of an individual's identity, with a critical intersection with quality of life and relationships (World Health Organization, 2006). The speech-language pathologist is careful to challenge their own assumptions that people after stroke and their current/future partners have no interest in sex and intimacy because they are either older, disabled, or both (Shakespeare et al., 2009). To clarify and get a better understanding of personal values and beliefs, the speech-language pathologist participates in both individual and group value clarification exercises and seeks clinical supervision when recognizing any values conflict (Geldard et al., 2017). The speech-language pathologist is also aware that the proportion of people having strokes under 45 years is increasing, and that those individuals may have additional or different needs compared to older survivors such as planning a family/having children (Béjot et al., 2016; Keating et al., 2021). The speech-language pathologist is careful not to assume either that because Liam is a young man, that sex is more important to him than other survivors who are women, or from sexual or cultural minorities. There is also a keen awareness from the speech-language pathologist that the socio-cultural-political context of the topic means that clients may not feel comfortable asking about it and may take any silence as tacit instructions to *not* raise it (McGrath et al., 2019). The speech-language pathologist also knows that it is possible that a client's own unconscious, ableist perspectives of not seeing sexuality as possible after stroke may influence how Liam and Beth approach the issue. The speech-language pathologist acknowledges that there could be many different priorities for Liam and Beth, but Liam and Beth are the ones to decide those priorities. The speech-language pathologist is somewhat uncomfortable with the topic, as they are with other difficult conversations, and understand that being aware of this discomfort helps them to monitor their reactions and practice patterns. The speech-language pathologist and team are aware of relevant guideline recommendations and participate in audits to monitor their implementation of those recommendations (Royal College of Physicians Intercollegiate Stroke Working Party, 2016; Stroke Foundation, 2017; Winstein et al., 2016).

In this rehabilitation service there is an essential, interdisciplinary team approach and responsibility to address the issue, which is shared by all team members in the interest of client-centered care as well as from the unique perspective of each profession (McGrath et al., 2021). This rehabilitation service acknowledges the research that indicates that individuals with stroke or their partners can have questions about sexuality and intimacy, or dissatisfaction with their sexuality (Lemieux et al., 2001; McGrath et al., 2019; Rosenbaum et al., 2014). There is an awareness that some education for Liam and Beth is required so they can even say they *do not* need assistance at that time. Additionally, this education extends to reminding Liam and Beth that they can re-enter the conversation after discharge from hospital along with provision of outpatient referral sources that Liam and Beth may consider once more medically related priorities are resolved.

As such, sexuality and intimacy are seen as a topics that can be proportionately raised along the continuum of care, and stroke survivors are clear that this should occur initially, prior to inpatient discharge but especially after discharge from hospital up to 1 to 2 years afterward (McGrath et al., 2019). One model of addressing sexual function, called the PLISSIT (Annon, 1976), helps to create a stepped-care type approach that sequentially addresses increasing degrees of need as required. In the first stage, the clinician seeks to give clients *Permission* to discuss sexual issues by raising the issue themselves through direct discussion with a client (e.g., "Stroke survivors may have questions about how the changes after stroke affect their sexual function, body image, intimacy, and relationships. Feel free to ask me about any questions or concerns you have."). Another method could be through embedding standardized needs assessments/checklists (and not skipping the sexuality question!) where stroke survivors can indicate whether they have concerns or not in a variety of domains including sexuality. Next, if required, *Limited Information* can be provided (e.g., brief detail about the topic or general overview of information, such as through a written handout). If further information is required in more detail, then *Specific Suggestions* are provided related to client

needs, and further sustained *Intensive Therapy* may be offered, which may include referral to specialized service providers (e.g., sex therapists). At each step, the clinician should check with their clients whether the clients have any further questions, or any unresolved issues.

In this speech-language pathologist's inpatient team (earlier in the continuum of care), they provided Liam and Beth *Permission,* raising the issue with them as part of the ward standard needs assessment. Sexuality and intimacy are treated as a topic like any other (e.g., continence, palliative care, mental health) to be raised without stigma. The couple were asked by a nurse whether they had any concerns about sexuality/intimacy because stroke can affect many physical, cognitive (including communication), and emotional functions and so each of these might affect sexuality, their identity, and their intimate relationships. Utilizing their specialized communication skills, the speech-language pathologist provided the nurse with a communication sheet to help the nurse support asking the questions with simple visual/written supports (Simmons-Mackie et al., 2010). Despite being overwhelmed, Liam and Beth listened and indicated they would take an information pamphlet on sexuality (Stroke Foundation, n.d.) but did not have questions yet as they were struggling with Liam's mobility and communication issues. The nurse reinforced that the Permission extended beyond that moment and indicated that they could ask questions at any time of any of the team and also re-establish the discussion with the outpatient service after they are discharged home.

Now at the outpatient service, the speech-language pathologist establishes the *Permission* level again with Liam and Beth, leading with more *Limited Information* specific to communication disability—"Liam and Beth, your aphasia may affect your intimacy and relationships [points to both Liam and Beth]. This is because communication can be important for saying how you feel and talk about intimacy and sex [points to supported communication board]." The speech-language pathologist also says that while communication can be an important part of intimacy itself (Lemieux et al., 2001), communication is important in discussions about intimacy between the couple and with their healthcare team, and they may need communication supports, which the speech-language pathologist can provide.

Beth indicates that they had wished to start a family and have children, and now they were not sure whether it was possible to have children at all, whether they could manage if they did, and how Beth could discuss this with Liam, then her doctor, and other team members. The speech-language pathologist and the couple decide that working on linguistic recovery of language and supported communication training for Beth will help them to talk more generally, thus helping their relationship; however, Liam and Beth wanted support to generate their thoughts about options for the future. In this way, the speech-language pathologist is providing more specialized support for conversation opportunity and success on the topic rather than *Specific Information* itself.

However, provision of this support to the couple will enable their *Specific Information* conversations to be more successful with other professionals on the team such as the occupational therapist, physiotherapist, physician, and social worker.

The speech-language pathologist knows they do not have extensive knowledge on sexuality but are also aware they do not need to be a sexuality expert to listen actively, problem-solve, and facilitate discussions. They are aware of some literature indicating that people with aphasia might expect their speech-language pathologist to have a greater role because of the important trust in the speech-language pathologist to facilitate communication (McGrath et al., 2019). The clinician is aware of the limitations to their knowledge and has referral sources, including sexual counsellors if required.

The speech-language pathologist schedules the next session to be a discussion on the topic and provides a variety of supported communication materials to facilitate the discussion. Materials from the Aphasia Institute intimacy support booklet (Aphasia Institute, 2005) help the speech-language pathologist convey concepts regarding sexuality with pictures and key words. The speech-language pathologist also provides supported materials for adjectives ("hard," "stressful," "rewarding," "complete"), emotions ("sad," "angry," "hopeful," "grateful"), and scales that support degree of feelings or importance of a concept ("not at all," "a bit," "a lot"). Cards that address different relevant functions associated with stroke such as: issues with getting an erection, feeling like a carer rather than partner, physical mobility (hemiplegia) for sex or looking after/keeping up with children, driving (driving kids around), communication (speaking to the kids and helping with homework) are also included. The speech-language pathologist then divides a line down the table into sections for "Why it is a good idea" and "Why it might not be a good idea." An additional, "What are our questions?" section provides opportunity to get further help. Liam and Beth sort their cards or written words scribed by the speech pathologist into the three sections, and then take a photo, to support their discussion. The speech-language pathologist uses techniques of Supported Conversation to verify Liam's responses, and ensure he understands and has opportunities to express himself. The speech-language pathologist then liaises with other key professionals and provides the support materials to them to aid their own discussions, along with an offer to support Liam specifically in those other health area discussions as the team take over more on *Specific Suggestions* and *Intensive Therapy*. Beth and Liam are able to tick off answers to their questions (e.g., options for mobility for Liam to actively look after any children) and also the team can refer on further to sexual therapists and/or doctor for answers they do not feel qualified to provide. Liam and Beth go on to have two children. Beth says it was not easy but a critical decision to make with Liam. Liam says, "it is really good" (thumbs up) but "tiring" and gestures pride (hand on heart with a giant smile).

Summary

Speech-language pathologists have a significant and valuable role to play in supporting people living with communication impairments to express their sexuality. While sexuality may appear to be different and more difficult than other aspects of stroke rehabilitation, it is important for speech-language pathologists to treat this topic as any other. In removing the taboo from sexuality, speech-language pathologists can use their core skills within an interdisciplinary team to support communication about sexuality for both clients and the team.

References

Annon, J. S. (1976). The PLISSIT model: A proposed conceptual scheme for the behavioral treatment of sexual problems. *Journal of Sex Education and Therapy, 2*(1), 1-15. https://doi.org/10.1080/01614576.1976.11074483

Aphasia Institute. (2005). *Intimacy and relationships: Talking to your doctor.* Aphasia Institute.

Béjot, Y., Delpont, B., & Giroud, M. (2016). Rising stroke incidence in young adults: More epidemiological evidence, more questions to be answered. *Journal of the American Heart Association, 5*(5), e003661. https://doi.org/10.1161/JAHA.116.003661

Chapey, R., Duchan, J. F., Elman, R. J., Garcia, L. J., Kagan, A., Lyon, J. G., & Simmons-Mackie, N. (2000). Life participation approach to aphasia: A statement of values for the future. *The ASHA Leader, 5*(3). https://doi.org/10.1044/leader.FTR.05032000.4

Cruz-Herranz, A., Illán-Gala, I., Martínez-Sánchez, P., Fuentes, B., & Díez-Tejedor, E. (2015). Recurrence of stroke amongst women of reproductive age: Impact of and on subsequent pregnancies. *European Journal of Neurology, 22*(4), 681-e42. https://doi.org/10.1111/ene.12630

Geldard, D., Geldard, K., & Foo, R. (2017). *Basic personal counselling: A training manual for counsellors.* Cengage Learning Australia.

Keating, J., Borschmann, K., Johns, H., Churilov, L., & Bernhardt, J. (2021). Young stroke survivors' preferred methods of meeting their unique needs: Shaping better care. *Neurology, 96*(13), e1701-e1710. https://doi.org/10.1212/WNL.0000000000011647

Kneebone, I. I. (2016). Stepped psychological care after stroke. *Disability and Rehabilitation, 38*(18), 1836-1843. https://doi.org/10.3109/09638288.2015.1107764

Lemieux, L., Cohen-Schneider, R., & Holzapfel, S. (2001). Aphasia and sexuality. *Sexuality and Disability, 19*(4), 253-266. https://doi.org/10.1023/A:1017953308761

Lepage, C., Auger, L. P., & Rochette, A. (2020). Sexuality in the context of physical rehabilitation as perceived by occupational therapists. *Disability and Rehabilitation, 43*(19), 2739-2749. https://doi.org/10.1080/09638288.2020.1715494

Lever, S., & Pryor, J. (2017). The impact of stroke on female sexuality. *Disability and Rehabilitation, 39*(20), 2011-2020. https://doi.org/10.1080/09638288.2016.1213897

McGrath, M., Lever, S., McCluskey, A., & Power, E. (2019a). Developing interventions to address sexuality after stroke: Findings from a four-panel modified Delphi study. *Journal of Rehabilitation Medicine, 51*(5), 352-360. https://doi.org/10.2340/16501977-2548

McGrath, M., Lever, S., McCluskey, A., & Power, E. (2019b). How is sexuality after stroke experienced by stroke survivors and partners of stroke survivors? A systematic review of qualitative studies. *Clinical Rehabilitation, 33*(2), 293-303. https://doi.org/10.1177/0269215518793483

McGrath, M., Low, M. A., Power, E., McCluskey, A., & Lever, S. (2021). Addressing sexuality among people living with chronic disease and disability: A systematic mixed methods review of knowledge, attitudes, and practices of health care professionals. *Archives of Physical Medicine and Rehabilitation, 102*(5), 999-1010. https://doi.org/10.1016/j.apmr.2020.09.379

Mellor, R. M., Greenfield, S. M., Dowswell, G., Sheppard, J. P., Quinn, T., & McManus, R. J. (2013). Health care professionals' views on discussing sexual wellbeing with patients who have had a stroke: A qualitative study. *PLoS ONE, 8*(10), e78802. https://doi.org/10.1371/journal.pone.0078802

Rose, T. A., Worrall, L. E., Hickson, L. M., & Hoffmann, T. C. (2012). Guiding principles for printed education materials: Design preferences of people with aphasia. *International Journal of Speech-Language Pathology, 14*(1), 11-23. https://doi.org/10.3109/17549507.2011.631583

Rosenbaum, T., Vadas, D., & Kalichman, L. (2014). Sexual function in post-stroke patients: Considerations for rehabilitation. *Journal of Sexual Medicine, 11*(1), 15-21. https://doi.org/10.1111/jsm.12343

Royal College of Physicians Intercollegiate Stroke Working Party. (2016). *National clinical guidelines for stroke.* The Stroke Program. https://www.rcplondon.ac.uk/guidelines-policy/stroke-guidelines

Shakespeare, T., Lezzoni, L. L., & Groce, N. E. (2009). The art of medicine: Disability and the training of health professionals. *The Lancet, 374*(9704), 1815-1816. https://doi.org/10.1016/S0140-6736(09)62050-X

Simmons-Mackie, N., Raymer, A., Armstrong, E., Holland, A., & Cherney, L. R. (2010). Communication partner training in aphasia: A systematic review. *Archives of Physical and Medical Rehabilitation, 97*(12), 2202-2221.e8. https://doi.org/10.1016/j.apmr.2016.03.023

Soriano, D., Carp, H., Seidman, D. S., Schiff, E., Langevitz, P., Mashiach, S., & Dulitzky, M. (2002). Management and outcome of pregnancy in women with thrombophylic disorders and past cerebrovascular events. *Acta Obstetricia et Gynecologica Scandinavica, 81*(3), 204-207. https://doi.org/10.1034/j.1600-0412.2002.810303.x

Stroke Foundation. (n.d.). *Sex and relationships after stroke fact sheet.* https://strokefoundation.org.au/what-we-do/for-survivors-and-carers/stroke-resources-and-fact-sheets/sex-and-relationships-after-stroke-fact-sheet#

Stroke Foundation. (2017). *Clinical guidelines for stroke management 2017.* https://informme.org.au/guidelines/living-clinical-guidelines-for-stroke-management

Winstein, C. J., Stein, J., Arena, R., Bates, B., Cherney, L. R., Cramer, S. C., . . . Zorowitz, R. D. (2016). Guidelines for adult stroke rehabilitation and recovery: A guideline for healthcare professionals from the American Heart Association/American Stroke Association. *Stroke, 47*(6), e98-e169. https://doi.org/10.1161/STR.0000000000000098

World Health Organization. (2006). *Defining sexual health—Report of a technical consultation on sexual health, 28-31 January 2002 Geneva.* Sexual Health Document Series, World Health Organization, Geneva.

World Health Organization. (2010). *Developing sexual health programmes: A framework for action.* https://apps.who.int/iris/handle/10665/70501

Financial Disclosures

Dr. Rebecca H. Affoo is a salaried assistant professor at Dalhousie University. She receives honoraria for continuing education and seminars. She serves on the editorial board of ASHA Perspectives and serves as a reviewer for several journals.

Wendy and Nick Allen reported no financial or proprietary interest in the materials presented herein.

Dr. Laura Arrington reported no financial or proprietary interest in the materials presented herein.

Dr. Miriam Carroll-Alfano reported no financial or proprietary interest in the materials presented herein.

Dr. Charlotte Clark reported no financial or proprietary interest in the materials presented herein.

Dr. Holly Damico reported no financial or proprietary interest in the materials presented herein.

Dr. Jack Damico reported no financial or proprietary interest in the materials presented herein.

Dr. Derek E. Daniels reported no financial or proprietary interest in the materials presented herein.

Dr. Natalie Douglas reported no financial or proprietary interest in the materials presented herein.

Dr. Julia M. Fischer reported no financial or proprietary interest in the materials presented herein.

Dr. Deborah Hersh reported no financial or proprietary interest in the materials presented herein.

Dr. Audrey Holland reported no financial or proprietary interest in the materials presented herein.

Dr. Dan Hudock reported no financial or proprietary interest in the materials presented herein.

Rebecca L. Jarzynski reported no financial or proprietary interest in the materials presented herein.

Sandra Lever reported no financial or proprietary interest in the materials presented herein.

Dr. Margaret McGrath reported no financial or proprietary interest in the materials presented herein.

Dr. Ryan Nelson reported no financial or proprietary interest in the materials presented herein.

Nancy Petersen reported no financial or proprietary interest in the materials presented herein.

Dr. Jack Pickering reported no financial or proprietary interest in the materials presented herein.

Dr. Laura Plexico reported no financial or proprietary interest in the materials presented herein.

Robin Pollens reported no financial or proprietary interest in the materials presented herein.

Dr. Emma Power reported no financial or proprietary interest in the materials presented herein.

Dr. Pamela Terrell reported no financial or proprietary interest in the materials presented herein.

Aspen Townsend reported no financial or proprietary interest in the materials presented herein.

Dr. Eva van Leer reported no financial or proprietary interest in the materials presented herein.

Dr. Christine Weill reported no financial or proprietary interest in the materials presented herein.

CeCelia and Wayne Zorn reported no financial or proprietary interest in the materials presented herein.

Index

To come.

Printed in the United States
by Baker & Taylor Publisher Services